T0226999

Surgical Advances in Female Pelvic Reconstruction

Editor

CRAIG V. COMITER

UROLOGIC CLINICS OF NORTH AMERICA

www.urologic.theclinics.com

Consulting Editor
SAMIR S. TANEJA

February 2019 • Volume 46 • Number 1

ELSEVIER

1600 John F. Kennedy Boulevard • Suite 1800 • Philadelphia, Pennsylvania, 19103-2899

http://www.theclinics.com

UROLOGIC CLINICS OF NORTH AMERICA Volume 46, Number 1
February 2019 ISSN 0094-0143, ISBN-13: 978-0-323-65525-5

Editor: Kerry Holland
Developmental Editor: Sara Watkins

© **2019 Elsevier Inc. All rights reserved.**

This periodical and the individual contributions contained in it are protected under copyright by Elsevier, and the following terms and conditions apply to their use:

Photocopying
Single photocopies of single articles may be made for personal use as allowed by national copyright laws. Permission of the Publisher and payment of a fee is required for all other photocopying, including multiple or systematic copying, copying for advertising or promotional purposes, resale, and all forms of document delivery. Special rates are available for educational institutions that wish to make photocopies for non-profit educational classroom use. For information on how to seek permission visit www.elsevier.com/permissions or call: (+44) 1865 843830 (UK)/(+1) 215 239 3804 (USA).

Derivative Works
Subscribers may reproduce tables of contents or prepare lists of articles including abstracts for internal circulation within their institutions. Permission of the Publisher is required for resale or distribution outside the institution. Permission of the Publisher is required for all other derivative works, including compilations and translations (please consult www.elsevier.com/permissions).

Electronic Storage or Usage
Permission of the Publisher is required to store or use electronically any material contained in this periodical, including any article or part of an article (please consult www.elsevier.com/permissions). Except as outlined above, no part of this publication may be reproduced, stored in a retrieval system or transmitted in any form or by any means, electronic, mechanical, photocopying, recording or otherwise, without prior written permission of the Publisher.

Notice
No responsibility is assumed by the Publisher for any injury and/or damage to persons or property as a matter of products liability, negligence or otherwise, or from any use or operation of any methods, products, instructions or ideas contained in the material herein. Because of rapid advances in the medical sciences, in particular, independent verification of diagnoses and drug dosages should be made.

Although all advertising material is expected to conform to ethical (medical) standards, inclusion in this publication does not constitute a guarantee or endorsement of the quality or value of such product or of the claims made of it by its manufacturer.

Urologic Clinics of North America (ISSN 0094-0143) is published quarterly by Elsevier Inc., 360 Park Avenue South, New York, NY 10010-1710. Months of issue are February, May, August, and November. Business and Editorial Offices: 1600 John F. Kennedy Blvd., Suite 1800, Philadelphia, PA 19103-2899. Periodicals postage paid at New York, NY and additional mailing offices. Subscription prices are $387.00 per year (US individuals), $757.00 per year (US institutions), $100.00 per year (US students and residents), $450.00 per year (Canadian individuals), $946.00 per year (Canadian institutions), $520.00 per year (foreign individuals), $946.00 per year (foreign institutions), and $240.00 per year (Canadian and foreign students/residents). Foreign air speed delivery is included in all *Clinics* subscription prices. All prices are subject to change without notice. **POSTMASTER:** Send address changes to *Urologic Clinics of North America*, Elsevier Health Sciences Division, Subscription Customer Service, 3251 Riverport Lane, Maryland Heights, MO 63043. **Customer Service: 1-800-654-2452 (US). From outside the United States, call 1-314-447-8871. Fax: 1-314-447-8029. E-mail: JournalsCustomerServiceusa@elsevier.com (for print support)** and **JournalsOnlineSupport-usa@elsevier.com (for online support)**.

Reprints. For copies of 100 or more, of articles in this publication, please contact the Commercial Reprints Department, Elsevier Inc., 360 Park Avenue South, New York, New York 10010-1710. Tel.: 212-633-3874; Fax: 212-633-3820; E-mail: reprints@elsevier.com.

Urologic Clinics of North America is covered in MEDLINE/PubMed (*Index Medicus*), *Excerpta Medica, Current Contents/Clinical Medicine, Science Citation Index,* and *ISI/BIOMED*.

PROGRAM OBJECTIVE

The goal of *Urologic Clinics of North America* is to keep practicing urologists and urology residents up to date with current clinical practice in urology by providing timely articles reviewing the state of the art in patient care.

TARGET AUDIENCE

Practicing urologists, urology residents and other healthcare professionals practicing in the discipline of urology.

LEARNING OBJECTIVES

Upon completion of this activity, participants will be able to:

- Review injection techniques, patient selection, and complications associated with urethral injections
- Discuss vaginal and abdominal surgical treatment options for patients with vesico vaginal fistula
- Recognize suture-based repair surgery for posterior vaginal prolapse and anterior compartment vaginal prolapse

ACCREDITATION

The Elsevier Office of Continuing Medical Education (EOCME) is accredited by the Accreditation Council for Continuing Medical Education (ACCME) to provide continuing medical education for physicians.

The EOCME designates this enduring material for a maximum of 15 *AMA PRA Category 1 Credit*(s)™. Physicians should claim only the credit commensurate with the extent of their participation in the activity.

All other healthcare professionals requesting continuing education credit for this enduring material will be issued a certificate of participation.

DISCLOSURE OF CONFLICTS OF INTEREST

The EOCME assesses conflict of interest with its instructors, faculty, planners, and other individuals who are in a position to control the content of CME activities. All relevant conflicts of interest that are identified are thoroughly vetted by EOCME for fair balance, scientific objectivity, and patient care recommendations. EOCME is committed to providing its learners with CME activities that promote improvements or quality in healthcare and not a specific proprietary business or a commercial interest.

The planning committee, staff, authors and editors listed below have identified no financial relationships or relationships to products or devices they or their spouse/life partner have with commercial interest related to the content of this CME activity:

Nitya Abraham, MD; Katherine Amin, MD; Jerry G. Blaivas, MD; Craig Comiter, MD; Melissa Daniel, MD; Linda Dayan, BA; Daniel S. Elliott, MD; Christopher S. Elliott, MD, PhD; Ekene A. Enemchukwu, MD, MPH; Michele Fascelli, MD; Joel T. Funk, MD, FACS; Laura L. Giusto, MD; Howard B. Goldman, MD; Zeynep Gul, MD; Juan M. Guzman-Negron, MD; Kerry Holland; Senad Kalkan, MD; Alison Kemp; Sunchin Kim, MD; Dominic Lee, MBBS(Hons), FRACS(Urology); Hanhan Li, MD; Brian J. Linder, MD; Elishia McKay, MD; Grant R. Pollock, MD; Vannita Simma-Chiang, MD; Ericka M. Sohlberg, MD; Raveen Syan, MD; Samir Taneja, MD; Christian O. Twiss, MD, FACS; Sandip P. Vasavada, MD; Vignesh Viswanathan; Shannon L. Wallace; Kara Watts, MD; Adi Y. Weintraub, MD; Patricia M. Zahner, MD; Philippe Zimmern, MD, FACS, FPMRS.

The planning committee, staff, authors and editors listed below have identified financial relationships or relationships to products or devices they or their spouse/life partner have with commercial interest related to the content of this CME activity:

Kathleen Kobashi, MD, FACS: is a consultant/advisor and serves on speakers' bureau for Allergan, Avadel, Axonics Modulation Technologies, Inc, and Medtronic.
Wai Lee, MD: Dr. Lee's spouse receives research support from Medtronic.
Una Lee, MD: is a consultant/advisor and serves on speakers' bureau for Medtronic.
Eric R. Sokol, MD: owns stock in Eclipse System and receives research support from ACell Inc., Coloplast Corp, and Cook
Justina Tam, MD: receives research support from Medtronic
Samir S. Taneja, MD: is a consultant/advisor for Elseiver and INSIGTEC, Ltd, and receives research support from MDxHealth. Dr. Taneja is a consultant/advisor and receives research support from Sophiris Bio Corp.
Ouida Lenaine Westney, MD: is a consultant/advisor for Boston Scientific Corporation

UNAPPROVED/OFF-LABEL USE DISCLOSURE

The EOCME requires CME faculty to disclose to the participants:

1. When products or procedures being discussed are off-label, unlabelled, experimental, and/or investigational (not US Food and Drug Administration [FDA] approved); and
2. Any limitations on the information presented, such as data that are preliminary or that represent ongoing research, interim analyses, and/or unsupported opinions. Faculty may discuss information about pharmaceutical agents that is outside of FDA-approved labelling. This information is intended solely for CME and is not intended to promote off-label use of these medications. If you have any questions, contact the medical affairs department of the manufacturer for the most recent prescribing information.

TO ENROLL

To enroll in the *Urologic Clinics of North America* Continuing Medical Education program, call customer service at 1-800-654-2452 or sign up online at http://www.theclinics.com/home/cme. The CME program is available to subscribers for an additional annual fee of USD $280.

METHOD OF PARTICIPATION

In order to claim credit, participants must complete the following:

1. Complete enrolment as indicated above.
2. Read the activity.
3. Complete the CME Test and Evaluation. Participants must achieve a score of 70% on the test. All CME Tests and Evaluations must be completed online.

CME INQUIRIES/SPECIAL NEEDS

For all CME inquiries or special needs, please contact elsevierCME@elsevier.com.

Contributors

CONSULTING EDITOR

SAMIR S. TANEJA, MD
The James M. Neissa and Janet Riha Neissa Professor of Urologic Oncology, Professor of Urology and Radiology, Director, Division of Urologic Oncology, Vice Chair, Department of Urology, NYU Langone Health, New York, New York, USA

EDITOR

CRAIG V. COMITER, MD
Professor, Departments of Urology, and Obstetrics and Gynecology (by Courtesy), Stanford University School of Medicine, Stanford, California, USA

AUTHORS

NITYA ABRAHAM, MD
Assistant Professor, Department of Urology, Montefiore Medical Center, Bronx, New York, USA

KATHERINE AMIN, MD
Fellow, Female Pelvic Medicine and Reconstructive Surgery, Section of Urology, Virginia Mason Medical Center, Seattle, Washington, USA

JERRY G. BLAIVAS, MD
Professor, Department of Urology, Icahn School of Medicine at Mount Sinai, New York, New York, USA

MELISSA DANIEL, MD
Resident, Department of Surgery, SUNY Downstate Medical Center, Brooklyn, New York, USA

LINDA DAYAN, BA
Research Coordinator, Institute for Bladder and Prostate Research, New York, New York, USA

CHRISTOPHER S. ELLIOTT, MD, PhD
Clinical Assistant Professor, Department of Urology, Stanford University, Stanford, California, USA; Division of Urology, Santa Clara Valley Medical Center, Valley Specialties Clinic, San Jose, California, USA

DANIEL S. ELLIOTT, MD
Professor, Department of Urology, Mayo Clinic, Rochester, Minnesota, USA

EKENE A. ENEMCHUKWU, MD, MPH
Assistant Professor, Departments of Urology, and Obstetrics and Gynecology (by Courtesy), Stanford University, Stanford, California, USA

MICHELE FASCELLI, MD
Glickman Urological and Kidney Institute, Lerner College of Medicine, Cleveland Clinic, Cleveland, Ohio, USA

JOEL T. FUNK, MD, FACS
Department of Surgery, Division of Urology, University of Arizona, Tucson, Arizona, USA

LAURA L. GIUSTO, MD
Glickman Urological and Kidney Institute, Cleveland Clinic, Cleveland, Ohio, USA

HOWARD B. GOLDMAN, MD
Glickman Urological and Kidney Institute, Cleveland Clinic, Cleveland, Ohio, USA

ZEYNEP GUL, MD
Resident, Department of Urology, Icahn School of Medicine at Mount Sinai, New York, New York, USA

JUAN M. GUZMAN-NEGRON, MD
Glickman Urological and Kidney Institute, Lerner College of Medicine, Cleveland Clinic, Cleveland, Ohio, USA

OSNAT ISRAELI, MD
Department of Obstetrics and Gynecology, Soroka University Medical Center, Faculty of Health Sciences, Ben-Gurion University of the Negev, Beer Sheva, Israel

SENAD KALKAN, MD
Assistant Professor, Department of Urology, Bezmialem Vakif University in Istanbul, Istanbul, Turkey

SUNCHIN KIM, MD
Department of Surgery, Division of Urology, University of Arizona, Tucson, Arizona, USA

KATHLEEN KOBASHI, MD, FACS
Virginia Mason Medical Center, Seattle, Washington, USA

DOMINIC LEE, MBBS (Hons), FRACS (Urology)
Department of Urology, St George Hospital, Kogarah, New South Wales, Australia

UNA LEE, MD
Surgeon, Female Pelvic Medicine and Reconstructive Surgery, Section of Urology, Virginia Mason Medical Center, Seattle, Washington, USA

WAI LEE, MD
Virginia Mason Medical Center, Seattle, Washington, USA

HANHAN LI, MD
Urinary Tract and Pelvic Reconstruction Fellow, Department of Urology, The University of Texas MD Anderson Cancer Center, Houston, Texas, USA

BRIAN J. LINDER, MD
Assistant Professor, Obstetrics and Gynecology, Department of Urology, Mayo Clinic, Rochester, Minnesota, USA

ELISHIA McKAY, MD
FPMRS Fellow, Department of Obstetrics and Gynecology, Montefiore Medical Center, Bronx, New York, USA

GRANT R. POLLOCK, MD
Department of Surgery, Division of Urology, University of Arizona, Tucson, Arizona, USA

VANNITA SIMMA-CHIANG, MD
Assistant Professor, Department of Urology, Icahn School of Medicine at Mount Sinai, New York, New York, USA

ERICKA M. SOHLBERG, MD
Department of Urology, Stanford University, Stanford, California, USA

ERIC R. SOKOL, MD
Associate Professor, Departments of Obstetrics and Gynecology, and Urology (by Courtesy), Division of Urogynecology and Pelvic Reconstructive Surgery, Stanford University School of Medicine, Stanford, California, USA

RAVEEN SYAN, MD
FPMRS Fellow, Department of Urology, Stanford University School of Medicine, Stanford, California, USA

JUSTINA TAM, MD
Department of Urology, Stony Brook Medicine, Stony Brook, New York, USA

CHRISTIAN O. TWISS, MD, FACS
Department of Surgery, Division of Urology, University of Arizona, Tucson, Arizona, USA

SANDIP P. VASAVADA, MD
Glickman Urological and Kidney Institute, Lerner College of Medicine, Cleveland Clinic, Cleveland, Ohio, USA

SHANNON L. WALLACE, MD
FPMRS Fellow, Department of Obstetrics and Gynecology, Division of Urogynecology and Pelvic Reconstructive Surgery, Stanford University School of Medicine, Stanford, California, USA

KARA WATTS, MD
Assistant Professor, Department of Urology, Montefiore Medical Center, Bronx, New York, USA

ADI Y. WEINTRAUB, MD
Consultant, Department of Obstetrics and Gynecology, Soroka University Medical Center, Faculty of Health Sciences, Ben-Gurion University of the Negev, Beer Sheva, Irsael

OUIDA LENAINE WESTNEY, MD
Professor, Fellowship Director, Urinary Tract and Pelvic Reconstruction, Department of Urology, The University of Texas MD Anderson Cancer Center, Houston, Texas, USA

PATRICIA M. ZAHNER, MD
Glickman Urological and Kidney Institute, Cleveland Clinic, Cleveland, Ohio, USA

PHILIPPE ZIMMERN, MD, FACS, FPMRS
Professor, Department of Urology, The University of Texas Southwestern Medical Center, Dallas, Texas, USA

Contents

Foreword: Reconstruction of the Female Pelvis: A Fundamental Pillar of Urology xv

Samir S. Taneja

Preface: Controversies in Vaginal Surgery xvii

Craig V. Comiter

Surgery for Stress Urinary Incontinence

Injection of Urethral Bulking Agents 1

Hanhan Li and Ouida Lenaine Westney

Urethral injection is a safe and minimally invasive method of treating female stress urinary incontinence with multiple bulking agents currently commercially available. Although there are numerous studies that demonstrate efficacy, long-term success is not yet proven. This article aims to describe the mechanism of action and properties of various agents, patient selection factors, available techniques for injection, outcomes of urethral injections, and complications associated with the procedure.

Synthetic Midurethral Slings: Roles, Outcomes, and Complications 17

Brian J. Linder and Daniel S. Elliott

Synthetic midurethral sling placement is the most studied anti-incontinence procedure available. Multiple randomized trials demonstrate its safety and efficacy, with results out to 5 years. With long-term follow-up, it seems there may be some benefit in efficacy to retropubic sling placement compared with the transobturator approach. Single-incision slings are a newer modification to multi-incision sling placement, and the data regarding safety and efficacy are not as mature as other forms of sling placement. Complications may occur with mesh midurethral sling placement and surgeons performing these procedures should be comfortable with the diagnosis and management of these issues.

Management of the Exposed or Perforated Midurethral Sling 31

Laura L. Giusto, Patricia M. Zahner, and Howard B. Goldman

The synthetic midurethral sling has become the gold standard for treatment of stress urinary incontinence since its introduction more than 20 years ago. With its utilization, the incidence of mesh-related complications has also increased. Mesh exposure and perforation are 2 common mesh complication scenarios that pelvic floor surgeons should be prepared to treat. This article highlights preoperative, perioperative, and postoperative factors to minimize the chance of vaginal wall mesh exposure or perforation of mesh into the lower urinary tract. It also summarizes common presenting symptoms, suggested evaluation and a range of treatment options.

Surgery for Stress Urinary Incontinence: Autologous Fascial Sling 41

Jerry G. Blaivas, Vannita Simma-Chiang, Zeynep Gul, Linda Dayan, Senad Kalkan, and Melissa Daniel

This article describes the operative technique of autologous fascial pubovaginal sling (AFPVS) surgery, examines the senior author's outcomes with AFPVS, compares these outcomes with those of other large studies and meta-analyses, and compares the safety and efficacy of AFPVS with those of the synthetic midurethral sling (SMUS). Recently, the SMUS has become the treatment of choice for most surgeons. The efficacy of the SMUS remains unchallenged and comparable with that of AFPVS, but SMUS are associated with more severe complications. In the author's opinion, the AFPVS should remain the gold standard for treating SUI.

Burch Colposuspension **53**

Ericka M. Sohlberg and Christopher S. Elliott

The Burch colposuspension has a 50-plus year history demonstrating strong long-term outcomes with minimal complications. Iterations of the procedure, including laparoscopic, robotic, and mini-incisional approaches, appear to have equal efficacy to the open procedure. Although the current use of the Burch colposuspension has waned with the growing shift toward sling surgery, it continues to have a role in the treatment of stress urinary incontinence. Specifically, a Burch procedure should be considered when vaginal access is limited, concurrent intra-abdominal surgery is planned, or mesh is contraindicated.

Surgery for Anterior Compartment Prolapse

Surgery for Anterior Compartment Vaginal Prolapse: Suture-Based Repair **61**

Katherine Amin and Una Lee

Native tissue anterior compartment prolapse repair remains an important surgical procedure for pelvic prolapse. Native tissue repair has been well-studied and is successful in relieving vaginal bulge symptoms and reducing prolapse within the vagina. Native tissue cystocele repair has been performed safely since the advent to modern vaginal surgery for prolapse. Reoperation rates are low and the contribution of apical support in the durability of vaginal wall defect repair surgery has been well-established. Native tissue cystocele repair addresses symptom relief for women, and should continue to be a part of pelvic floor reconstructive surgery.

Surgery for Anterior Compartment Prolapse Synthetic Graft-Augmented Repair **71**

Osnat Israeli and Adi Y. Weintraub

Pelvic organ prolapse is a common and bothersome problem that affects women's work, traveling, physical exercise, sleep, and sexual function. Synthetic implants show superiority in reducing recurrence of pelvic organ prolapse. However, inserting foreign materials carries an increased risk of complications. In this article containing the most updated available literature, we look back at the history of synthetic mesh repair, examine its efficacy and advantages, assess common complications, review current opinions, and look at the future for ways to improve the use of mesh for better results and fewer complications in an attempt to improve women's quality of life.

Surgery for Posterior Compartment Prolapse

Posterior Vaginal Wall Prolapse: Suture-Based Repair **79**

Juan M. Guzman-Negron, Michele Fascelli, and Sandip P. Vasavada

Pelvic organ prolapse is common in parous women, although few report symptoms. The incidence of posterior compartment prolapse, or rectocele, is less well-reported. Posterior vaginal wall prolapse is associated with pain, constipation, and splinting. Surgery is the mainstay of therapy for symptomatic rectoceles.

Though several surgical techniques have been described, no clear indications for type of repair have emerged. This article reviews the management strategies and draws conclusions about suture-based and site-specific techniques.

Surgery for Posterior Compartment Vaginal Prolapse: Graft Augmented Repair **87**

Sunchin Kim, Grant R. Pollock, Christian O. Twiss, and Joel T. Funk

Posterior compartment vaginal prolapse can be approached with multiple surgical techniques, including transvaginally, transperineally, and transanally, repaired with either native tissue or with the addition of an augment. Augment material for posterior compartment prolapse includes biologic graft (dermal, porcine submucosal), absorbable mesh (Vicryl polyglactin), or nonabsorbable synthetic mesh (polypropylene). Anatomic success rates for posterior compartment repair with augment has ranged from 54% to 92%. Augmented posterior compartment repair has not been shown to have superior outcome to native tissue repair. The focus of this article is on the transvaginal approach comparing native tissue repair with graft or mesh augmented repair.

Surgery for Apical Vaginal Prolapse

Transvaginal Suture-Based Repair **97**

Ekene A. Enemchukwu

An estimated 300,000 women undergo pelvic organ prolapse (POP) surgery in the United States every year at a cost of more than 1 billion dollars per year. The prevalence of POP is approximately 2.9% to 8%, and increases with age. Apical support is required to achieve successful prolapse repair. As the search for the safest, most durable, surgical repair continues, transvaginal native tissue repairs have the advantage of providing minimally invasive surgical repairs without the added risk of abdominal, laparoscopic, or robotic surgery while avoiding the risk of mesh augmentation.

Surgery for Apical Vaginal Prolapse after Hysterectomy: Transvaginal Mesh-Based Repair **103**

Shannon L. Wallace, Raveen Syan, and Eric R. Sokol

Several transvaginal mesh products have been marketed to address vaginal vault prolapse. Although data are limited, prolapse recurrence rates and subjective outcome measures seem to be equivalent for vaginal mesh compared with native tissue apical prolapse repair, and the different vaginal meshes have not proven superior to one another. Given the known unique complications specific to vaginal mesh with equivalent outcomes for the apical vaginal prolapse, it is reasonable to reserve mesh use for specific high-risk cases, such as patients with large apical prolapse recurrence after native tissue repair who are not candidates for sacrocolpopexy.

Surgery for Apical Vaginal Prolapse After Hysterectomy: Abdominal Sacrocolpopexy **113**

Wai Lee, Justina Tam, and Kathleen Kobashi

The number of surgeries for pelvic organ prolapse in the United States is increasing. Abdominal sacrocolpopexy has become the gold standard for women desiring a restorative repair of their apical pelvic organ prolapse. Despite the associated morbidity of abdominal sacrocolpopexy, advances in minimally invasive approaches have safely increased the number of these surgeries performed, especially among urologists. Moreover, a number of studies have demonstrated superior objective outcomes after abdominal sacrocolpopexy when compared with vaginal approaches. Variations in the technique are described, but no consensus exists on a standard approach.

Surgery for Vesicovaginal Fistula

Vaginal Approach to Vesicovaginal Fistula 123

Dominic Lee and Philippe Zimmern

 Video content accompanies this article at http://www.urologic.theclinics.com.

Vesicovaginal fistula is the most commonly encountered sequela of genitourinary trauma. Although the etiology differs between developed and developing countries, the principles of fistula repair must be strictly adhered to for success. Timing and route of repair remain contentious, because of a lack of randomized data. Evaluation and management is dictated by the surgeon's experience. Minimally invasive techniques with laparoscopy and robotic technology are generating wider interest with reduced postoperative morbidity, but a transvaginal technique should be in the arsenal of all pelvic reconstructive surgeons. More research is required to evaluate the optimal surgical route and technique for successful outcomes.

Abdominal Approach to Vesicovaginal Fistula 135

Elishia McKay, Kara Watts, and Nitya Abraham

 Video content accompanies this article at https://www.urologic.theclinics.com/.

Principles of abdominal vesicovaginal fistula (VVF) repair include good exposure of the fistulous tract, double-layer bladder closure, retrograde fill of the bladder to ensure a water-tight seal, tension-free closure and continuous postoperative bladder drainage. Minimally invasive approaches, particularly robot-assisted laparoscopy, have demonstrated shorter operative times, decreased blood loss, improved visibility, and similar cure rates without increased adverse events. These techniques are therefore rising in popularity among surgeons. Ultimately, surgical approach to VVF repair depends upon the individual characteristics of the patient and fistula, as well as the preference and experience of the surgeon.

UROLOGIC CLINICS OF NORTH AMERICA

FORTHCOMING ISSUES

May 2019
Emerging Technologies in Renal Stone Management
Ojas Shah and Briana Matlaga, *Editors*

August 2019
Modern Management of Testicular Cancer
Sia Daneshmand, *Editor*

November 2019
Considerations in Gender Reassignment Surgery
Lee C. Zhao and Rachel Bluebond-Langner, *Editors*

RECENT ISSUES

November 2018
Pediatric Urology
Anthony Caldamone, Hillary L. Copp, Aseem R. Shukla, and Armando J. Lorenzo, *Editors*

August 2018
Advances in Urologic Imaging
Samir S. Taneja, *Editor*

May 2018
Current Management of Invasive Bladder and Upper Tract Urothelial Cancer
Jeffrey M. Holzbeierlein, *Editor*

THE CLINICS ARE AVAILABLE ONLINE!
Access your subscription at:
www.theclinics.com

Foreword

Reconstruction of the Female Pelvis: A Fundamental Pillar of Urology

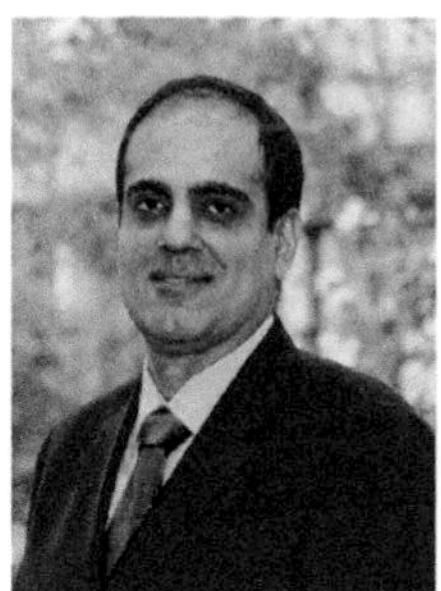

Samir S. Taneja, MD
Consulting Editor

Female pelvic medicine has evolved from a niche subspecialty practiced by a few urologists in select programs to a fundamental component of urology, essential for comprehensive training in the "core curriculum" of urologic surgery. The subspecialty has gracefully negotiated the overlapping interests of gynecologists and urologists in the field and has emerged with a fully integrated subspecialty, recognized by both specialties and their boards. In this way, the field has benefited greatly from a diversity of perspective in surgical approach to female incontinence and pelvic dysfunction.

For those in training, the concepts emerging from the study of female pelvic dysfunction and reconstruction are highly translatable to urologic disease in general. Much of the current management of male bladder dysfunction, as an example, has emerged from early observations made in the introduction and implementation of urodynamic studies by experts in the female pelvic medicine field. In the practice of radical prostatectomy, an understanding of the anatomic and mechanical forces that provide continence has allowed an evolution in surgical approach. In the rapidly expanding field of male pelvic reconstructive surgery, concepts are borrowed in creating strategic approaches to incontinence, pelvic pain, and obstructive urinary dysfunction.

In this issue of *Urologic Clinics* devoted to female pelvic reconstruction, the breadth and diversity of reconstructive techniques are well demonstrated. The simple needle suspension for bladder hypermobility, taught in the days that I trained, has been replaced with elegant pelvic floor reconstructive techniques that allow individualized approaches to select forms of incontinence, prolapse, and combinations thereof. The authors have elegantly conveyed the critical elements of each technique, the inherent benefits, the limitations, and the comparative outcomes. I believe this issue will be highly useful to the practicing urologist in formulating a plan for surgical approaches to the individual patient and particularly useful to residents in training as they master the ever-growing complexity of the field of female pelvic reconstruction. I am indebted to the Guest Editor, Dr Craig Comiter, and to the individual authors for both the incredible effort they have put forward and the high quality of the issue they have created.

Samir S. Taneja, MD
Division of Urologic Oncology
Department of Urology
NYU Langone Health
222 East 41st Street, 12th Floor
New York, NY 10017, USA

E-mail address:
samir.taneja@nyumc.org

Urol Clin N Am 46 (2019) xv
https://doi.org/10.1016/j.ucl.2018.09.003
0094-0143/19/© 2018 Published by Elsevier Inc.

Preface
Controversies in Vaginal Surgery

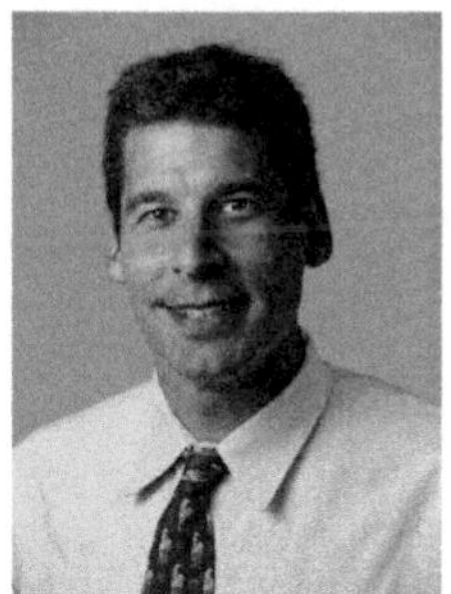

Craig V. Comiter, MD
Editor

Over the past 20 years, there has been a substantial rise in the use of surgery for the treatment of stress urinary incontinence and pelvic organ prolapse. While the incidence of stress incontinence and vaginal prolapse does increase with age, and the proportion of senior citizens has increased steadily during that time period, the use of surgery has increased more dramatically than is explained by simple increase in disease prevalence.

The establishment of an entire field devoted to the surgical management of incontinence and vaginal prolapse, Female Pelvic Medicine and Reconstructive Surgery, and the graduation of more than 100 new fellowship-trained specialists each year from more than 50 fellowship programs, has created a group of surgeons who possess the unique skills needed to manage these previously undertreated issues. In addition to an ever-growing and improving corps of surgeons, and an increased patient awareness through direct to consumer advertising and on-line patient-directed education, a plethora of surgical kits have hit the market: all combining to create an entire industry around the utilization of surgery for women with bothersome urinary incontinence and pelvic organ prolapse.

As with much of surgery, and health care in general, there are choices for both the patient and the provider, and each choice comes with its own set of risks, benefits, costs, and alternatives. Even with high-level scientific evidence regarding these risks and benefits, it is still not clear which treatment represents the best option for a particular patient. This issue of the *Urologic Clinics* focuses on Surgical Advances in Female Pelvic Reconstructive Surgery and provides up-to-date data and recommendations regarding the most common surgical treatments offered for stress incontinence and pelvic organ prolapse. For the treatment of stress urinary incontinence, the authors compare the risks and benefits of periurethral bulking agents versus midurethral synthetic sling versus pubovaginal sling using autologous fascia. With respect to pelvic organ prolapse, the authors compare the risks and benefits of suture-based repair versus mesh-augmented repair for the treatment of anterior, posterior, and apical prolapse surgery. For the treatment of vesicovaginal fistulas, the authors compare the vaginal and abdominal approaches.

Craig V. Comiter, MD
Department of Urology
Department of Obstetrics and Gynecology
Stanford University School of Medicine
300 Pasteur Drive
Room S-287
Stanford, CA 94305-5118, USA

E-mail address:
ccomiter@stanford.edu

Urol Clin N Am 46 (2019) xvii
https://doi.org/10.1016/j.ucl.2018.09.002
0094-0143/19/© 2018 Published by Elsevier Inc.

Surgery for Stress Urinary Incontinence

Injection of Urethral Bulking Agents

Hanhan Li, MD[a], Ouida Lenaine Westney, MD[b,*]

KEYWORDS

• Urethral injections • Female stress urinary incontinence • Urethral bulking agents

KEY POINTS

- Urethral injections are a safe and minimally invasive method to treat female stress urinary incontinence (SUI).
- Urethral injections should be offered to patients desiring nonsurgical treatment of SUI with the understanding of decreasing long-term success and the need for retreatment.
- Urethral injections are indicated in patients who are not surgical candidates or as second-line therapy in patients with prior failed SUI surgery.

INTRODUCTION

Stress urinary incontinence (SUI) is characterized by involuntary loss of urine associated with exertion, effort, or coughing/sneezing.[1] The classification of SUI includes urethral hypermobility (type 1), intrinsic sphincter deficiency (ISD, type 3), or both (type 2).[2] SUI is common with a prevalence of 10% to 30% in all women and is associated with significant cost to patients and society.[3] The average annual direct medical cost to the individual for treatment of SUI is estimated at $751 to $1277, whereas the total annual cost has been estimated at $13.12 billion.[4]

Several nonoperative and operative options are available in the treatment of female SUI. Urethral injections are a well-described, minimally invasive technique and represent the second most commonly performed procedure for SUI behind urethral slings.[5] Several urethral bulking agents (UBAs) are available for injection with no definitive evidence for superiority.[6] Furthermore, controversy surrounds the specific indications and patient selection for the use of urethral injections. The purpose of this article is to describe the mechanism of action and properties of various UBAs, patient selection factors, available techniques for injection, outcomes of urethral injections, and complications associated with the procedure.

HISTORY

Although the first descriptions of urinary incontinence were attributed to the Egyptians, treatment with urethral injection was described in 1938. Bryan C. Murless, a British obstetrician, injected sodium morrhuate (a sclerosing agent) into the anterior vaginal wall of 20 women in order to promote urethrovaginal scarring, thereby preventing urinary leaking.[7] Several other sclerosing agents were subsequently described; but their use was complicated by excessive scarring, vaginal sloughing, and pulmonary embolism.[8]

Later attempts at urethral injections were made in the 1980s with polytetrafluoroethylene. Treatment was complicated by migration of the agent (regional lymph nodes, lungs, and brain) and granulomatous reaction resulting in urinary tract erosion and obstruction.[9] Polytetrafluoroethylene was ultimately abandoned as a UBA. In the 1990s, the suitability of autologous fat was studied. Because of its low immunogenic potential

Disclosures: Dr O.L. Westney is a consultant for Boston Scientific.
[a] Department of Urology, MD Anderson Cancer Center, Unit 1373, 1515 Holcombe Boulevard, Houston, TX 77030, USA; [b] Urinary Tract and Pelvic Reconstruction, Department of Urology, MD Anderson Cancer Center, Unit 1373, 1515 Holcombe Boulevard, Houston, TX 77030, USA
* Corresponding author.
E-mail address: owestney@mdanderson.org

Urol Clin N Am 46 (2019) 1–15
https://doi.org/10.1016/j.ucl.2018.08.012
0094-0143/19/© 2018 Elsevier Inc. All rights reserved.

urologic.theclinics.com

and availability, autologous fat was an appealing agent; however, its efficacy was questioned in a randomized control trial that showed no difference to placebo along with a poor safety profile associated with fat embolism.[10,11]

In 1993, glutaraldehyde cross-linked bovine collagen was approved by the Food and Drug Administration (FDA) for use as an UBA. Collagen became the gold standard against which newly developed UBAs were compared.[12] At a minimum of 1-year follow-up, the average cure rate for collagen was reported at 40% to 60% with 33% of patients requiring repeat injections at the 50-month follow-up.[13] Although collagen is no longer commercially available for urologic applications in the United States after 2010, its role in understanding the efficacy of newer UBAs is historically relevant.

MECHANISM OF ACTION

Urethral injections add bulk to the proximal urethra, allowing for coaptation of the urethral wall and ultimately resulting in resistance to the passive outflow of urine in patients with SUI.[14] In one study using urethral pressure reflectometry, Klarskov and Lose[15] found that the mean squeeze opening pressure was significantly higher in patients who benefited from urethral injections. They concluded that urethral injections increase the central volume of the urethra, allowing for an increase in the power of the sphincter when it contracts. As a result, urinary outflow control is more effective. In an ultrasound study of urethral injections, Unger and colleagues[16] found that increased injection volume and percentage of urethral coaptation were positively correlated with improved outcomes. These findings further support the proposed mechanism of urethral injections in SUI.

INDICATIONS FOR URETHRAL INJECTIONS

Patients with a low leak point pressure (<60 cm H_2O) suggesting an incompetent urethra, stable bladder, and no evidence of urethral hypermobility were thought to be most suitable for urethral injections.[17,18] Nevertheless, many investigators questioned the criterion for absent urethral hypermobility. Bent and colleagues[19] administered 1 to 3 injections in patients with urethral hypermobility who wished to avoid surgery or were too medically fragile for surgery. After the 12-month follow-up, maintenance of improvement was observed in 44% of patients; the investigators concluded that patients with hypermobility also benefit from urethral injections. In another study of 187 patients, Herschorn and colleagues[20] found that collagen injection was associated with cure in 23% and improvement in 52% at a mean of 22 months of follow-up. No difference in outcome was noted between patients with and without hypermobility, and the investigators concluded that hypermobility was not a contraindication to injection. Urethral injections are also commonly indicated for patients who are not able to tolerate surgical intervention. In addition, urethral injections may be an option in patients with ISD who failed a suspension procedure. In one series, collagen injection resulted in subjective improvement in 93% of patients.[21]

Although radiation therapy was previously thought to be a contraindication, patients with radiation therapy and a fixed urethra may also benefit from injection therapy. In a study of patients with SUI who underwent radiation therapy for gynecologic cancer, Krhut and colleagues[22] found that women receiving polyacrylamide injections had reduced leakage and decreased scores on the International Consultation on Incontinence Questionnaire. The investigators concluded that urethral injection is a promising avenue for treatment in patients with SUI and prior radiation treatment.

Contraindications include mucosal fragility, urinary tract infection, and hypersensitivity to the bulking agent. Although studies showed decreased success rate in patients with detrusor overactivity,[20] one study showed no difference between patients with and without detrusor overactivity.[23] The investigators recommended that patients should not be excluded from treatment with urethral injections simply because of the presence of detrusor overactivity.

URETHRAL BULKING AGENTS

Agent Properties

An ideal UBA should be biocompatible and nonimmunogenic in order to avoid an inflammatory and fibrotic response. In addition, the agent should not migrate, which requires a particle diameter greater than 80 μm.[24] Furthermore, UBAs should be hypoallergenic and should not be subject to degradation. However, no past or current agent meets all of these criteria. Many UBAs were brought to the market, although only a few are still available. They may be classified into 3 main categories: synthetic, xenograft, and human autograft or allograft (**Table 1**).

Table 1
Urethral bulking agents

Composition	Mechanism of Action	FDA Approval	Injection System	Success Rate	Special Considerations
Polyacrylamide gel (2.5% cross-linked polyacrylamide and 97.5% water)	There is an initial macrophage and giant cell invasion followed by fibroblasts, which create a fibrous network.	Investigational device in United States European use starting in 2006	Proprietary urethroscope with 23-gauge injection needle	Significant improvement in incontinence episodes and quality of life at 1-y follow-up	Investigational device only in the United States
Calcium hydroxyapatite in a water-based carrier gel (sodium carboxymethylcellulose)	There is a minimal inflammatory response (calcium hydroxyapatite is normal constituent of teeth and bones) with absent ingrowth of collagen and fibrous tissue.	2005	Standard or injection cystoscope; 21-gauge injection needle	63.4% at 12-mo follow-up	Radiopaque, allowing radiographic follow-up of injection
Glutaraldehyde cross-linked bovine collagen	It provides scaffold in which host fibroblasts deposit collagen.	1993–2010	Standard or injection cystoscope; 21-gauge rigid needle	Average 40%–60% cure rate at minimum of 1-y follow-up	Skin testing required because of hypersensitivity (4%); contraindicated in patients with multiple allergies, celiac disease, and prior allergic reaction to collagen
Carbon-coated zirconium beads in a water-based carrier gel consisting of 2.8% glucan	—	1999	Standard cystoscope; 18–20 periurethral (1.5 in) and transurethral (15.0 in) injection needles (pencil and spinal tip)	66.1% experienced improvement in one or more incontinence grade at 12-mo follow-up	Clogging of carbon beads in syringe with loss of carrier gel resulting in higher injection pressure, creating risk for extrusion

(*continued on next page*)

Table 1
(continued)

Composition	Mechanism of Action	FDA Approval	Injection System	Success Rate	Special Considerations
Polydimethylsiloxane particles (silicone) suspended in a water-soluble carrier gel (polyvinylpyrrolidone)	Fibroblasts surround the silicone particles with collagen-forming nodules.	2006	Injection scope combined with proprietary injection device	76.1% cured or improved at 12-mo follow-up	Somewhat cumbersome injection device
Ethylene vinyl alcohol copolymer dissolved in dimethyl sulfoxide	Dimethyl sulfoxide dissolves, and the ethylene vinyl alcohol solidifies, creating a bulking effect. Phase change occurs at 66°F. Agent does not undergo degradation.	2004–2006	Standard cystoscope with injection needle	59% dry or improved at 12-mo follow-up	1 mL/min injection rate at 30°–45° angle to submucosa in order to allow ethylene vinyl alcohol to escape the dimethyl sulfoxide carrier
Non-animal stabilised hyaluronic acid/ Dextronomer gel (NASHA/Dx gel)	Dextranomer microspheres slowly undergo hydrolysis with delayed deposition of extracellular matrix and collagen.	High rate of pseudoabscess formation led to removal from market.	Standard cystoscope with 22- to 23-gauge need approach or Implacer device	76% at 12-mo follow-up	Used successfully in the treatment of vesicoureteral reflux in children

Types of Urethral Bulking Agents

Bovine cross-linked collagen, FDA approved in 1993, contains at least 95% type I collagen and 1% to 5% type III collagen. After injection, a local inflammatory reaction replaces the collagen with endogenous collagen. Because of the inflammatory reaction and subsequent resorption of collagen, repeat injections were required, often 3 separate injections.[14] Cure rates between 40% and 60% were previously reported.[25,26] Cross and colleagues[27] showed substantial improvement in 74% and improvement in 20% of patients receiving collagen injection at a median 18-month follow-up. Long-term results of collagen injection were questioned by Gorton and colleagues[28] who reported subjective improvement in only 26% of women 5 years after treatment. Complications included delayed skin reactions, arthralgias, osteitis pubis, pulmonary embolism,[29] and periurethral mass.[30] Because of the local immune response and allergic reaction in 2% to 3% of patients, skin testing was required before administration.

Porcine dermal implant is a nonreconstituted porcine dermal collagen.[31] The collagen is in its original shape and can provide permanent support for ingrowth of native tissue because of its similarity to human dermis. This product is nonallergenic, in contrast to collagen. Production of injectable Porcine dermis was phased out by the manufacturer in favor of grafts for abdominal wall reconstruction.

A fully cross-linked polyvinylpyrrolidone, a type of silicone, suspended in polyvinylpyrrolidine gel, an excretable low-molecular-weight carrier is FDA-approved Most Macroplastique particles are greater than 100 μm, which reduces the risk of migration. However, particle size is variable from less than 50 μm to greater than 400 μm. In a retrospective review of 21 patients receiving a silicone injection with a median 31-month follow-up, 48% of patients were dry or improved, whereas 52% had failures.[32] Another multicenter study evaluated the durability of a silicone injection among women with documented success 12 months after injection.[33] Among patients who had at least one Stamey grade improvement from baseline at the 12-month follow-up, 84% of patients had sustained improvement at 24 months and 67% of patients were dry (Stamey grade 0). In a meta-analysis, Ghoniem and Miller[34] demonstrated improvement in 75% after short-term follow-up (<6 months), 73% at midterm follow-up (6–18 months), and 64% at long-term follow-up (>18 months). The investigators concluded that silicone is a safe and durable injection agent for the treatment of ISD. Although silicone is thought to be inert, a recent report of 2 patients with rapid failure of their injection after initial success was attributed to an immune rejection.[35] Another case study reported suburethral mass formation requiring excision after Silicon injection.[36]

The zirconium oxide bead in polysaccharide gel was approved by the FDA in 1999. It consists of smaller particles (95–200 μm), allowing for lower pressure injection but maintaining the target size threshold of 80 μm. In an initial report of results, Madjar and colleagues[37] reported that 30 of 46 patients were cured or improved at a mean of 9 months' follow-up. Periurethral mass formation, manifested by obstructive urinary symptoms, was noted in 2.9% of patients (4 of 135) 12 to 18 months after receiving the injection.[38] In addition, migration of beads into local lymph nodes was observed with radiographic evaluation and associated with declining success rates from 6 months to 12 months.[39]

Ethylene vinyl alcohol copolymer was FDA approved in 2004 but voluntarily withdrawn in 2006, possibly because of the high rates of urethral erosion. From an efficacy standpoint, the agent was evaluated at a median 51-month follow-up; 69% of patients reported being very satisfied or satisfied.[40]

Hyaluronic acid with dextranomer is a combination of hydrophilic dextran polymer in hyaluronic acid base and the dextronomer was used successfully in vesicoureteral reflux in children.[41] The dextranomer is the bulking agent with particle size measurements ranging from 80 to 200 μm. An optional placement technique used a proprietary device at the midurethra, thus, not requiring cystoscopic equipment. Concerns due to high rates of pseudoabscess formation led to its withdrawal as an UBA. A case study also reported the development of a large pseudocyst after injection in a patient with SUI. The mass caused urinary retention, which resulted in excision and persistence of SUI.[42] In a larger cases series of 35 patients with ISD receiving injection of the dextronomer, Lightner and colleagues[43] observed 4 patients with pseudoabscess formation and obstruction requiring operative intervention.

Calcium hydroxyapatite in an aqueous gel carrier was FDA approved in 2005 for ISD. This UBA is nonimmunogenic because it is a normal constituent of bone. Early reports suggested decreased pad use 1 year after injection.[44] Particles are uniform in size (between 75 and 125 μm) and shape. Radiographs and ultrasound may localize this agent. Prior case reports suggest that granulomas are possible with calcium hydroxyapatite injection.[45,46]

Polyacrylamide gel consists of 2.5% cross-linked polyacrylamide and 97.5% water. European utilization of Bulkamid as an UBA started in 2006 but is currently not commercially available in the United States.[47] In a prospective multicenter study of 135 patients with SUI receiving transurethral injections, 64% of patients had subjective improvement, whereas objective improvement in urine leakage was also demonstrated.[48,49] In a systematic review of 8 studies enrolling 767 patients, Kasi and colleagues[50] showed decreased incontinence at 1 year after injection with polyacrylamide gel. At the 8-year follow-up, Mouritsen and colleagues[51] reported that 44% of patients were cured or much improved. In a novel application, Krause and colleagues[52] used the injection for SUI after closure of a vesicovaginal fistula caused by obstetric trauma. They reported 3 of 4 patients were continent after injection and concluded that the material can be a treatment option in this patient cohort. Most common complications included pain (4%–14%) and urinary tract infection (3%–7%). One case report describes periurethral abscess formation after injection requiring transvaginal drainage.[53]

Experimental Agents

Because the ideal UBA is yet to be developed, research efforts continue toward developing UBAs. Polymethyl methacrylate was previously shown to be a promising agent in a pig model.[54] In another multicenter study with a 12-month follow-up, Bent and colleagues[55] harvested autologous auricular chondrocytes from 32 patients with SUI. The chondrocytes were cultured and injected into the urethra 81.2% of patients remaining dry or improved at 12 months. The investigators concluded that the chondrocytes had a low likelihood of migrating or biodegrading. Another study reported the use of a gel infused with nerve growth factor and fibroblast growth factor was associated with a bulking effect with no migration in a rat model.[56] The investigators suggested this agent was a promising avenue for the development of future UBAs.

METHODS OF INJECTION

Procedural Considerations

Urethral injections may be administered in the office setting, without the risk of general anesthesia and greatly enhancing patient convenience. Important considerations include the storage requirements for the UBA, such as refrigeration, and whether special proprietary equipment is required for the injection. Because of the risk of infection associated with manipulation of the urinary tract, patients are given a dose of antibiotics before the injection.[57] Patients should also void before discharge from the office. Postvoid residuals should be measured; if residuals are high, patients should be instructed on self-catheterization.

Injection Route

Periurethral and transurethral routes of administration are available with most urologists reporting a preference for transurethral injections because of familiarity with the approach.[58] Prior studies suggest no differences in outcomes and complications between the two injection techniques with collagen[59] and hyaluronic acid.[60] Of note, these studies suggest that periurethral injections require higher volumes, which is associated with higher cost. In a randomized control trial, Schulz and colleagues[60] showed increased urinary retention for periurethral injection but no difference in urinary tract infections. They concluded that periurethral and transurethral injections were equally effective and safe. In another study examining combined periurethral injection of zirconium beads and transurethral collagen to transurethral collagen alone, Sokol and colleagues[61] found a higher cure rate at 2 weeks for the combined injection group (72.7% vs 39.2%, respectively, $P = .003$). However, this difference did not persist at 6 months (33.3% vs 29.4%, respectively, $P = .700$). The investigators concluded that a combined transurethral and periurethral approach did not improve outcomes. Regardless of the injection route, a high variance in localization of the injection agent in the urethra (even with a systematic approach to injection) was demonstrated in a study using 3-dimensional ultrasound.[62]

Another area of interest is the location of injection along the course of the urethra. One study suggested that midurethral injection is beneficial in patients with urethral hypermobility.[63] In a study evaluating bladder neck and midurethral injections with collagen, Kuhn and colleagues[64] found a small benefit for midurethral injections. However, in a study evaluating silicone injection with 3-dimensional endo-vaginal examination, Hegde and colleagues[65,66] found that both circumferential and proximal urethral injections were individually associated with successful outcomes. Furthermore, the investigators found that proximal urethral injections were more likely to be associated with circumferential injections.

Therefore, the investigators concluded that proximal urethral injections are preferred over midurethral injections.

TECHNIQUES

Periurethral Injection

The bladder is first emptied, and patients are placed in the lithotomy position. Local anesthesia (0.5–1.0 mL of 1% lidocaine) is injected on both sides of the urethra. The cystoscope is then introduced to the level of the urethrovesical junction. A 22-gauge spinal needle attached to a 5-mL syringe is then placed at the injection site and advanced parallel to the urethra. During advancement of the spinal needle, small volumes of local anesthesia with indigo carmine is injected to facilitate visualization. The needle is advanced to the desired level, and the syringe is replaced with the UBA. The material is administered, and the effect is noted through the cystoscope (**Fig. 1**). This process is then repeated on the other side of the urethra.

Transurethral Injection

Performance of transurethral injections requires a needle for delivery of the material into the submucosal space. The size of the needle depends on the characteristics of the agent. Materials composed of a larger mean particle size and higher viscosity will require a larger-gauge needle. In general, however, dedicated injection needles range in size from 18 to 23 gauge. A standard rigid cystoscope or an injection scope with a working element can be used. Injection systems are currently available from the following cystoscopic equipment manufacturers: Karl Storz (Tuttlingen, Germany) (**Fig. 2**A) and Richard Wolf (Vernon Hills, IL) (**Fig. 2**B). These systems allow for more precise guidance of the needle using a resectoscope element rather than making manual adjustments via the working channel.

After obtaining consent, patients are positioned into dorsal lithotomy. The vagina and urethra are prepped and draped in a standard fashion. The urethra is infused with 20 mL of 2% lidocaine jelly and allowed to dwell in the bladder for at least 10 minutes. To improve analgesia, 1% lidocaine solution (0.25–0.5 mL) is injected in the planned injection locations. Attempted recannulation of these needle sites for the bulking agent delivery decreases the likelihood of material extravasation from additional punctures in the urethral mucosa. For all agents, with the exception of silicone, it is possible to use the same needle for the local anesthetic and injectable agent in series, thus, reducing the possibility of creating multiple mucosal defects. Before placing the scope, the needle should be primed with local anesthetic and passed through the working channel.

After intubating the urethra, the bladder should be drained to decrease discomfort from overdistension during the procedure. The bladder neck is visualized, and the scope is withdrawn 1.5 to 2.0 cm distally. The injection sites are planned after reassessing the quality of the bladder neck tissue. In the patient with no prior urethral surgery or injections, the urethral mucosal should be pliable and receptive. A standard location using a clock reference would be 3 and 9 o'clock; however, in some injection-naïve female patients, the material may dissect circumferentially only requiring a single injection site. Before mucosal penetration, confirm that the needle has been primed with local anesthetic. Patients should be instructed that they will feel a "stick followed by a burning sensation then nothing." Advance the needle through the urethral mucosa at a 45° angle to the lumen. The bevel of the needle should be

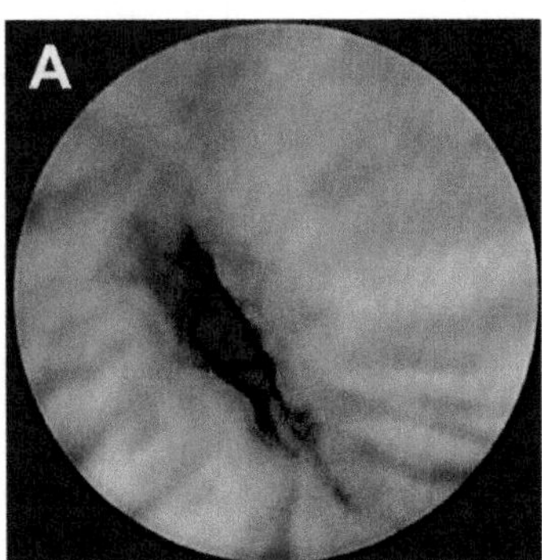

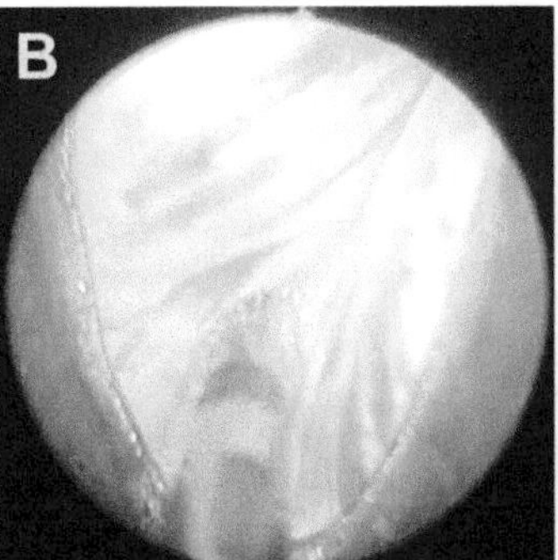

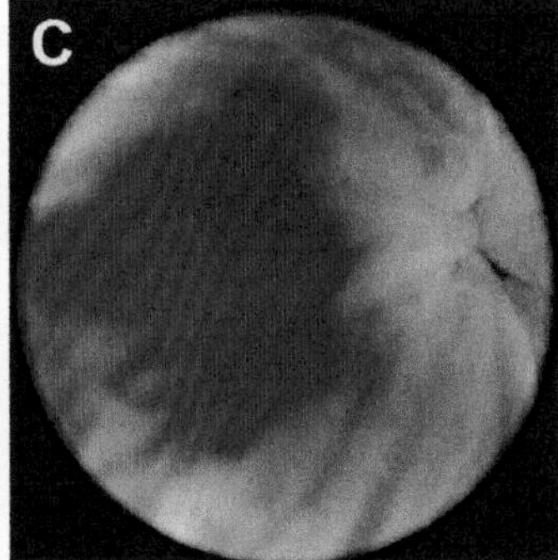

Fig. 1. Endoscopic view of before, during, and after urethral injection. A patient with previous urethral injection is noted to have incomplete coaptation of the urethra with residual bulge on the left side of the urethra (*A*). After injecting the right side of the urethra (*B*), coaptation is noted (*C*).

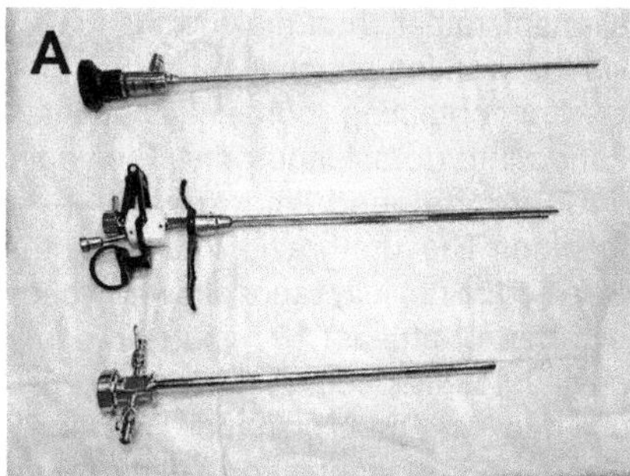

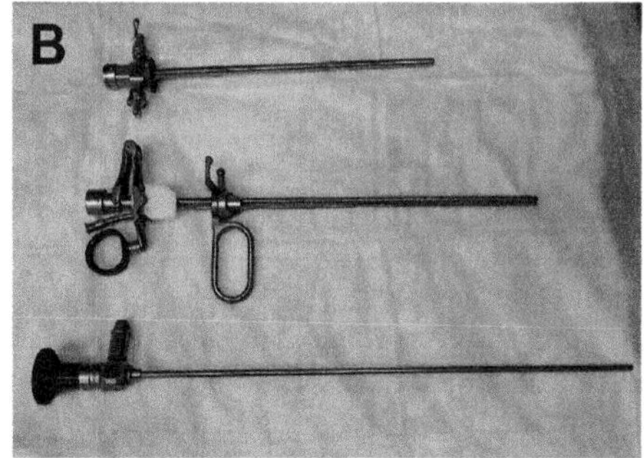

Fig. 2. Injection cystoscopes used for urethral injections. Karl Storz injection cystoscope with lens, resectoscope-type working element, and sheath (*A*). Richard Wolf cystoscope with sheath, working element, and lens (*B*). (*Courtesy of* Karl Storz, Tuttlingen, Germany; and Richard Wolf, Co, Vernon Hills, IL. with permission.)

directed toward the lumen. Because of the limited potential volume in the submucosal space, it is necessary to be judicious about the amount of local injected. Thus, limit the injected volume per site to 0.5 mL or less, if possible. After injection, request verbal feedback from patients regarding when the discomfort has dissipated before proceeding with the UBA. At this point, the local anesthetic syringe is switched for the injectable agent of choice (with the exception of the silicone injectable).

Insertion/Proprietary Devices

Silicone and dextronomer preparations are two UBAs that have been delivered with urethral insertion devices. These devices obviated cystourethroscopy. For the latter, the insertion device had 4 angled ports allowing for 4 needles. After measuring the urethral length, the Implacer is positioned at the appropriate depth and the UBA is injected. In the past, a similar device was available for silicone injection. However, this option is no longer available in favor of the cystoscopic approach.

Silicone Injectable

Injection of silicone requires a reusable administration device, which includes a syringe adapter (**Fig. 3**A). The physician can choose one of 2 needles to attach to the adapter for product delivery; Rigid Endoscopic Needle 3.8-F shaft × 14.5 in (370 mm) long with a 20-gauge tip × 0.54 in (14 mm) long or Rigid Endoscopic Needle 5-F shaft × 15 in (380 mm) long with 18-gauge tip × 0.54 in (14 mm) long (**Fig. 3**B). Recent modifications in the dimensions and weight of the administration device make it possible for a single person to manage the scope and the device in comparison with earlier models.[63] For details regarding the assembly of the administration device, please refer to the manufacturer's insert.

Silicone Injection Technique

Before bulking, adequate analgesia must be established. The most efficient manner to achieve this consists of injecting the local anesthetic in all planned injection sites before starting with the UBA. As previously mentioned, it is necessary

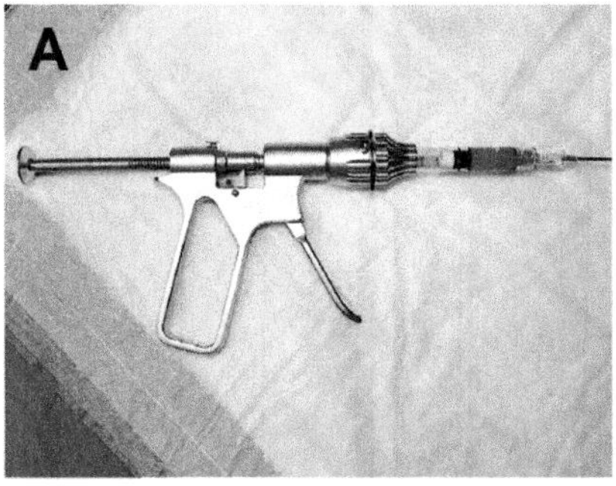

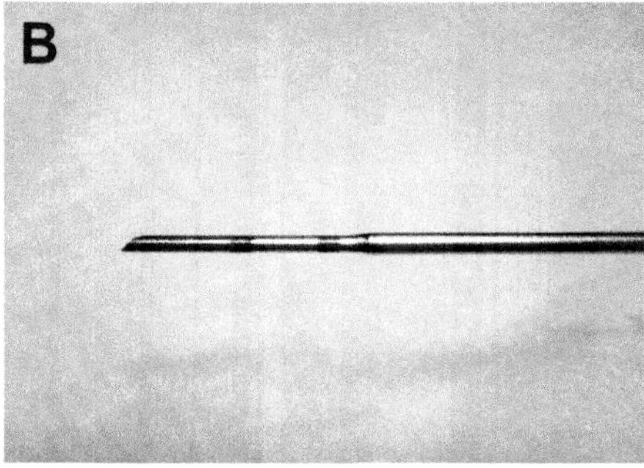

Fig. 3. Macroplastique syringe adaptor and uroplasty injection needle. Reusable administration device with a syringe adapter (*A*) connected to the Uroplasty Rigid Endoscopic Needle (*B*). (*Courtesy of* Cogentix, Minnetonka, MN.)

to attempt to reutilize the same sites for the bulking agent to prevent additional areas for extravasation.

During placement of the needle and administration device through the working channel, it may be necessary for an assistant to stabilize the cystoscope. Advance the scope into the bladder while pushing the needle forward to confirm orientation of the bevel toward the lumen. Retract the needle tip and scope back into the urethra 1.5 to 2.0 cm distal from the bladder neck. For injection, the manufacturer describes a tissue tunneling technique that is similar to the ideal placement technique for all injectables. The needle enters the tissue at a 30° to 45° angle followed by advancement of the needle for 0.5 cm. The angle is flattened to be parallel with the urethra, and the needle is advanced for another 0.5 cm.

The administration device lever should be deployed slowly to prevent rapid egress of the agent into the submucosa. Pause a few seconds between each pull to allow for equilibration of the pressure within the submucosal space. Continue until the syringe is completed at each location and/or satisfactory coaptation has been achieved. In all positions, wait approximately 30 seconds before withdrawing the needle from the tissue to limit product loss from the implantation site. It is suggested that further injections not be attempted until after 12 weeks from the prior injection.

Injection of polyacrylamide gel uses a proprietary urethroscope with 0° lens. Additional disposables unique to the UBA are also used in the injection system. Further details on this system can be found from the manufacturer, as this UBA is not available in the United States.

OUTCOMES

Studies examining urethral injections are limited by the lack of consensus in outcome instruments. Objective evaluation of outcomes requires physical examination and urodynamic testing but are not always used or reported. Subjective outcomes are frequently reported but often are not standardized between studies. Owing to the retrospective nature and limited cohort size of many studies, investigators question the overall quality of the available evidence. In a recent Cochrane Review, Kirchin and colleagues[67] identified 14 randomized controlled trials evaluating urethral injections, rated as moderate quality. They concluded that the evidence was insufficient to guide practice. They also suggested that further trials using placebo as a control were necessary because of one trial demonstrating similar outcomes between saline injection and autologous fat.[10]

Urethral Injections as Compared with Surgical Intervention

Prior investigations comparing urethral injections with surgical intervention has not demonstrated superiority. In a randomized controlled trial of collagen injection compared with surgery (needle suspensions, Burch colposuspension, and slings), Corcos and colleagues[68] showed a success rate of 72.2% after surgery versus 53.1% after urethral injections. However, no differences were detected on the Rand Medical Outcomes Study 36-Item Health Survey and Incontinence Impact Questionnaire. The investigators concluded that urethral injections are a viable alternative to surgery. In comparing open surgical treatment with injection, Maher and colleagues[69] showed that the cure rate was higher for the pubovaginal sling (81%) versus transurethral injection with silicone (9%). Cure was defined as absence of urinary leaking due to SUI on urodynamics. Furthermore, injection therapy was found to be more expensive over time. At the 5-year follow-up, 69% of patients were noted to be satisfied with the pubovaginal sling. In contrast, only 29% of patients receiving the silicone injection were found to be satisfied. These results suggest that patient satisfaction with subjective outcomes are not comparable with objective measurements of success, but both are necessary measurements of intervention outcomes.

Urethral Injections in Patients with Prior Stress Urinary Incontinence Surgeries

The association between prior surgery and the subsequent success of urethral injections is another area of investigation. In a study of patients with a failed midurethral sling, Lee and colleagues[70] found a low cure rate with injection of silicone but a satisfaction rate of 77%. One study showed an improved success rate in patients receiving urethral injections after previously failed surgery compared with patients who did not have prior surgery.[25] Another retrospective review of factors associated with successful urethral injections only identified previous surgery as predictive of success after injection.[71] Other factors, including age, parity, hypermobility, detrusor overactivity, and low maximal urethral pressure, were not predictive.

However, another study failed to show a difference in outcomes between patients with and without prior surgery.[26] Furthermore, a retrospective review of 165 patients who failed midurethral slings showed that 11.2% of patients who had repeat midurethral sling failed, whereas 38.8% of patients who had injections failed.[72] A study reporting survey results of the International Urogynecology Association demonstrated that surgeons prefer treating most patients with recurrent SUI after midurethral sling with a retropubic sling, whereas surgeons prefer intervention with urethral injections in patients who do not have urethral hypermobility.[73] The relationship between injections and subsequent surgeries requires further delineation. In a retrospective study of 43 patients with SUI, Koski and colleagues[74] found no association between prior urethral injections and the success of surgery.

Comparison with Conservative Treatment Modalities

Home pelvic floor exercise remains an option for conservative therapy.[75] In a comparison between silicon injection and home pelvic exercises, ter Meulen and colleagues[76] showed improved outcomes at the 3-month follow-up with injection therapy with a higher percentage of patients reporting cure or marked improvement. A high rate of complications was associated with injection, including urinary retention in 73% and dysuria in 47%.

Age

Although urethral injections are appealing in elderly patients who are medically fragile, previous study demonstrates no difference in outcomes among patients 50 years of age and younger, 51 to 70 years of age, and greater than 70 years old.[20] Nevertheless, another study examining collagen urethral injections showed that younger women receiving urethral injections were more likely to eventually require surgery than older women.[77] This association may be confounded by the fact that younger women may be more likely to pursue surgical intervention than older women. The impact of age on the success of urethral injections has not been well studied.

Trials Comparing Urethral Bulking Agents

Although many of these agents are not commercially available, these studies are notable, as they demonstrate the wide variety of study outcomes. Most trials evaluating UBAs used collagen as the control arm. In contrast, one randomized controlled trial compared autologous fat with placebo. In this study, Lee and colleagues[10] terminated the trial early because of a death secondary to fat embolism 3 days after injection. Only 56 of the planned 90 participants were enrolled, resulting in an underpowered study. However, no difference in subjective and objective outcomes were detected between the autologous fat injection group and the placebo (saline injection) group. Because of the poor safety profile and lack of efficacy, autologous fat is no longer used as a UBA. The investigators also found improved pad use in patients receiving saline injections. This finding suggests that more trials should include a placebo group as a comparison arm. In a nonrandomized, prospective comparison of collagen with autograft fat injection, Haab and colleagues[78] found significantly more improvement in patients with collagen injection (70.9%) compared with fat injection (31.2%, $P<.001$) at 7 months of follow-up. The investigators concluded that collagen was more effective for the treatment of SUI associated with ISD as compared with autologous fat.

In 2 studies comparing carbon particles with collagen, no differences were noted between the UBAs.[79,80] Lightner and colleagues[79] had a follow-up to 12 months and showed increased complications with carbon particles. Andersen[80] had a longer follow-up at 32.3 months.[80] In another study comparing silicone particles with collagen, Ghoniem and colleagues[81] showed an improved cure (36.9% vs 24.8%, $P<.05$) and symptom improvement for silicone particles. Next, a comparison of hyaluronic acid with collagen demonstrated a lower cure rate for hyaluronic acid at 12 months compared with collagen.[82] In a different study, Bano and colleagues[83] compared porcine dermis injection with silicone particles in a study with a 6-month follow-up. They found no difference in objective results, but injectable dermis was associated with improved subjective outcomes. However, no *P* values were provided in comparisons of the two treatment options. Finally, in a randomized controlled trial comparing polyacrylamide gel with collagen, Sokol and colleagues[84] found no difference in incontinence episodes at 12 months. Because the superiority of a single UBA was not established in the literature, the decision to use a certain type of agent should be based on physician experience and the cost to patients.

Cost

In a retrospective study of cost associated with a suburethral sling compared with collagen injection performed in 1995, Berman and Kreder[85] found that the average cost per patient treated with a sling was $10,382 compared with $4996 for urethral injections. Despite the higher cost, the investigators noted higher efficacy at 15 months in the sling group at 71% compared with 27% in the collagen group. The investigators concluded that despite the higher cost, a sling was more cost-effective because of the improved outcomes. In contrast, another cost-utility study performed a decision-tree analysis of previous studies to compare the midurethral sling with injection.[86] The investigators found that a midurethral sling was $436,465 more than injection for every 100 women treated in 1 year. In addition, the investigators found that the sling was associated with an incremental cost-effectiveness ratio of $70,400 per utility gained compared with injection. The investigators, therefore, concluded that urethral injections are more cost-effective than surgery.

COMPLICATIONS

The overall safety track record of urethral injections is very strong.[58] However, a more recent study reports a complication rate of 32%.[87] In this review of 117 studies, de Vries and colleagues[87] compiled the incidence of complications, treatment required by the complication, and follow-up time for various types of injections. Among the 6095 patients, 2095 complications were recorded. Most complications required noninvasive treatment, whereas 46 patients required an incision and drainage procedure and 21 required invasive surgery. This study, however, is limited by heterogeneity and a bias toward a higher complication rate by introducing case reports of complications associated with specific UBAs. The investigators conclude that the overall safety profile of injections is acceptable and that further study is required to determine which product offers the best outcomes and lowest complication rate.

The most common overall complication of urethral injections is pain, which can be attenuated by local anesthesia. After the urethral injections are performed, the most common complication is urinary retention. Pseudocyst formation and urinary retention are associated with injection of dextronomer. Simple aspiration was shown to effectively decompress the mass in one case series,[88] but this treatment failed in another case report.[42] Urinary tract infections are also common, occurring in 10% of patients. Prophylactic antibiotics are administered to prevent urinary tract infections. Less common complications include suburethral abscesses. Abscesses are associated with voiding dysfunction that slowly worsens. In addition, urethral diverticula have previously been reported as a complication of collagen injections.[89]

Periurethral masses are also a known complication, usually presenting within 18 months of injection. In a case report of a patient receiving a zirconium bead injection, Berger and Morgan[90] described a periurethral mass in a patient 5 years after the injection. The investigators concluded that although most masses manifest shortly after injection, clinical suspicion of a periurethral mass should be maintained several years after injection. In another case report, injection of calcium hydroxyapatite was associated with a 2-cm prolapse of the mucosa through the external urethra.[91] The investigators attributed this complication to excessive force during injection and turning the bevel toward the mucosa, rather than away from the mucosa. A similar clinical outcome was reported with the same agent by another group secondary to granuloma formation.[45] Urethral erosion is also a rare complication and has been reported with the use of ethyl vinyl alcohol (**Fig. 4**).

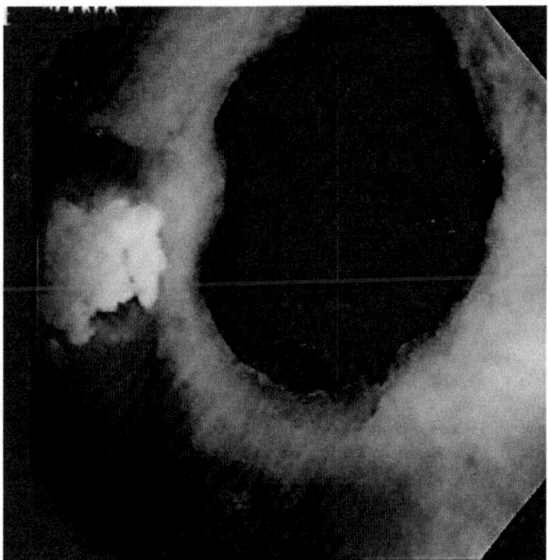

Fig. 4. Urethral erosion of a UBA. A rare complication whereby the UBA (Tegress) has eroded through the submucosa into the urethral lumen. (*Courtesy of* C.R. Bard, Murray Hill, NJ.)

SUMMARY

Despite several decades of experience, several UBAs are available; but a clearly superior UBA has yet to emerge. Several experimental agents are also under investigation. In addition, questions remain regarding the exact role of urethral injections in the management of SUI. Certainly, patients who refuse surgery or are poor surgical candidates benefit from urethral injections. However, the role of urethral injections in failed surgery or younger patients remains unclear. Many of these questions likely remain because of the lack of high-quality evidence and uniform outcome measures in the literature. Moving forward, randomized prospective studies of UBAs should incorporate a placebo arm, although all studies should include both objective and validated subjective outcome measures. Even though much remains to be studied, the current literature shows that urethral injections are a safe and minimally invasive modality available in the treatment armamentarium against SUI.

REFERENCES

1. Haylen BT, de Ridder D, Freeman RM, et al. An International Urogynecological Association (IUGA)/International Continence Society (ICS) joint report on the terminology for female pelvic floor dysfunction. Int Urogynecol J 2010;21(1):5–26.
2. Blaivas JG, Olsson CA. Stress incontinence: classification and surgical approach. J Urol 1988;139(4): 727–31.
3. Thomas TM, Plymat KR, Blannin J, et al. Prevalence of urinary incontinence. Br Med J 1980;281(6250): 1243–5.
4. Chong EC, Khan AA, Anger JT. The financial burden of stress urinary incontinence among women in the United States. Curr Urol Rep 2011;12(5):358–62.
5. Rogo-Gupta L, Litwin MS, Saigal CS, et al, Urologic Diseases in America Project. Trends in the surgical management of stress urinary incontinence among female Medicare beneficiaries, 2002-2007. Urology 2013;82(1):38–41.
6. Starkman JS, Scarpero H, Dmochowski RR. Emerging periurethral bulking agents for female stress urinary incontinence: is new necessarily better? Curr Urol Rep 2006;7(5):405–13.
7. Dmochowski RR, Appell RA. Injectable agents in the treatment of stress urinary incontinence in women: where are we now? Urology 2000;56(6 Suppl 1): 32–40.
8. Sachse H. Treatment of urinary incontinence with sclerosing solutions. Indications, results, complications. Urol Int 1963;15:225–44 [in German].
9. Ferro MA, Smith JH, Smith PJ. Periurethral granuloma: unusual complication of Teflon periurethral injection. Urology 1988;31(5):422–3.
10. Lee PE, Kung RC, Drutz HP. Periurethral autologous fat injection as treatment for female stress urinary incontinence: a randomized double-blind controlled trial. J Urol 2001;165(1):153–8.
11. Currie I, Drutz HP, Deck J, et al. Adipose tissue and lipid droplet embolism following periurethral injection of autologous fat: case report and review of the literature. Int Urogynecol J Pelvic Floor Dysfunct 1997;8(6):377–80.
12. Dmochowski R, Appell RA. Advancements in minimally invasive treatments for female stress urinary incontinence: radiofrequency and bulking agents. Curr Urol Rep 2003;4(5):350–5.
13. Corcos J, Fournier C. Periurethral collagen injection for the treatment of female stress urinary incontinence: 4-year follow-up results. Urology 1999; 54(5):815–8.
14. Winters JC, Appell R. Periurethral injection of collagen in the treatment of intrinsic sphincteric deficiency in the female patient. Urol Clin North Am 1995;22(3):673–8.
15. Klarskov N, Lose G. Urethral injection therapy: what is the mechanism of action? Neurourol Urodyn 2008; 27(8):789–92.
16. Unger CA, Barber MD, Walters MD. Ultrasound evaluation of the urethra and bladder neck before and after transurethral bulking. Female Pelvic Med Reconstr Surg 2016;22(2):118–22.
17. Appell RA. Collagen injection therapy for urinary incontinence. Urol Clin North Am 1994;21(1):177–82.
18. McGuire EJ, Appell RA. Transurethral collagen injection for urinary incontinence. Urology 1994;43(4): 413–5.
19. Bent AE, Foote J, Siegel S, et al. Collagen implant for treating stress urinary incontinence in women with urethral hypermobility. J Urol 2001;166(4): 1354–7.
20. Herschorn S, Steele DJ, Radomski SB. Followup of intraurethral collagen for female stress urinary incontinence. J Urol 1996;156(4):1305–9.
21. Isom-Batz G, Zimmern PE. Collagen injection for female urinary incontinence after urethral or periurethral surgery. J Urol 2009;181(2):701–4.
22. Krhut J, Martan A, Jurakova M, et al. Treatment of stress urinary incontinence using polyacrylamide hydrogel in women after radiotherapy: 1-year follow-up. Int Urogynecol J 2016;27(2):301–5.
23. Monga AK, Robinson D, Stanton SL. Periurethral collagen injections for genuine stress incontinence: a 2-year follow-up. Br J Urol 1995;76(2):156–60.
24. Malizia AA Jr, Reiman HM, Myers RP, et al. Migration and granulomatous reaction after periurethral injection of polytef (Teflon). JAMA 1984;251(24):3277–81.
25. Eckford SD, Abrams P. Para-urethral collagen implantation for female stress incontinence. Br J Urol 1991;68(6):586–9.
26. Khullar V, Cardozo LD, Abbott D, et al. GAX collagen in the treatment of urinary incontinence in elderly women: a two year follow up. Br J Obstet Gynaecol 1997;104(1):96–9.
27. Cross CA, English SF, Cespedes RD, et al. A followup on transurethral collagen injection therapy for urinary incontinence. J Urol 1998;159(1):106–8.
28. Gorton E, Stanton S, Monga A, et al. Periurethral collagen injection: a long-term follow-up study. BJU Int 1999;84(9):966–71.
29. Sweat SD, Lightner DJ. Complications of sterile abscess formation and pulmonary embolism following periurethral bulking agents. J Urol 1999; 161(1):93–6.

30. Malabarey O, Walter JE. Collagenoma and voiding dysfunction as complications of periurethral bulking. Int Urogynecol J 2015;26(7):1077–8.
31. Harper C. Permacol: clinical experience with a new biomaterial. Hosp Med 2001;62(2):90–5.
32. Barranger E, Fritel X, Kadoch O, et al. Results of transurethral injection of silicone micro-implants for females with intrinsic sphincter deficiency. J Urol 2000;164(5):1619–22.
33. Ghoniem G, Corcos J, Comiter C, et al. Durability of urethral bulking agent injection for female stress urinary incontinence: 2-year multicenter study results. J Urol 2010;183(4):1444–9.
34. Ghoniem GM, Miller CJ. A systematic review and meta-analysis of Macroplastique for treating female stress urinary incontinence. Int Urogynecol J 2013; 24(1):27–36.
35. Bennett AT, Lukacz ES. Two cases of suspected rejection of polydimethylsiloxane urethral bulking agent. Female Pelvic Med Reconstr Surg 2017; 23(3):e10–1.
36. Wasenda EJ, Nager CW. Suburethral mass formation after injection of polydimethylsiloxane (Macroplastique(R)) urethral bulking agent. Int Urogynecol J 2016;27(12):1935–6.
37. Madjar S, Covington-Nichols C, Secrest CL. New periurethral bulking agent for stress urinary incontinence: modified technique and early results. J Urol 2003;170(6 Pt 1):2327–9.
38. Madjar S, Sharma AK, Waltzer WC, et al. Periurethral mass formations following bulking agent injection for the treatment of urinary incontinence. J Urol 2006; 175(4):1408–10.
39. Pannek J, Brands FH, Senge T. Particle migration after transurethral injection of carbon coated beads for stress urinary incontinence. J Urol 2001;166(4): 1350–3.
40. Kuhn A, Stadlmayr W, Sohail A, et al. Long-term results and patients' satisfaction after transurethral ethylene vinyl alcohol (Tegress) injections: a two-centre study. Int Urogynecol J Pelvic Floor Dysfunct 2008;19(4):503–7.
41. Lackgren G, Wahlin N, Skoldenberg E, et al. Long-term followup of children treated with dextranomer/hyaluronic acid copolymer for vesicoureteral reflux. J Urol 2001;166(5):1887–92.
42. Abdelwahab HA, Ghoniem GM. Obstructive suburethral mass after transurethral injection of dextranomer/hyaluronic acid copolymer. Int Urogynecol J Pelvic Floor Dysfunct 2007;18(11):1379–80.
43. Lightner DJ, Fox J, Klingele C. Cystoscopic injections of dextranomer hyaluronic acid into proximal urethra for urethral incompetence: efficacy and adverse outcomes. Urology 2010; 75(6):1310–4.
44. Mayer R, Lightfoot M, Jung I. Preliminary evaluation of calcium hydroxylapatite as a transurethral bulking agent for stress urinary incontinence. Urology 2001; 57(3):434–8.
45. Palma PC, Riccetto CL, Martins MH, et al. Massive prolapse of the urethral mucosa following periurethral injection of calcium hydroxylapatite for stress urinary incontinence. Int Urogynecol J Pelvic Floor Dysfunct 2006;17(6):670–1.
46. Gafni-Kane A, Sand PK. Foreign-body granuloma after injection of calcium hydroxylapatite for type III stress urinary incontinence. Obstet Gynecol 2011; 118(2 Pt 2):418–21.
47. Lose G, Mouritsen L, Nielsen JB. A new bulking agent (polyacrylamide hydrogel) for treating stress urinary incontinence in women. BJU Int 2006;98(1): 100–4.
48. Toozs-Hobson P, Al-Singary W, Fynes M, et al. Two-year follow-up of an open-label multicenter study of polyacrylamide hydrogel (Bulkamid(R)) for female stress and stress-predominant mixed incontinence. Int Urogynecol J 2012;23(10):1373–8.
49. Lose G, Sorensen HC, Axelsen SM, et al. An open multicenter study of polyacrylamide hydrogel (Bulkamid(R)) for female stress and mixed urinary incontinence. Int Urogynecol J 2010;21(12):1471–7.
50. Kasi AD, Pergialiotis V, Perrea DN, et al. Polyacrylamide hydrogel (Bulkamid(R)) for stress urinary incontinence in women: a systematic review of the literature. Int Urogynecol J 2016;27(3):367–75.
51. Mouritsen L, Lose G, Moller-Bek K. Long-term follow-up after urethral injection with polyacrylamide hydrogel for female stress incontinence. Acta Obstet Gynecol Scand 2014;93(2):209–12.
52. Krause HG, Lussy JP, Goh JT. Use of periurethral injections of polyacrylamide hydrogel for treating post-vesicovaginal fistula closure urinary stress incontinence. J Obstet Gynaecol Res 2014;40(2): 521–5.
53. Gopinath D, Smith AR, Reid FM. Periurethral abscess following polyacrylamide hydrogel (Bulkamid) for stress urinary incontinence. Int Urogynecol J 2012;23(11):1645–8.
54. Lemperle G, Lappin PB, Stone C, et al. Urethral bulking with polymethylmethacrylate microspheres for stress urinary incontinence: tissue persistence and safety studies in miniswine. Urology 2011; 77(4):1005.e1-7.
55. Bent AE, Tutrone RT, McLennan MT, et al. Treatment of intrinsic sphincter deficiency using autologous ear chondrocytes as a bulking agent. Neurourol Urodyn 2001;20(2):157–65.
56. Oh SH, Bae JW, Kang JG, et al. Dual growth factor-loaded in situ gel-forming bulking agent: passive and bioactive effects for the treatment of urinary incontinence. J Mater Sci Mater Med 2015;26(1):5365.
57. American Urological Association. Urologic surgery antimicrobial prophylaxis. 2012. Available at: http://www.auanet.org/guidelines/antimicrobial-prophylaxis-

(2008-reviewed-and-validity-confirmed-2011-amended-2012). Accessed May 29, 2018.
58. Lightner DJ. Review of the available urethral bulking agents. Curr Opin Urol 2002;12(4):333–8.
59. Faerber GJ, Belville WD, Ohl DA, et al. Comparison of transurethral versus periurethral collagen injection in women with intrinsic sphincter deficiency. Tech Urol 1998;4(3):124–7.
60. Schulz JA, Nager CW, Stanton SL, et al. Bulking agents for stress urinary incontinence: short-term results and complications in a randomized comparison of periurethral and transurethral injections. Int Urogynecol J Pelvic Floor Dysfunct 2004;15(4):261–5.
61. Sokol ER, Aguilar VC, Sung VW, et al. Combined trans- and periurethral injections of bulking agents for the treatment of intrinsic sphincter deficiency. Int Urogynecol J Pelvic Floor Dysfunct 2008;19(5):643–7.
62. Yune JJ, Quiroz L, Nihira MA, et al. The Location and distribution of transurethral bulking agent: 3-dimensional ultrasound study. Female Pelvic Med Reconstr Surg 2016;22(2):98–102.
63. Petros PE, Ulmsten UI. An integral theory and its method for the diagnosis and management of female urinary incontinence. Scand J Urol Nephrol Suppl 1993;153:1–93.
64. Kuhn A, Stadlmayr W, Lengsfeld D, et al. Where should bulking agents for female urodynamic stress incontinence be injected? Int Urogynecol J Pelvic Floor Dysfunct 2008;19(6):817–21.
65. Hegde A, Smith AL, Aguilar VC, et al. Three-dimensional endovaginal ultrasound examination following injection of Macroplastique for stress urinary incontinence: outcomes based on location and periurethral distribution of the bulking agent. Int Urogynecol J 2013;24(7):1151–9.
66. van Kerrebroeck P, ter Meulen F, Farrelly E, et al. Treatment of stress urinary incontinence: recent developments in the role of urethral injection. Urol Res 2003;30(6):356–62.
67. Kirchin V, Page T, Keegan PE, et al. Urethral injection therapy for urinary incontinence in women. Cochrane Database Syst Rev 2017;(7):CD003881.
68. Corcos J, Collet JP, Shapiro S, et al. Multicenter randomized clinical trial comparing surgery and collagen injections for treatment of female stress urinary incontinence. Urology 2005;65(5):898–904.
69. Maher CF, O'Reilly BA, Dwyer PL, et al. Pubovaginal sling versus transurethral Macroplastique for stress urinary incontinence and intrinsic sphincter deficiency: a prospective randomised controlled trial. BJOG 2005;112(6):797–801.
70. Lee HN, Lee YS, Han JY, et al. Transurethral injection of bulking agent for treatment of failed mid-urethral sling procedures. Int Urogynecol J 2010;21(12):1479–83.
71. Koduri S, Goldberg RP, Kwon C, et al. Factors influencing the long-term success of periurethral collagen therapy in the office. Int Urogynecol J Pelvic Floor Dysfunct 2006;17(4):346–51.
72. Gaddi A, Guaderrama N, Bassiouni N, et al. Repeat midurethral sling compared with urethral bulking for recurrent stress urinary incontinence. Obstet Gynecol 2014;123(6):1207–12.
73. Giarenis I, Thiagamoorthy G, Zacche M, et al. Management of recurrent stress urinary incontinence after failed midurethral sling: a survey of members of the International Urogynecological Association (IUGA). Int Urogynecol J 2015;26(9):1285–91.
74. Koski ME, Enemchukwu EA, Padmanabhan P, et al. Safety and efficacy of sling for persistent stress urinary incontinence after bulking injection. Urology 2011;77(5):1076–80.
75. Berghmans LC, Hendriks HJ, Bo K, et al. Conservative treatment of stress urinary incontinence in women: a systematic review of randomized clinical trials. Br J Urol 1998;82(2):181–91.
76. ter Meulen PH, Berghmans LC, Nieman FH, et al. Effects of Macroplastique Implantation System for stress urinary incontinence and urethral hypermobility in women. Int Urogynecol J Pelvic Floor Dysfunct 2009;20(2):177–83.
77. Groutz A, Blaivas JG, Kesler SS, et al. Outcome results of transurethral collagen injection for female stress incontinence: assessment by urinary incontinence score. J Urol 2000;164(6):2006–9.
78. Haab F, Zimmern PE, Leach GE. Urinary stress incontinence due to intrinsic sphincteric deficiency: experience with fat and collagen periurethral injections. J Urol 1997;157(4):1283–6.
79. Lightner D, Calvosa C, Andersen R, et al. A new injectable bulking agent for treatment of stress urinary incontinence: results of a multicenter, randomized, controlled, double-blind study of Durasphere. Urology 2001;58(1):12–5.
80. Andersen RC. Long-term follow-up comparison of durasphere and contigen in the treatment of stress urinary incontinence. J Low Genit Tract Dis 2002;6(4):239–43.
81. Ghoniem G, Corcos J, Comiter C, et al. Cross-linked polydimethylsiloxane injection for female stress urinary incontinence: results of a multicenter, randomized, controlled, single-blind study. J Urol 2009;181(1):204–10.
82. Lightner D, Rovner E, Corcos J, et al. Randomized controlled multisite trial of injected bulking agents for women with intrinsic sphincter deficiency: mid-urethral injection of Zuidex via the Implacer versus proximal urethral injection of Contigen cystoscopically. Urology 2009;74(4):771–5.
83. Bano F, Barrington JW, Dyer R. Comparison between porcine dermal implant (Permacol) and silicone injection (Macroplastique) for urodynamic

stress incontinence. Int Urogynecol J Pelvic Floor Dysfunct 2005;16(2):147–50 [discussion: 150].

84. Sokol ER, Karram MM, Dmochowski R. Efficacy and safety of polyacrylamide hydrogel for the treatment of female stress incontinence: a randomized, prospective, multicenter North American study. J Urol 2014;192(3):843–9.
85. Berman CJ, Kreder KJ. Comparative cost analysis of collagen injection and fascia lata sling cystourethropexy for the treatment of type III incontinence in women [see comments]. J Urol 1997;157(1):122–4.
86. Kunkle CM, Hallock JL, Hu X, et al. Cost utility analysis of urethral bulking agents versus midurethral sling in stress urinary incontinence. Female Pelvic Med Reconstr Surg 2015;21(3):154–9.
87. de Vries AM, Wadhwa H, Huang J, et al. Complications of urethral bulking agents for stress urinary incontinence: an extensive review including case reports. Female Pelvic Med Reconstr Surg 2017. [Epub ahead of print].
88. Petrou SP, Pak RW, Lightner DJ. Simple aspiration technique to address voiding dysfunction associated with transurethral injection of dextranomer/hyaluronic acid copolymer. Urology 2006;68(1):186–8.
89. Kumar D, Kaufman MR, Dmochowski RR. Case reports: periurethral bulking agents and presumed urethral diverticula. Int Urogynecol J 2011;22(8): 1039–43.
90. Berger MB, Morgan DM. Delayed presentation of pseudoabscess secondary to injection of pyrolytic carbon-coated beads bulking agent. Female Pelvic Med Reconstr Surg 2012;18(5):303–5.
91. Lai HH, Hurtado EA, Appell RA. Large urethral prolapse formation after calcium hydroxylapatite (Coaptite) injection. Int Urogynecol J Pelvic Floor Dysfunct 2008;19(9):1315–7.

Synthetic Midurethral Slings

Roles, Outcomes, and Complications

Brian J. Linder, MD, Daniel S. Elliott, MD*

KEYWORDS

- Stress urinary incontinence • Anti-incontinence surgery • Female • Midurethral sling
- Retropubic sling • Transobturator sling

KEY POINTS

- Synthetic midurethral sling placement is the most extensively studied anti-incontinence procedure available, with multiple randomized studies demonstrating its safety and efficacy.
- Retropubic and transobturator multi-incision slings have similar short-term efficacy, although 5-year follow-up data suggest lower recurrence rates with a retropubic approach.
- In cases with concomitant urethral reconstruction, synthetic midurethral sling placement should be avoided.
- Surgeons implanting midurethral slings should be comfortable diagnosing and managing potential complications that may arise.

INTRODUCTION

Female stress urinary incontinence (SUI) is a highly prevalent condition that will likely expand as the population ages. The estimated lifetime prevalence of a woman undergoing surgery for SUI is 13.6%.[1] Presently, synthetic midurethral sling placement represents most anti-incontinence procedures performed in the United States.[2,3] Synthetic midurethral sling placement is the most extensively researched surgical treatment of SUI, with more than 2000 published articles establishing its effectiveness and describing their safety profile.[4,5] This article evaluates the current role of synthetic midurethral slings in managing female SUI, techniques for placement, long-term outcomes for various slings, and the most frequently encountered complications and their management.

BRIEF BACKGROUND AND HISTORY

Originally introduced in 1996, synthetic midurethral sling placement has rapidly expanded in volume, and supplanted other anti-incontinence procedures in volume performed nationally among urologists.[2,6] Since the initial report multiple modifications to the technique for sling placement have been made, including introduction of the transobturator approach to sling placement in 2001,[7] and single incision slings in 2006.[8] The expansion of midurethral sling placement has likely been secondary to the ability to perform them on an outpatient basis, with limited morbidity, durable efficacy, and in a less invasive manner than other traditional options (eg, pubovaginal sling placement or Burch retropubic urethropexy).[5]

SURGICAL TECHNIQUE FOR SLING PLACEMENT

As with all surgical procedures one cannot overstate the importance of proper patient selection and thorough preoperative counseling, including discussion of the potential benefits, risks, details related to the use of mesh materials in pelvic surgeries, and reviewing the nonmesh alternatives

Disclosure: The authors have no conflicts of interest or disclosures.
Department of Urology, Mayo Clinic, 200 First Street Southwest, Rochester, MN 55905, USA
* Corresponding author.
E-mail address: Elliott.Daniel@mayo.edu

Urol Clin N Am 46 (2019) 17–30
https://doi.org/10.1016/j.ucl.2018.08.013
0094-0143/19/© 2018 Elsevier Inc. All rights reserved.

that are available. Shared decision making with patients is of utmost importance. Although multiple routes and techniques for midurethral sling placement exist, they all share several surgical principals. Common features for these procedures include: dorsolithotomy positioning, prophylactic perioperative antibiotics, placement of a transurethral Foley catheter, and performing intraoperative cystoscopy. For low-risk patients, the American Urologic Association (AUA) best practice statement notes that early ambulation is sufficient thromboembolic prophylaxis for synthetic midurethral sling placement.[9]

Retropubic Techniques

Retropubic midurethral sling placement can either be performed with trocar passage from the vagina to the abdomen (ie, bottom-up, **Fig. 1**A, B) or from the abdomen to the vagina (ie, top-down, **Fig. 1**C). Regardless of the approach, the vaginal dissection is similar for each. Using the indwelling Foley catheter balloon as a guide, the bladder neck is palpated and marked. The vaginal epithelium is injected in the midline for hydrodissection, either with local anesthetic or normal saline. Likewise, hydrodissection is performed in the periurethral tissues where the dissection will be carried out. A roughly 2-cm midline incision is made over the midurethral portion of the anterior vaginal wall. The vaginal epithelium is then dissected away from the underlying periurethral tissues, and the dissection carried to the level of the ischial rami bilaterally. We perform adequate dissection in these channels to permit passage of the surgeon's index finger. The retropubic space is then injected with additional local anesthetic. Two small stab incisions are made immediately above the pubic symphysis, roughly 2 cm lateral to the midline on each side, to allow for trocar passage. Trocar passage is performed, either in a top-down or bottom-up fashion, per surgeon preference. Careful attention is paid to making sure the trocar passes immediately adjacent to the back of the pubic symphysis, to decrease the risk of bladder perforation. Before trocar passage, some surgeons use a Mandarin placed inside of the Foley catheter, which is intended to deflect the bladder from the path of the trocar. When using this technique, the handle of the Mandarin is moved toward the ipsilateral side of trocar passage. In one study, a median bladder displacement of 1.4 cm was seen on ultrasound with this technique.[10]

Following trocar passage, cystoscopy is performed to evaluate for urinary tract injury. This includes careful evaluation of the urethra with a 0-degree lens. Likewise, the bladder is fully distended and thoroughly inspected using a 70-degree lens to evaluate for perforation by the trocar. Adequate distention is necessary to remove any folds from the bladder mucosa and allow for complete evaluation. If a bladder perforation has occurred, it typically does so at the 1- or 11-o'clock positions. In that instance, the trocar is removed and repassed.

The vaginal dissection is inspected to evaluate for thinned areas of dissection or "button holes," because these would lead to vaginal mesh exposures. Following this, the sling is passed, tensioned per the surgeon's discretion, and deployed. There is wide variation in tensioning techniques (eg, intraoperative stress testing, cystoscopic evaluation of urethral coaptation, subjective tensioning over a surgical instrument),[11] although regardless of technique, the result typically includes the sling being placed in a tension-free manner. The midline vaginal incision is then closed with an absorbable suture, the suprapubic sling tails are trimmed to below the skin level, and the suprapubic stabs incisions are closed.

Transobturator Techniques

Transobturator sling placement can be performed using a helical or C-shaped trocar, and either in a path from the medial thigh to the vagina (ie, outside-in; **Fig. 2**A) or vice versa (ie, inside-out; **Fig. 2**B). Hydrodissection and a midline vaginal incision are made, similar to that described for the retropubic technique. Following this, the dissection is carried at roughly a 45-degree angle laterally until the obturator membrane is encountered. Care is taken during this dissection to ensure that the dissection is carried beyond the level of the vaginal fornix to avoid sulcal mesh exposures and focal pain following sling placement. A small stab incision is made on the medial thigh, at the superior and medial portion of the obturator foramen, as determined from palpation of the pubic ramus. This should be below the adductor longus tendon and at the level of the clitoris. For transobturator sling placement we typically use a reusable C-shaped passer in an outside-in fashion. Initially, the trocar is aligned vertically (perpendicular to the floor) and the obturator membrane is perforated. The trocar is then turned roughly 45° (clockwise or counterclockwise, depending on the side of placement) and the tip of the trocar is passed on to the surgeon's index finger, which is in the vaginal dissection bed. With this approach the surgeon's index finger in the dissection bed prevents vaginal perforation or urethral injury. The vaginal epithelium is inspected and the sling deployed. Cystoscopy is

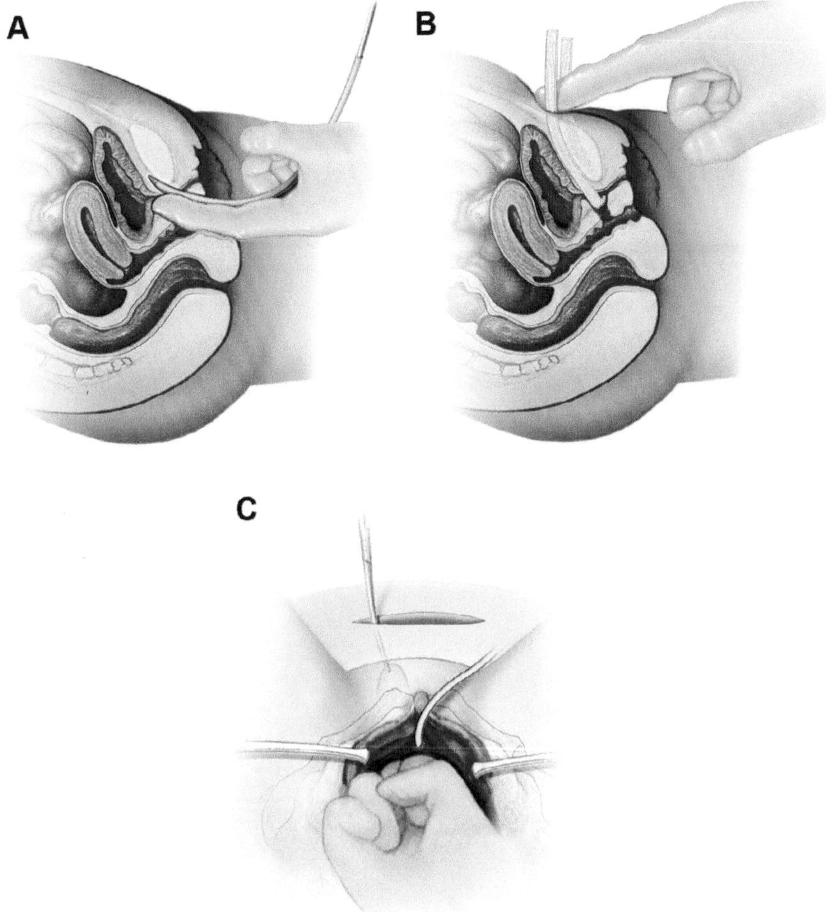

Fig. 1. Illustration of synthetic retropubic midurethral sling placement via (*A, B*) the bottom-up approach and (*C*) the top-down approach. (*Courtesy of* Mayo Foundation for Medical Education and Research, all rights reserved; with permission.)

performed to rule out urinary tract injury. The sling should be placed in a tension-free manner, the sling tails are trimmed, the vaginal epithelium is closed with an absorbable suture, and the skin incisions are closed.

Single incision slings are modeled after the inside-out transobturator technique for midurethral sling placement. These slings differ in that they are not full length and the mesh sling material does not perforate the obturator membrane or thigh muscles. Instead, an anchoring mechanism is deployed in the obturator externis muscle and membrane to provide secure mesh attachment. Thus, the procedure only involves a single vaginal incision, with no exit incision in the medial thigh. As with all sling placements, passage of the trocar and sling deployment should be performed as per the manufacturer instructions (**Fig. 3**).

MESH MATERIALS AND BODY REACTION

Ideally, an implanted material for stress incontinence would lead to incorporation by the body's connective tissue, be permanent, resistant to infection, and inert. It has been identified that several qualities of the implanted material, such as pore size, weave, and fiber diameter, were important in determining the body's reaction to the material.[12] Currently, the ideal mesh should be large pore (>75 μm) and monofilament (type I), to allow for the body's immune responses to penetrate the interstices and collagen fiber incorporation. Previous use of smaller pore size meshes (type III) was associated with mesh encapsulation and high rates of mesh exposure and infection.[12]

In studies to date, the use of type I polypropylene mesh in pelvic surgery has not been associated with an increased risk of cancer

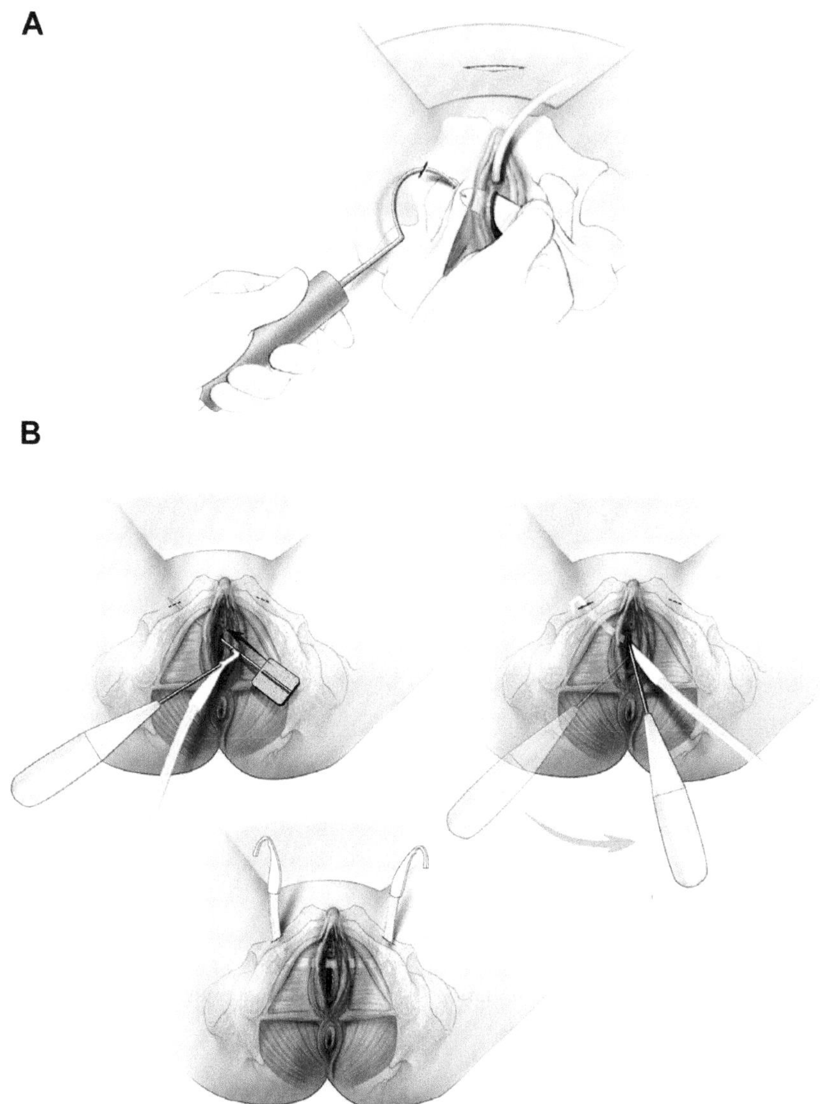

Fig. 2. Illustration of synthetic transobturator midurethral sling placement via (*A*) the outside-in approach and (*B*) the inside-out approach. (*Courtesy of* Mayo Foundation for Medical Education and Research, all rights reserved; with permission.)

formation or systemic disease.[13–16] In a Swedish nationwide study of 5.4 million women, including 20,905 that underwent midurethral sling placement, having undergone midurethral sling placement was not associated with an increased risk of cancer later in life.[16] Likewise, in review of a New York state registry of 2102 patients undergoing mesh implantation, no increased risk of autoimmune disorders was identified in women that underwent sling placement as compared with a matched control cohort undergoing nonmesh surgery (ie, colonoscopy or hysterectomy).[14]

FOOD AND DRUG ADMINISTRATION AND MESH USE

A contemporary discussion of midurethral sling placement is not complete without reviewing the current environment and climate for the use of mesh in pelvic floor surgery.[17] As background, in 2008 the Food and Drug Administration (FDA) released a public notification informing clinicians and patients of adverse events related to use of surgical mesh in pelvic floor surgeries. They noted "serious complications associated with transvaginal placement of surgical mesh in repair of pelvic

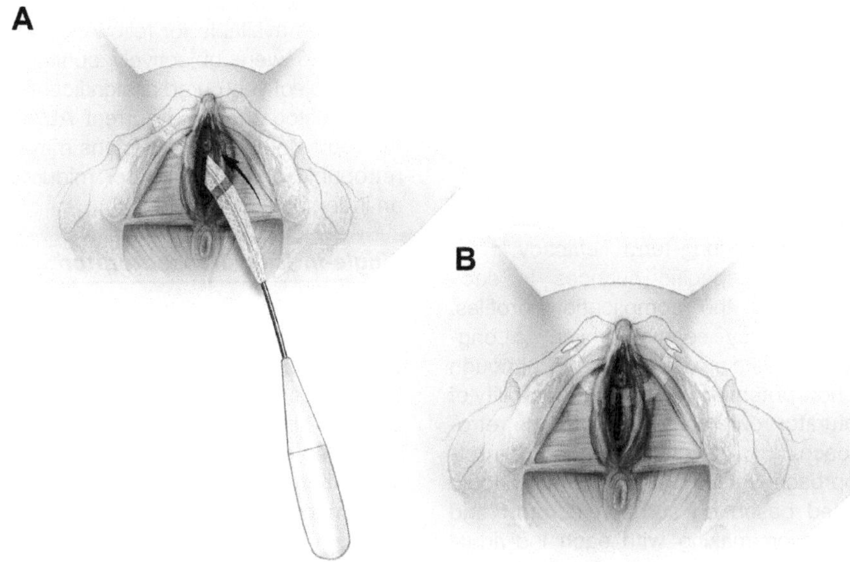

Fig. 3. Illustration of synthetic single-incision sling placement, including: (*A*) trocar positioning and trajectory (*arrow*), (*B*) completed single-incision sling placement. (*Courtesy of* Mayo Foundation for Medical Education and Research, all rights reserved; with permission.)

organ prolapse and stress urinary incontinence."[18] Following this, the FDA continued to monitor outcomes for pelvic floor surgeries involving mesh and later issued an update in 2011. In this statement, the FDA noted that risks of serious complications associated with transvaginal pelvic organ prolapse repair with mesh are not rare, and that further updates regarding stress incontinence surgeries would be provided.[19] In 2013, an additional update was released reporting that "the safety and effectiveness of multi-incision slings is well-established in clinical trials that followed patients for up to 1 year."[20]

Despite this, use of synthetic urethral slings has been subject to dramatically increased scrutiny.[17] Many patients have exposure and preconceived notions regarding mesh placement even before consultation with a pelvic floor surgeon.[21] For instance, in one study, before consultation with a pelvic floor surgeon 62% of patients reported knowledge of mesh, with the main source of information coming from television advertisements for legal counsel.[21] Notably, 22% of patients reported that they would not consider implantation of a mesh product. In addition, there was a degree of misinformation, with 28% of patients reporting mesh products had all been recalled.[21]

More recently, in 2016 multiple national subspecialty organizations whose primary focus is the care of women with pelvic floor disorders, including the Society for Urodynamics, Female Pelvic Medicine, and Reconstructive Surgery and the American Urogynecologic Society, have released a joint position statement supporting the use of synthetic midurethral sling placement in the treatment of women with SUI.[5] They note that "polypropylene mesh midurethral slings are a standard of care for the surgical treatment of SUI and represent a great advance in the treatment of this condition."

Likewise, guidelines including comments regarding the safety and efficacy of synthetic midurethral slings exist from the European Urologic Association and AUA.[12,22] Synthetic midurethral sling placement remains a surgical treatment option for the index female patient with bothersome stress incontinence in the 2017 AUA guideline on the subject (alongside other options, such as autologous fascia pubovaginal sling, Burch colposuspension, and urethral bulking agent injection).[22] That being said, with the concerns of vaginal mesh placement for prolapse, synthetic midurethral sling placement has also received increased scrutiny.[17] In one study evaluating the type of slings placed at eight academic centers, over a 7-year period that included the 2011 and 2013 FDA notification, there was a trend toward decreasing use of synthetic mesh slings, although this was not significant.[23] Likewise, there was increased use of autologous fascial slings, although this may represent a referral bias in academic centers.[23]

OUTCOMES FOLLOWING SYNTHETIC MIDURETHRAL SLING PLACEMENT

Multi-incision Retropubic and Transobturator Slings

Whether using a transobturator or retropubic approach to multi-incision midurethral sling placement, high-quality evidence exists to support excellent short-term outcomes, with increasing evidence for their long-term efficacy.[4,24–26] Although there are specific nuances to each approach, such as the complication profiles, medium-term efficacy seems similar.[22] Long-term comparative data are less available, although starting to show potentially decreased durability of the transobturator route compared with the retropubic approach.[25,27,28] Overall, selection of a retropubic approach versus transobturator should be determined based on surgeon comfort and in shared decision making with each individual patient.[22]

In short- and medium-term follow-up retropubic and transobturator sling seem to have comparable efficacy.[4,26,29,30] In a large systematic review and meta-analysis, including 12,113 women in 81 trials, the 1-year subjective cure rates ranged between 62% and 98% for transobturator slings and 71% and 97% for retropubic slings.[4] Objective cure rates were similar between the two approaches.[4] In a separate systematic review and meta-analysis including 15,855 women, the retropubic approach was associated with higher subjective (odds ratio, 0.83; P = .03) and objective (odds ratio, 0.82; P = .01) cure rate compared with the transobturator route.[24]

With regard to longer term follow-up, the 5-year results of some randomized trials are now available, as is further extended follow-up in retrospective series.[25,27,31] In the 5-year longitudinal follow-up from the Trial of Mid-Urethral Slings (ToMUS), the retropubic and transobturator groups had a decrease in success rates over time, and the treatments no longer met the prespecified criteria for equivalence, with the retropubic sling showing a slight benefit (51.3% vs 43.4%).[25] Likewise, a nationwide Danish study, including 5820 women treated with a midurethral sling, found that the transobturator approach was associated with a two-fold higher risk of reoperation within 5 years compared with the retropubic approach.[27]

Several smaller cohort studies with extended follow-up to 17 years after retropubic midurethral sling placement are also available.[32,33] In one prospective series, including 52 women initially, 42 of 46 patients (91%) with an office visit documented were objectively continent at 17-year evaluation.[32] In the other, 90 women underwent surgery and 78% were available for follow-up. Of those, more than 90% were objectively continent, and 87% were subjectively cured or significantly improved.[33]

Taken together, the current AUA guideline on the topic notes that physicians may offer either a retropubic or transobturator midurethral sling to an index patient.[22]

Single-Incision Transobturator Slings

Single-incision slings are a more recent addition to the surgical armamentarium in treating stress incontinence, and as such data regarding their efficacy are immature.[22] Furthermore, the available data are hindered in that many of the early studies evaluated the use of the TVT-Secur, which was later withdrawn from clinical use. For instance, in systematic reviews and meta-analyses evaluating these early studies, the TVT-Secur was found inferior to standard full-length midurethral slings.[26,34]

More recently, there have been several publications with 1- to 2-year follow-up evaluating the efficacy of other single-incision slings.[35,36] Over time, modifications to the anchoring mechanism may impact the treatment efficacy. In a recent single center randomized trial of 98 women, at 1-year follow-up there was no significant difference in the rate of a positive cough stress test between the MiniArc single-incision sling and the Monarc sling (29% vs 21%; P = .5).[35] Likewise, in a single-center randomized trial including 201 women, at the 2-year end point similar cure rates were seen with the Contasure single incision sling compared with the full-length sling.[36] The AUA guideline on SUI comments that single-incision sling may be offered to index patients, as long as providers discuss the immaturity of the evidence regarding efficacy and safety with the patient.[22]

Situations to Avoid Synthetic Midurethral Sling Placement

There are contraindications to placement of urethral mesh, including patients undergoing concomitant urethral diverticulectomy, urethrovaginal fistula repair, or mesh excision and concomitant SUI surgery.[22] This is secondary to potential impact of a foreign body near the suture line impacting healing, which may lead to urethral mesh perforation. Additionally, the recent AUA guideline notes surgeons should consider avoiding mesh placement in patients at risk for poor wound healing (eg, those with prior radiation therapy, local scarring, poor tissue quality),[22] and in those taking high-dose systemic corticosteroids. In such settings, other anti-incontinence procedures, such as a pubovaginal sling, urethral bulking agent injection, or Burch retropubic colposuspension, may remain viable options. Recently, given the risk of voiding dysfunction following autologous pubovaginal sling placement, techniques relying on midurethral positioning of the fascial sling, via a transobturator[37,38] and a retropubic approach,[39] have been reported.

COMPLICATIONS FOLLOWING SYNTHETIC MIDURETHRAL SLING PLACEMENT

As with any procedure, it is important for the surgeon to be aware of and comfortable managing potential surgical complications that may arise. Although we review several specific complications and their management, it is important to contextualize these with their frequency and the overall safety of midurethral sling placement, and recognize that this is not an exhaustive list of all potential complications.[25,30,40,41] Additionally, it is worth noting that although managed in a similar fashion, the risks of some specific complications vary between the type of sling used (eg, retropubic vs transobturator).[24,26]

Using a national dataset including 8772 women undergoing isolated midurethral sling placement in the United States, the overall 30-day complication rate was roughly 3.5%, with urinary tract infection the most common adverse event (2.9%).[40] In this study using the National Surgical Quality Improvement Program dataset, the 30-day readmission rate was 0.9% and the 30-day reoperation rate was 0.7%.[40] With regard to interventions for mesh-related complications, a population-based cohort from Ontario, Canada including 59,887 women undergoing midurethral sling placement (including concomitant procedures) found that with 10-year follow-up, 3% of women may undergo a procedure for mesh removal or revision.[42] In this study, lower surgeon volume was associated with a 37% greater risk of complications and repeat mesh-related surgeries.[42]

Bladder Perforation

Bladder perforation is possible with any route of sling placement, although it is more common with retropubic trocar passage.[26,30] Universal intraoperative cystoscopy is useful for early identification of bladder perforation, should it occur (**Fig. 4**). During cystoscopy, adequate bladder distention is needed for appropriate visualization. In addition to evaluating for bladder perforations, cystoscopy at the time of sling may detect other abnormalities, with a reported incidence that 5% of cystoscopies following sling placement had pertinent findings.[43]

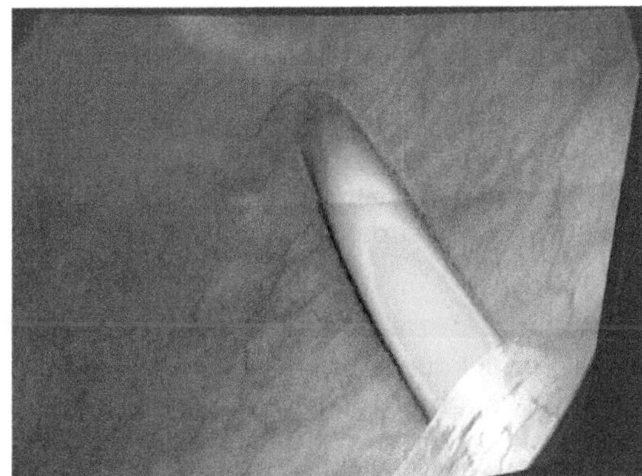

Fig. 4. Intraoperative cystoscopy image showing trocar bladder perforation.

The reported frequency of bladder perforation is variable, from 1% to 34%, and there is some evidence that this rate decreases with increasing surgical experience.[44] Other potential risk factors for bladder perforation that have been reported include prior cesarean section, colposuspension, body mass index less than 30 kg/m^2, rectocele, and local anesthesia.[45]

Typically, trocar bladder perforation is managed with removal and repassage of the offending trocar. Postoperative management is variable among surgical practices, ranging from observation to temporary indwelling Foley catheter placement. In one series of 25 patients with bladder perforation, who subsequently passed their voiding trial, and were discharged without a catheter, no significant adverse events were reported.[46] Others report leaving a catheter in for 1 to several days.[44] Aside from the potential short-term catheter use, trocar bladder perforation has not been associated with decreased efficacy, or long-term sequela following sling placement in several series.[43,47] In contrast, one study noted a higher rate of intraoperative trocar perforations among patients that subsequently had a mesh perforation (bladder or urethra) when compared with those with vaginal mesh exposures.[48] In this study, of the 27 women with postoperative mesh perforations 15 were urethral and 12 involved the bladder, and it is unclear where the area of injury was during trocar placement. Patients with a mesh perforation were also more likely to have a perioperative hematoma or require a blood transfusion.[48]

Urethral Injury

Urethral injury, although rare, is possible during midurethral sling placement, either during the initial dissection or with trocar passage. In these cases, recognition is important to prevent further complications (such as urethrovaginal fistula or urethral mesh erosion) and allow for appropriate repair. In this setting we repair the urethra primarily using absorbable suture, and delay sling placement.[22] A Foley catheter is left in place to facilitate healing, and a repeat attempt at sling placement is performed at a later date.

Vascular Injury

Vascular injury during synthetic midurethral sling placement is a broad category of complications, with severity ranging from a hematoma, which is self-contained and managed with observation, to those necessitating blood transfusion, or even major vascular injury leading to hemodynamic instability. Although vascular injury is possible with all approaches to sling placement, it is more common with retropubic sling placement.[4,24,26,49,50]

Clinically identified pelvic hematomas have been reported in 0.7% to 8% of women after retropubic midurethral sling placement, and 0% to 2% of women after transobturator sling placement.[4,51,52] This may be an underestimation of the occurrence rate, because routine imaging to evaluate for this is not typically performed. For instance, in a small prospective series where an MRI was performed 6 to 8 hours after sling placement, hematomas were detected in 25% of patients (6 of 24) undergoing retropubic sling placement (either mesh or porcine dermis).[53] Most hematomas involve the retropubic space and can be managed conservatively, with transfusion as needed, if the patient is hemodynamically stable and has adequate symptom control (**Fig. 5**A, B). It is important to recognize that resolution of the hematoma can take several months, as seen in a study including serial ultrasounds to follow five patients with a retropubic hematoma.[51] In cases of massive hematomas, described as 8 to 12 cm, successful management via drainage (laparotomy, vaginal, or suprapubic) has been reported.[54]

Intraoperative bleeding from the periurethral connective tissues is typically mild or moderate and is controlled with cautery, suture ligature, or compression (either with a vaginal packing at the end of the case, or slight tension on the Foley catheter, which uses the balloon to help tamponade bleeding).[51] Major vessel injury is rare and necessitates prompt recognition, surgical exploration, and repair.[55] Some have reported use of endovascular intervention, including embolization in such cases.[49,56]

Bowel Injury

Bowel perforation is a rare, although potentially life-threatening complication of sling placement, typically when placed via a retropubic approach. Several case reports exist, although the estimated overall incidence is 0.03% to 0.07%.[4,57–60] It is thought that patients with prior abdominal or pelvic surgery, and those with prior inguinal hernia repair are at increased risk for bowel injury.[59,61] Potential techniques to decrease the risk of bowel injury include use of Trendelenburg positioning and using a transobturator approach.[62]

Bowel perforation is a serious potential complication and prompt recognition is crucial. Bowel injury should be suspected in cases of persistent abdominal pain with fever and feculent or purulent drainage from the abdominal sling exit incisions. If suspected, radiographic imaging (either upright abdominal radiograph or computed tomography) should be pursued, with abdominal exploration and management of the bowel injury.

Postoperative Pain

Postoperative discomfort and pain are not uncommon after most surgical procedures, and following

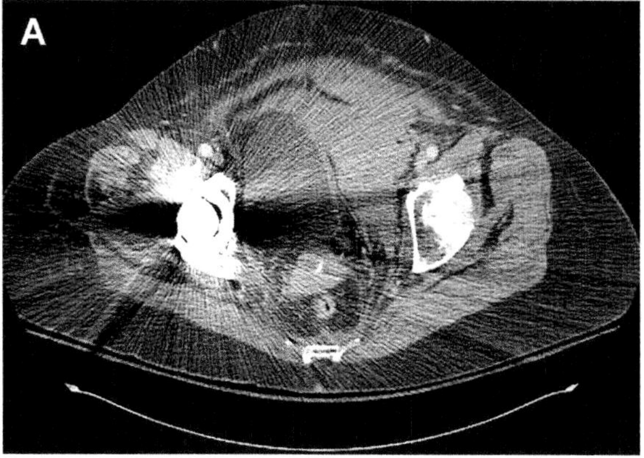

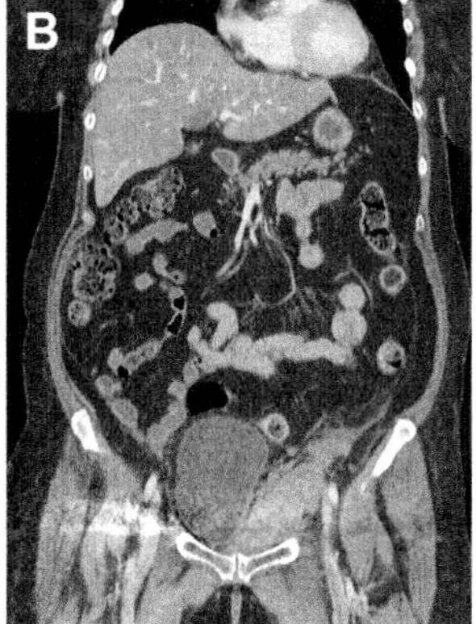

Fig. 5. Retropubic hematoma formation following retropubic sling placement on (*A*) axial computed tomography imaging and (*B*) coronal computed tomography imaging.

sling placement is typically self-limited, although persistent pain can occur. In a recent secondary analysis of the ToMUS trial data, the presence of any surgical pain, pain severity, and pain medication use was not different between retropubic and transobturator approaches.[63] Overall, 70% of patients were pain-free by 2 weeks after midurethral sling placement, and 90% by 6 weeks.[63] Not surprisingly, at 2 weeks, groin pain was more common in the transobturator group and suprapubic pain was more common in the retropubic group.[63] At 1 year, 1.7% of patients (5 of 299) in the transobturator group and 1% of patients (3 of 298) patients in the retropubic group reported any pain related to the operation.[63] Depending on the severity and duration of the pain, patients may be managed with observation, medical management, pelvic floor physical therapy, and less commonly mesh excision.

Postoperative Voiding Dysfunction

Voiding dysfunction following midurethral sling placement may occur secondary to persistent urinary urgency (which was present preoperatively), de novo urinary urgency, and/or bladder outlet obstruction. Patients with postoperative voiding dysfunction should be assessed for urinary tract infection, and for potential bladder outlet obstruction. If there is no evidence of infection or obstruction, management of persistent urinary urgency follows the clinical principles of over active bladder management.[64]

Patients with slings causing bladder outlet obstruction may present with de novo or worsening urinary urgency, or with elevated postvoid residuals. This is more commonly seen with the retropubic approach midurethral sling placement, as opposed to transobturator approach.[4,24,26,30] In the ToMUS trial the rate of surgical intervention for voiding dysfunction with 24-month follow-up was 3% for retropubic slings and 0% for transobturator sling.[30] Other potential predictors for voiding dysfunction after midurethral sling placement include concomitant prolapse surgery, a lower peak flow rate on unintubated uroflow, voiding by a mechanism other detrusor contraction, and Charlson Comorbidity Index score.[65–69]

Urinary retention following sling placement most commonly presents as a failed initial voiding trial.[67] In the early postoperative setting, this is typically managed with bladder drainage (either indwelling Foley catheter, or clean intermittent self-catheterization), with repeat voiding trial. In a multicenter study of 464 isolated sling placements, 21.8% failed the initial voiding trial.[67] At the follow-up visit, 90% passed a second voiding trial and 38.5% of the remainder passed on the third attempt.[67] Likewise, in a secondary analysis of the ToMUS trial, the frequency of voiding dysfunction decreased from 20% on postoperative Day 1, to 6% on Day 14, and 2% by 6 weeks.[70] Similarly, in a population-based cohort, including 18,8454 women, the rate of midurethral sling revision or removal for voiding dysfunction was 1.3%.[71]

Variable management of persistent voiding dysfunction has been reported, including continued observation, sling loosening, and sling lysis/partial excision.[72–74] The optimal timing of surgical intervention is debated. Early sling loosening (up to 10–14 days postoperatively) has been reported, and has the benefit of keeping the original sling intact, with subsequently fewer positive cough stress tests than sling incision.[72,75,76] The downside of early sling loosening is the potential for overtreatment. For instance, in a small prospective series, 52% of women (11 of 21) needing intermittent catheterization for 7 days or more, and managed with observation, ultimately did not need surgical intervention (ie, sling incision).[72]

For those managed conservatively that do have persistent symptoms at 4 to 6 weeks, typically sling revision is performed, either in the form of sling lysis or partial sling excision (**Fig. 6**). In these cases, we attempt to limit the extent of periurethral mobilization to preserve sling fixation, which may aid in maintaining continence.[77,78] It is important to counsel patients that with either technique there is a risk of SUI recurring, which may be severe enough to necessitate undergoing additional treatment, even a repeat anti-incontinence surgery.[78]

Vaginal Mesh Exposure

Vaginal mesh exposure occurs when the mesh material protrudes through the vaginal epithelial lining (**Fig. 7**).[79] Patients may present with vaginal

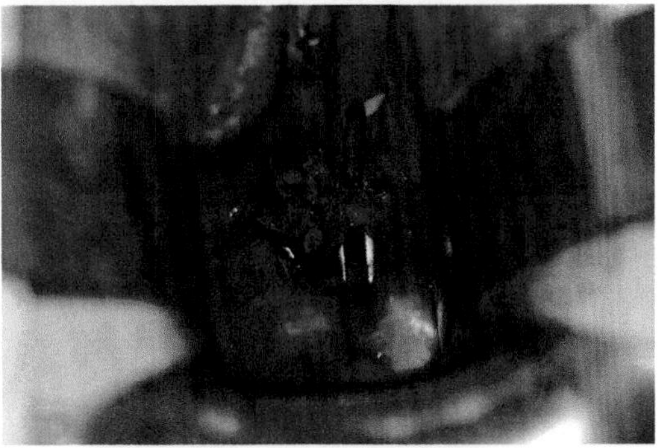

Fig. 6. Sling revision surgery for postoperative voiding dysfunction, a right angle is shown behind the sling following dissection away from the urethra.

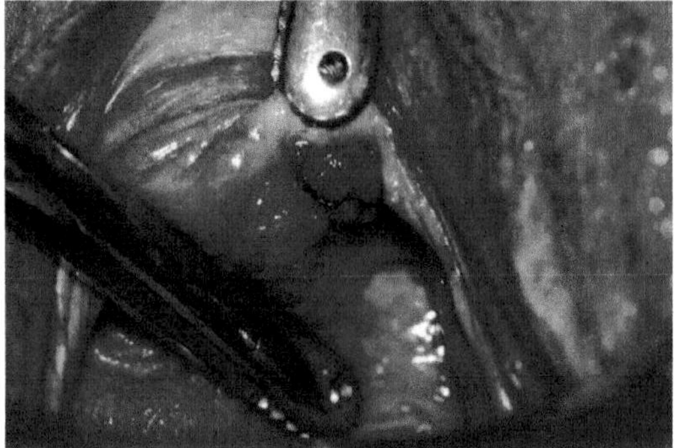

Fig. 7. Periurethral vaginal mesh exposure following midurethral sling.

bleeding, discharge, irritation, dyspareunia, or pain for their partner during intercourse. With the use of type I polypropylene mesh materials vaginal mesh exposure is reported to occur in roughly 1.5% to 2% of cases, including long-term follow-up.[25] In addition to technical considerations and atrophic vaginal tissues, risk factors for vaginal mesh exposure have been reported including younger age, concomitant prolapse repair, diabetes mellitus, prior bariatric surgery, retropubic approach to sling placement, and preoperative anemia.[71,80,81]

Management options for vaginal mesh exposure include observation, topical estrogen use, or surgical revision. Observation may be used if the exposure is small and the patient is not symptomatic. Topical vaginal estrogen has been reported to be successful in cases of small-volume exposures.[82] Failing more conservative therapy, surgery to revise the mesh may be needed. In these cases, we typically excise a portion of the mesh and reclose the vaginal epithelium over the dissected area. Extensive mesh removal is less commonly needed in cases of vaginal exposure of a type I mesh. In contrast, in patients with a type III mesh in place, complete mesh removal is warranted given the tissue encapsulation that typically occurs (**Fig. 8**A–C). The more aggressive the mesh revision/removal, the greater the likelihood of recurrent urinary incontinence.

Bladder or Urethral Mesh Perforation/Extrusion

Bladder or urethral mesh erosion may be the result of a missed injury during initial placement, or secondary to true erosion over time. The former of these scenarios highlights the importance of recognizing these injuries at the time of the initial sling, because delayed management has greater morbidity. In cases of intravesical or intraurethral mesh, patients may present with dysuria, urinary tract infections, hematuria, irritative voiding symptoms, or voiding difficulty. On cystoscopy, mesh in the bladder may be directly visible or it may be associated with stone formation (**Fig. 9**A–C).

The management of mesh in the bladder or urethra involves excision of the mesh and

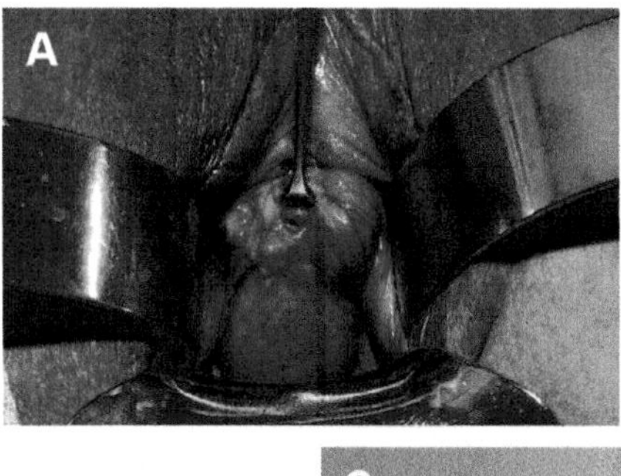

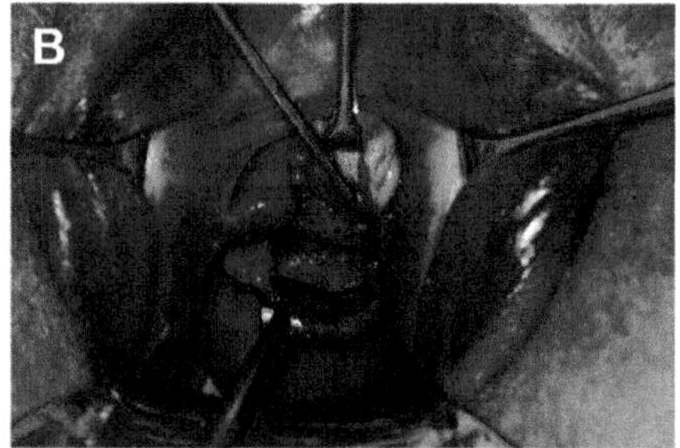

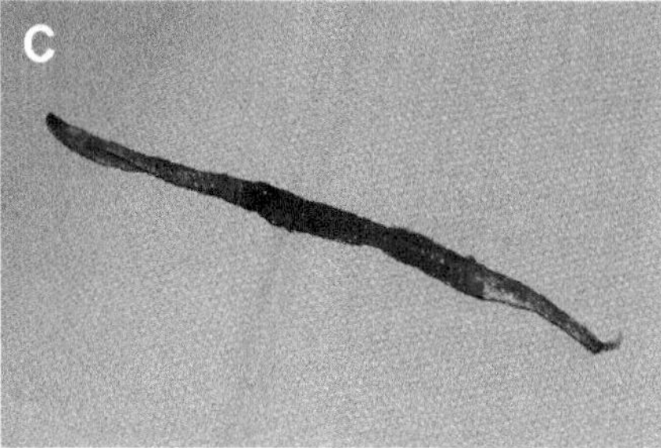

Fig. 8. Vaginal mesh exposure of a type III mesh. (*A*) a small area of mesh exposure is seen. (*B*) The tissue response demonstrates encapsulation with minimal tissue ingrowth, as opposed to incorporation seen with type I mesh materials. (*C*) Completed removal of the entire sling.

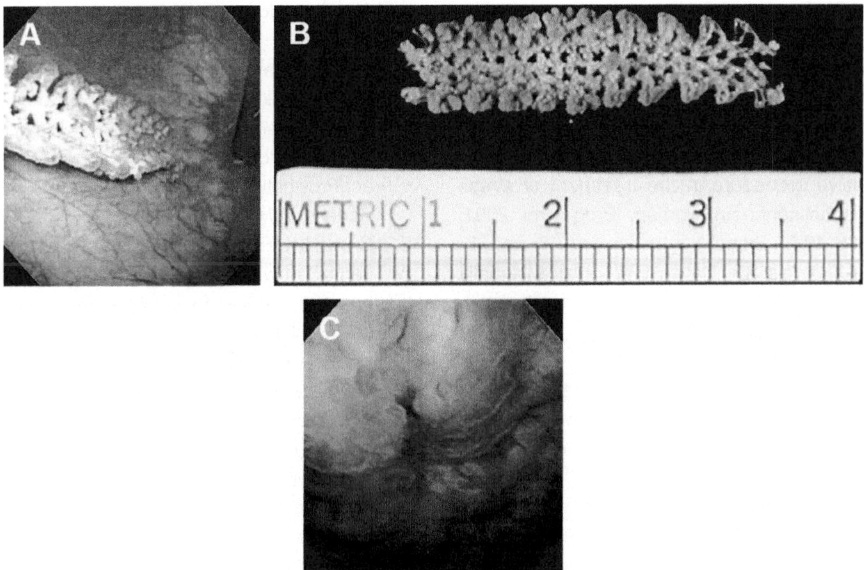

Fig. 9. Bladder perforation by a midurethral sling managed endoscopically with holmium laser excision. (*A*) Extent of the bladder perforation. (*B*) Mesh specimen removed following transection with the laser. (*C*) Bladder on cystoscopy 6-week after the procedure, no residual mesh is identified.

reconstruction. Endoscopic approaches, including use of the holmium laser, have been reported in this setting.[83–85] Success rates for endoscopic management are higher for midurethral sling mesh in the bladder, rather than the urethra.[83] Long-term follow-up is needed to ensure adequate epithelialization over the resection site.[86] An endoscopic approach avoids the potentially larger morbidity of reconstructive surgery, although likely with somewhat lower long-term success rates. In cases with more severe erosions, failed endoscopic management, concomitant fistula formation, or where the patient prefers a more definitive approach, excision via a transabdominal or transvesical approach with bladder reconstruction or urethroplasty may be necessary.[87,88] Prospective data following such reconstructions are limited, and one small series (n = 5) found that many of the patients continued to have incontinence despite the use of physical therapy/salvage autologous sling placement.[88]

SUMMARY

Synthetic midurethral sling placement is the most studied anti-incontinence procedure available, with multiple randomized trials describing its safety and efficacy, with results out to 5 years. With longer follow-up it seems there may be some benefit in efficacy to retropubic sling placement as compared with the transobturator approach. Single-incision slings are a newer modification to multi-incision sling placement, and the data regarding safety and efficacy are not as mature as with other forms of sling placement. Complications may occur with the use of synthetic midurethral slings and surgeons performing these should be comfortable with the diagnosis and management of these issues.

REFERENCES

1. Wu JM, Matthews CA, Conover MM, et al. Lifetime risk of stress urinary incontinence or pelvic organ prolapse surgery. Obstet Gynecol 2014;123(6):1201–6.
2. James MB, Theofanides MC, Sui W, et al. Sling procedures for the treatment of stress urinary incontinence: comparison of national practice patterns between urologists and gynecologists. J Urol 2017;198(6):1386–91.
3. Jonsson Funk M, Levin PJ, Wu JM. Trends in the surgical management of stress urinary incontinence. Obstet Gynecol 2012;119(4):845–51.
4. Ford AA, Rogerson L, Cody JD, et al. Mid-urethral sling operations for stress urinary incontinence in women. Cochrane Database Syst Rev 2017;(7):CD006375.
5. American Urogynecologic Society, Society of Urodynamics, Female pelvic medicine & urogenital reconstruction. Position statement: mesh midurethral slings for stress urinary incontinence. 2018. Available at: https://www.augs.org/assets/1/6/AUGS-SUFU_MUS_Position_Statement.pdf.

6. Chughtai BI, Elterman DS, Vertosick E, et al. Midurethral sling is the dominant procedure for female stress urinary incontinence: analysis of case logs from certifying American urologists. Urology 2013; 82(6):1267–71.
7. Delorme E. Transobturator urethral suspension: mini-invasive procedure in the treatment of stress urinary incontinence in women. Prog Urol 2001; 11(6):1306–13 [in French].
8. Moore RD, Serels SR, Davila GW, et al. Minimally invasive treatment for female stress urinary incontinence (SUI): a review including TVT, TOT, and mini-sling. Surg Technol Int 2009;18:157–73.
9. Forrest JB, Clemens JQ, Finamore P, et al. AUA best practice statement for the prevention of deep vein thrombosis in patients undergoing urologic surgery. J Urol 2009;181(3):1170–7.
10. Abbasy SA, Kenton K, Brubaker L, et al. Measurement of transurethral bladder neck displacement during tension-free vaginal tape procedure. Int Urogynecol J 2011;22(6):721–4.
11. Borazjani A, Pizarro-Berdichevsky J, Li J, et al. Surgeons' views on sling tensioning during surgery for female stress urinary incontinence. Int Urogynecol J 2017;28(10):1489–95.
12. Chapple CR, Cruz F, Deffieux X, et al. Consensus Statement of the European Urology Association and the European Urogynaecological Association on the use of implanted materials for treating pelvic organ prolapse and stress urinary incontinence. Eur Urol 2017;72(3):424–31.
13. Linder BJ, Trabuco EC, Carranza DA, et al. Evaluation of the local carcinogenic potential of mesh used in the treatment of female stress urinary incontinence. Int Urogynecol J 2016;27(9):1333–6.
14. Chughtai B, Sedrakyan A, Mao J, et al. Is vaginal mesh a stimulus of autoimmune disease? Am J Obstet Gynecol 2017;216(5):495.e1-e7.
15. King AB, Zampini A, Vasavada S, et al. Is there an association between polypropylene midurethral slings and malignancy? Urology 2014;84(4): 789–92.
16. Altman D, Rogers RG, Yin L, et al. Cancer risk after midurethral sling surgery using polypropylene mesh. Obstet Gynecol 2018;131(3):469–74.
17. Chapple CR, Raz S, Brubaker L, et al. Mesh sling in an era of uncertainty: lessons learned and the way forward. Eur Urol 2013;64(4):525–9.
18. United States Food and Drug Administration. Complications associated with transvaginal placement of surgical mesh in repair of pelvic organ prolapse and stress urinary incontinence. 2008.
19. United States Food and Drug Administration. Serious complications associated with transvaginal placement of surgical mesh for pelvic organ prolapse: FDA safety communication. 2011. Available at: http://www.fda.gov/MedicalDevices/Safety/AlertsandNotices/ucm262435.htm. Accessed April 15, 2014.
20. United States Food and Drug Administration. Considerations about surgical mesh for SUI. 2013. Available at: https://www.fda.gov/MedicalDevices/ProductsandMedicalProcedures/ImplantsandProsthetics/UroGynSurgicalMesh/ucm345219.htm. Accessed March 1, 2018.
21. Brown LK, Fenner DE, Berger MB, et al. Defining patients' knowledge and perceptions of vaginal mesh surgery. Female Pelvic Med Reconstr Surg 2013; 19(5):282–7.
22. Kobashi KC, Albo ME, Dmochowski RR, et al. Surgical treatment of female stress urinary incontinence: AUA/SUFU guideline. J Urol 2017;198(4):875–83.
23. Rac G, Younger A, Clemens JQ, et al. Stress urinary incontinence surgery trends in academic female pelvic medicine and reconstructive surgery urology practice in the setting of the Food and Drug Administration public health notifications. Neurourol Urodyn 2017;36(4):1155–60.
24. Fusco F, Abdel-Fattah M, Chapple CR, et al. Updated systematic review and meta-analysis of the comparative data on colposuspensions, pubovaginal slings, and midurethral tapes in the surgical treatment of female stress urinary incontinence. Eur Urol 2017;72(4):567–91.
25. Kenton K, Stoddard AM, Zyczynski H, et al. 5-year longitudinal followup after retropubic and transobturator mid urethral slings. J Urol 2015;193(1):203–10.
26. Schimpf MO, Rahn DD, Wheeler TL, et al. Sling surgery for stress urinary incontinence in women: a systematic review and metaanalysis. Am J Obstet Gynecol 2014;211(1):71.e1-e27.
27. Foss Hansen M, Lose G, Kesmodel US, et al. Reoperation for urinary incontinence: a nationwide cohort study, 1998-2007. Am J Obstet Gynecol 2016; 214(2):263.e1-e8.
28. Schierlitz L, Dwyer PL, Rosamilia A, et al. Three-year follow-up of tension-free vaginal tape compared with transobturator tape in women with stress urinary incontinence and intrinsic sphincter deficiency. Obstet Gynecol 2012;119(2 Pt 1):321–7.
29. Barber MD, Kleeman S, Karram MM, et al. Transobturator tape compared with tension-free vaginal tape for the treatment of stress urinary incontinence: a randomized controlled trial. Obstet Gynecol 2008; 111(3):611–21.
30. Richter HE, Albo ME, Zyczynski HM, et al. Retropubic versus transobturator midurethral slings for stress incontinence. N Engl J Med 2010;362(22): 2066–76.
31. Tommaselli GA, Di Carlo C, Formisano C, et al. Medium-term and long-term outcomes following placement of midurethral slings for stress urinary incontinence: a systematic review and metaanalysis. Int Urogynecol J 2015;26(9):1253–68.

32. Braga A, Caccia G, Sorice P, et al. Tension-free vaginal tape for treatment of pure urodynamic stress urinary incontinence: efficacy and adverse effects at 17-year follow-up. BJU Int 2018;122(1): 113–7.
33. Nilsson CG, Palva K, Aarnio R, et al. Seventeen years' follow-up of the tension-free vaginal tape procedure for female stress urinary incontinence. Int Urogynecol J 2013;24(8):1265–9.
34. Nambiar A, Cody JD, Jeffery ST, et al. Single-incision sling operations for urinary incontinence in women. Cochrane Database Syst Rev 2017;(7): CD008709.
35. Tieu AL, Hegde A, Castillo PA, et al. Transobturator versus single incision slings: 1-year results of a randomized controlled trial. Int Urogynecol J 2017; 28(3):461–7.
36. Dogan O, Kaya AE, Pulatoglu C, et al. A randomized comparison of a single-incision needleless (Contasure-needleless(R)) mini-sling versus an inside-out transobturator (Contasure-KIM(R)) mid-urethral sling in women with stress urinary incontinence: 24-month follow-up results. Int Urogynecol J 2018. [Epub ahead of print].
37. Linder BJ, Elliott DS. Autologous transobturator urethral sling placement for female stress urinary incontinence. J Urol 2015;193(3):991–6.
38. Linder BJ, Elliott DS. Autologous transobturator urethral sling placement for female stress urinary incontinence: short-term outcomes. Urology 2016;93: 55–9.
39. Khan ZA, Nambiar A, Morley R, et al. Long-term follow-up of a multicentre randomised controlled trial comparing tension-free vaginal tape, xenograft and autologous fascial slings for the treatment of stress urinary incontinence in women. BJU Int 2015; 115(6):968–77.
40. Cohen AJ, Packiam VT, Nottingham CU, et al. 30-day morbidity and reoperation following midurethral sling: analysis of 8772 cases using a national prospective database. Urology 2016;95:72–9.
41. Propst K, O'Sullivan DM, Tulikangas PK. Suburethral sling procedures in the United States: complications, readmission, and reoperation. Int Urogynecol J 2017;28(10):1463–7.
42. Welk B, Al-Hothi H, Winick-Ng J. Removal or revision of vaginal mesh used for the treatment of stress urinary incontinence. JAMA Surg 2015;150(12): 1167–75.
43. Zyczynski HM, Sirls LT, Greer WJ, et al. Findings of universal cystoscopy at incontinence surgery and their sequelae. Am J Obstet Gynecol 2014;210(5): 480.e1-8.
44. McLennan MT, Melick CF. Bladder perforation during tension-free vaginal tape procedures: analysis of learning curve and risk factors. Obstet Gynecol 2005;106(5 Pt 1):1000–4.
45. Stav K, Dwyer PL, Rosamilia A, et al. Risk factors for trocar injury to the bladder during mid urethral sling procedures. J Urol 2009;182(1):174–9.
46. Crosby EC, Vilasagar S, Duecy EE, et al. Expectant management of cystotomy at the time of midurethral sling placement: a retrospective case series. Int Urogynecol J 2013;24(9):1543–6.
47. Gold RS, Groutz A, Pauzner D, et al. Bladder perforation during tension-free vaginal tape surgery: does it matter? J Reprod Med 2007;52(7):616–8.
48. Osborn DJ, Dmochowski RR, Harris CJ, et al. Analysis of patient and technical factors associated with midurethral sling mesh exposure and perforation. Int J Urol 2014;21(11):1167–70.
49. Jung YS, Lee JH, Shin TS, et al. Arterial injury associated with tension-free vaginal tapes-secur procedure successfully treated by radiological embolization. Int Neurourol J 2010;14(4):275–7.
50. Sun MJ. A life-threatening hematoma after the single-incision sling MiniArc procedure: a case report. J Minim Invasive Gynecol 2013;20(4): 529–32.
51. Flock F, Reich A, Muche R, et al. Hemorrhagic complications associated with tension-free vaginal tape procedure. Obstet Gynecol 2004;104(5 Pt 1): 989–94.
52. Kolle D, Tamussino K, Hanzal E, et al. Bleeding complications with the tension-free vaginal tape operation. Am J Obstet Gynecol 2005;193(6):2045–9.
53. Giri SK, Wallis F, Drumm J, et al. A magnetic resonance imaging-based study of retropubic haematoma after sling procedures: preliminary findings. BJU Int 2005;96(7):1067–71.
54. Balachandran A, Curtiss N, Duckett J. The management of massive haematomas after insertion of retropubic mid-urethral slings. Int Urogynecol J 2015; 26(10):1449–52.
55. Abouassaly R, Steinberg JR, Lemieux M, et al. Complications of tension-free vaginal tape surgery: a multi-institutional review. BJU Int 2004;94(1):110–3.
56. Ko JK, Ku CH. Embolization for pelvic arterial bleeding following a transobturator tape procedure. J Obstet Gynaecol Res 2014;40(3):865–8.
57. Agostini A, Bretelle F, Franchi F, et al. Immediate complications of tension-free vaginal tape (TVT): results of a French survey. Eur J Obstet Gynecol Reprod Biol 2006;124(2):237–9.
58. Kascak P, Kopcan B. Fatal Injury of the Small Intestine during Retropubic Sling Placement. Case Rep Obstet Gynecol 2015;2015:164545.
59. Meschia M, Busacca M, Pifarotti P, et al. Bowel perforation during insertion of tension-free vaginal tape (TVT). Int Urogynecol J Pelvic Floor Dysfunct 2002;13(4):263–5 [discussion: 265].
60. Anger JT, Litwin MS, Wang Q, et al. Complications of sling surgery among female Medicare beneficiaries. Obstet Gynecol 2007;109(3):707–14.

61. Castillo OA, Bodden E, Olivares RA, et al. Intestinal perforation: an infrequent complication during insertion of tension-free vaginal tape. J Urol 2004;172(4 Pt 1):1364.
62. Rooney KE, Cholhan HJ. Bowel perforation during retropubic sling procedure. Obstet Gynecol 2010; 115(2 Pt 2):429–31.
63. Thomas TN, Siff LN, Jelovsek JE, et al. Surgical pain after transobturator and retropubic midurethral sling placement. Obstet Gynecol 2017;130(1):118–25.
64. Gormley EA, Lightner DJ, Faraday M, et al. Diagnosis and treatment of overactive bladder (non-neurogenic) in adults: AUA/SUFU guideline amendment. J Urol 2015;193(5):1572–80.
65. Linder BJ, Trabuco EC, Gebhart JB, et al. Can urodynamic parameters predict sling revision for voiding dysfunction in women undergoing synthetic midurethral sling placement? Female Pelvic Med Reconstr Surg 2017. [Epub ahead of print].
66. Hong B, Park S, Kim HS, et al. Factors predictive of urinary retention after a tension-free vaginal tape procedure for female stress urinary incontinence. J Urol 2003;170(3):852–6.
67. Ripperda CM, Kowalski JT, Chaudhry ZQ, et al. Predictors of early postoperative voiding dysfunction and other complications following a midurethral sling. Am J Obstet Gynecol 2016;215(5):656.e1-e6.
68. Salin A, Conquy S, Elie C, et al. Identification of risk factors for voiding dysfunction following TVT placement. Eur Urol 2007;51(3):782–7 [discussion: 787].
69. Wheeler TL 2nd, Richter HE, Greer WJ, et al. Predictors of success with postoperative voiding trials after a mid urethral sling procedure. J Urol 2008;179(2): 600–4.
70. Ferrante KL, Kim HY, Brubaker L, et al. Repeat post-op voiding trials: an inconvenient correlate with success. Neurourol Urodyn 2014;33(8):1225–8.
71. Jonsson Funk M, Siddiqui NY, Pate V, et al. Sling revision/removal for mesh erosion and urinary retention: long-term risk and predictors. Am J Obstet Gynecol 2013;208(1):73.e1-7.
72. Brennand EA, Tang S, Birch C, et al. Early voiding dysfunction after midurethral sling surgery: comparison of two management approaches. Int Urogynecol J 2017;28(10):1515–26.
73. Goldman HB. Simple sling incision for the treatment of iatrogenic urethral obstruction. Urology 2003; 62(4):714–8.
74. Nitti VW, Carlson KV, Blaivas JG, et al. Early results of pubovaginal sling lysis by midline sling incision. Urology 2002;59(1):47–51 [discussion: 51–2].
75. Moksnes LR, Svenningsen R, Schiotz HA, et al. Sling mobilization in the management of urinary retention after mid-urethral sling surgery. Neurourol Urodyn 2017;36(4):1091–6.
76. Price N, Slack A, Khong SY, et al. The benefit of early mobilisation of tension-free vaginal tape in the treatment of post-operative voiding dysfunction. Int Urogynecol J Pelvic Floor Dysfunct 2009; 20(7):855–8.
77. Kim-Fine S, El-Nashar SA, Linder BJ, et al. Patient satisfaction after sling revision for voiding dysfunction after sling placement. Female Pelvic Med Reconstr Surg 2016;22(3):140–5.
78. Clifton MM, Linder BJ, Lightner DJ, et al. Risk of repeat anti-incontinence surgery following sling release: a review of 93 cases. J Urol 2014;191(3): 710–4.
79. Haylen BT, Freeman RM, Swift SE, et al. An International Urogynecological Association (IUGA)/International Continence Society (ICS) joint terminology and classification of the complications related directly to the insertion of prostheses (meshes, implants, tapes) & grafts in female pelvic floor surgery. Int Urogynecol J 2011;22(1):3–15.
80. Chen HY, Ho M, Hung YC, et al. Analysis of risk factors associated with vaginal erosion after synthetic sling procedures for stress urinary incontinence. Int Urogynecol J Pelvic Floor Dysfunct 2008;19(1): 117–21.
81. Linder BJ, El-Nashar SA, Carranza Leon DA, et al. Predictors of vaginal mesh exposure after midurethral sling placement: a case-control study. Int Urogynecol J 2016;27(9):1321–6.
82. Kobashi KC, Govier FE. Management of vaginal erosion of polypropylene mesh slings. J Urol 2003; 169(6):2242–3.
83. Ogle CA, Linder BJ, Elliott DS. Holmium laser excision for urinary mesh erosion: a minimally invasive treatment with favorable long-term results. Int Urogynecol J 2015;26(11):1645–8.
84. Hodroff M, Portis A, Siegel SW. Endoscopic removal of intravesical polypropylene sling with the holmium laser. J Urol 2004;172(4 Pt 1):1361–2.
85. Lee CH, Ku JY, Lee K, et al. Clinical application of a transurethral holmium laser excision of exposed polypropylene mesh at lower urinary tract: single surgeon experience with long-term follow-up. Female Pelvic Med Reconstr Surg 2018;24(1):26–31.
86. Cohen SA, Goldman HB. Mesh perforation into a viscus in the setting of pelvic floor surgery-presentation and management. Curr Urol Rep 2016;17(9):64.
87. Blaivas JG, Sandhu J. Urethral reconstruction after erosion of slings in women. Curr Opin Urol 2004; 14(6):335–8.
88. Colhoun A, Rapp DE. Long-term outcomes after repair of transurethral perforation of midurethral sling. Female Pelvic Med Reconstr Surg 2016; 22(4):272–5.

Management of the Exposed or Perforated Midurethral Sling

Laura L. Giusto, MD*, Patricia M. Zahner, MD,
Howard B. Goldman, MD

KEYWORDS

• Midurethral sling • MUS • Stress urinary incontinence • SUI • Mesh complication • Exposure
• Perforation

KEY POINTS

- Evolution of mesh midurethral slings as the gold standard for treatment of stress urinary incontinence has led to an increased incidence of mesh-related complications, including an approximate 2% risk of mesh exposure.
- Risk factors for mesh exposure or perforation include comorbidities and behaviors associated with poor wound healing, including diabetes, smoking, nutritional deficiency, and advanced age, as well intraoperative factors, such as bleeding/hematoma formation and trocar perforation.
- Diagnosis of mesh exposure or perforation requires focused history taking, pelvic examination with half speculum and careful palpation, and in certain situations, cystourethroscopy, vaginoscopy, and/or translabial/vaginal ultrasound.
- For small mesh exposures with minimal symptoms, less-invasive management options may be offered.
- For symptomatic or large mesh exposure, treatment options are typically more invasive.

INTRODUCTION

Stress urinary incontinence (SUI) is a common condition that affects close to one-third of all adult women in the United States and when untreated is associated with depression, anxiety, social isolation, and decreased quality of life.[1] The cause of SUI has been attributed to intrinsic sphincter deficiency and/or hypermobility of the urethra, with contributing factors such as parity, body mass index, tobacco use, and collagen disorders. Patients with symptomatic SUI have several choices regarding treatment options, ranging from noninvasive to surgical interventions. For those considering surgical intervention, level A evidence supports treatments such as synthetic midurethral sling (MUS), autologous fascia pubovaginal sling, Burch colposuspension, and urethral bulking agents.[2]

Historically, autologous fascial pubovaginal slings and Burch colposuspension were the surgeries of choice for SUI. The synthetic MUS was introduced in 1995, and as a minimally invasive technique, it eventually became the most popular option for treatment of SUI, stress predominant urinary incontinence, and occult SUI associated with pelvic organ prolapse.[3] The principles of all synthetic MUSs are similar, which involves transvaginal placement of a small piece of mesh at the midurethral position in a tension-free fashion. The MUS can be placed retropubically, either top-down or bottom-up, or via an inside-out or outside-in transobturator (TO) approach. Techniques and choice of manufacturer are typically

Disclosures: None.
Glickman Urological and Kidney Institute, Cleveland Clinic, 9500 Euclid Avenue/Q10, Cleveland, OH 44195, USA
* Corresponding author.
E-mail address: giustol@ccf.org

Urol Clin N Am 46 (2019) 31–40
https://doi.org/10.1016/j.ucl.2018.08.003
0094-0143/19/© 2018 Elsevier Inc. All rights reserved.

based on surgeon preference or training, although recent 5-year longitudinal data from the TOMUS trial comparing retropubic (RP) to TO MUSs show increased success rates in patients who underwent an RP MUS.[4] Although the utilization of synthetic mesh has offered a reliable, efficacious long-term treatment option for SUI, its use has also introduced novel mesh-related complications. Two of the most common complications include pain and "mesh erosion," a catch-all description that is defined in later discussion.

Recent focus has therefore been drawn to the use of synthetic mesh materials, particularly in its transvaginal use for MUSs and its associated complications. In response to this, the Food and Drug Administration conducted a systematic review in 2011 of all published literature from 1996 to 2011 and concluded that the rate of mesh erosion through the vagina is 2% at 1 year following surgery and that the safety and effectiveness at 1 year after MUS is well established.[5] Based on this report, the Society of Urodynamics, Female Pelvic Medicine and Urogenital Reconstruction (SUFU) and the American Urogynecologic Society (AUGS) published a joint position statement stating that "polypropylene mesh midurethral slings are a standard of care for the surgical treatment of SUI," which is also repeated and supported by the European Commission enquiry.[3,6]

Despite its level A evidence and recommendations for use by the major American and European Gynecologic and Urologic associations, the use of transvaginal synthetic mesh for SUI is not without risk. To better classify the various mesh complications, the International Urogynecological Association and the International Continence Society published a joint classification to standardize the terminology and complications related to mesh-related surgery.[7] This language has largely been used in the literature since its publication. They emphasize the avoidance of the term mesh "erosion" due to the implication that the mesh inherently wears away through adjacent tissue. Instead, a mesh "exposure" is described as the ability to identify vaginal mesh, either visibly or by palpation at the surgical incision site. Alternately, an "extrusion" is the passage directly out of a body structure or tissue and represents a delayed process whereby mesh gradually passes through the vaginal wall. A "perforation" represents a delayed event of mesh entering a viscus organ, such as the urethra, bladder, or bowel. For simplicity and standardization within this article, the term mesh exposure describes visible or palpable mesh at the incision site *or* vaginal wall. Perforation will continue to be used as defined above, but may also describe an intraoperative event, such as trocar injury through the vaginal mucosa or lower urinary tract.

As the synthetic MUS will likely remain the gold-standard treatment of SUI with continued risk of mesh complications, this article focuses on the preoperative, perioperative, and postoperative factors that may influence mesh exposure or perforation due to MUS placement. Typical patient presentation, recommended evaluation for diagnosis, as well as treatment options for mesh complications are also discussed.

PREVALENCE OF MESH EXPOSURE AND PERFORATION

It has been estimated that more than 3 million synthetic MUSs have been placed for treatment of SUI since they were introduced.[8] Synthetic grafts are produced with some degree of variance by different manufacturers, but all synthetic slings currently in use are composed of large-pore monofilament polypropylene mesh, also known as a type 1 mesh. Because this mesh is commonly used in general surgery and in hernia repairs, much of the research on the safety and efficacy of the human use of synthetic mesh comes from literature published in this area. The ideal mesh material is porous enough to allow for adequate tissue ingrowth. It should be permanent, nonabsorbable, inert, and resistant to infection and have the ability to completely incorporate into the host tissue.[9,10]

Despite this ideal material, the rate of mesh sling exposure, as discussed above, occurs in approximately 2% of sling placements, with a range in the literature from 0% to 8.1%.[8,11] A 2017 Cochrane Review of MUS operations in women for SUI reported the overall rate of erosion/exposure/extrusion to be 24/1000 with a TO approach versus 21/1000 for a RP approach.[12] Older slings, which were not as porous as type 1 mesh and did not allow for adequate tissue ingrowth, such as the Obtape and Uratape, have been known to have a higher rate of exposure and are no longer in use.

PREOPERATIVE CONSIDERATIONS AND PATIENT FACTORS CONTRIBUTING TO MESH EXPOSURE AND PERFORATION

While evaluating whether a patient is a good candidate for synthetic MUS placement, there are many preoperative factors to consider that may influence surgical outcomes. Various retrospective reviews have been performed in women who have had vaginal mesh exposures in an effort to determine preoperative risk factors that may increase a patient's likelihood of such an event occurring. In general, risk factors for mesh exposure or perforation include comorbidities and behaviors associated with poor wound healing, including diabetes, smoking, nutritional deficiency, and advanced age as well as intraoperative factors, such as bleeding/hematoma formation and trocar perforation.

Linder and colleagues[13] performed a case-control study of 2123 women who underwent MUS sling placement and then identified predictive clinical risk factors of the 1.3% necessitating surgical repair for mesh exposure. They found that previous bariatric surgery and preoperative hemoglobin (<13 g/dL), premenopausal status, and age less than 50 were all significant risk factors for postoperative mesh exposure. The association with bariatric surgery and anemia may be suggestive of poor nutritional state. Complications from a younger, premenopausal cohort may be secondary to increased periurethral vascularity and risk of bleeding/hematoma formation intraoperatively, being sexually active with increased likelihood of mesh exposure becoming symptomatic, as well as likelihood to have more invasive surgery than an older cohort.

Another case control study by Kolkanali and colleagues[14] demonstrated in a multivariate analysis of their study population that older age, diabetes mellitus, current smoking, length of vaginal incision greater than 2 cm, recurrent vaginal incision for postoperative complications, and previous pelvic organ prolapse or incontinence surgery were independent risk factors for mesh exposure. Unlike the previous study, older age was found to be a contributing risk factor, likely due to increased comorbidities in this population, including vaginal atrophy.

Vaginal atrophy is typically seen in the postmenopausal state and advanced age. Atrophy is manifested by thin, poorly perfused tissue that in theory may increase the likelihood of postoperative mesh exposure. Topical vaginal estrogen is known to accelerate reepithelialization and stimulate angiogenesis and wound contraction.[15] Therefore, some surgeons anecdotally pretreat patients with vaginal atrophy before performing surgery for incontinence, although there are few studies that evaluate vaginal estrogen on perioperative outcome. A report by the Society of Gynecologic Surgeons Systematic Review Group assessed the literature on vaginal estrogen and the management of pelvic floor disorders in postmenopausal women and determined no studies were powered to determine the effect of postoperative vaginal estrogen on surgical complications.[16]

In another retrospective review, Osborn and colleagues[11] noted an increased association of mesh perforation in patients with a trocar injury, bleeding complications, and diabetes and a decreased risk of mesh perforation of the bladder or urethra in those with an increased body mass index. It is postulated that increased perivesical fat deposition separates the bladder from the pubic symphysis, allowing space for passage of trocars without injury.

Appropriate preoperative counseling of increased risk of mesh complication would therefore be appropriate for patients with diabetes, active smokers, and patients with deficient nutritional status. The 2017 AUA/SUFU Guidelines on Surgical Treatment of SUI also emphasize proper healing of vaginal epithelium to prevent mesh exposures. Patients at risk for poor healing include those with scar tissue from previous pelvic surgery, history of pelvic radiation therapy, severe atrophy, as well as chronic states such as immunosuppression, collagen, and autoimmune disorders.[2] If patients with these risk factors or comorbidities are seeking surgical intervention, care must be taken to discuss chance of complications and alternatives to synthetic mesh.

PERIOPERATIVE CONSIDERATIONS AND TECHNICAL FACTORS CONTRIBUTING TO MESH EXPOSURE AND PERFORATION

Most intraoperative complications are due to injury of adjacent structures either during the dissection to place the trocar or during trocar passage. Bleeding and/or hematoma formation secondary to vascular injury is common.[17] Although not uncommon due to the nature of the procedure, and typically only a complication if unrecognized, vaginal skin, bladder, and urethral perforation not addressed during time of surgery may also lead to postoperative complications. Patient positioning, hydrodissection, and vigilant inspection for mesh exposure or perforation at time of surgery are key technical factors to minimizing immediate as well as delayed mesh complications.

Patient positioning is an often underestimated factor in minimizing surgical complications. The patient is typically placed in the dorsal lithotomy position with the table in the Trendelenburg position to help bowel fall out of the way of trocar trajectory, with legs padded carefully to prevent neuropraxia.

Hydrodissection may also be used throughout the case to minimize injury to adjacent tissue. RP hydrodissection is a technique used in placement of top-down or bottom-up MUS to minimize chance of bladder perforation. A spinal needle is used to inject dilute local anesthesia posterior to the pubic symphysis and lateral to the bladder, and in doing so, displaces the bladder away from the pelvic sidewall allowing a wider space for unobstructed trocar passage. Vaginal wall hydrodissection with local anesthesia plus epinephrine into the submucosa at the level of the midurethra is also used to find the optimal plane for dissection between the vaginal wall and periurethral fascia.[18] Blanching of vaginal mucosa with injection suggests a superficial plane, whereas no evidence of distension suggests injection might be too deep. Extending hydrodissection toward bilateral vaginal sulci also allows the vaginal skin to be elevated off the pelvic bone.

Bladder perforation with trocar placement is more common with RP sling placement, and there are various techniques to minimize the chance of perforation depending on the surgical technique. To decrease trocar perforation when placing a tension-free vaginal tape using bottom-up RP approach, it is recommended to use a catheter with stylet or cystoscope sheath to deviate the bladder neck to the opposite side of trocar placement.[19] In a top-down RP approach, many surgeons have found that taking care to place the trocar in close proximity to the pubic symphysis while maintaining fingertip control of the trocar during its entry into the periurethral space can minimize the incidence of bladder perforation with the trocar.

Vigilant inspection for mesh complications begins with careful vaginal palpation and cystoscopy after trocar passage. Inspection of the anterior vaginal wall is crucial to rule out a buttonhole injury. If the trocar passes through the vaginal skin, remove the trocar, form a new, slightly deeper passage, repass the trocar, and close the vaginal defect with a 3-0 absorbable suture. Missing a vaginal skin injury will lead to mesh exposure, which may not be noted until follow-up.

Cystoscopy should be performed with a 70° lens to rule out trocar perforation. Recognition of trocar perforation intraoperatively is imperative. The bladder should be fully distended because folds in the mucosa of an underfilled bladder may impair visualization of an injury. Drainage of cystoscopic irrigation emanating from the suprapubic trocar sites is also a sign of bladder perforation. If a perforation is noted, the trocar should be removed and placed again. A Foley catheter may be placed at the surgeon's discretion. Perforation into the urethra calls for delay of synthetic sling placement at a future time and management of the urethra, with either Foley placement or urethral repair depending on the degree of laceration.

Placement of a TO versus RP MUS sling may also influence the eventual location of delayed mesh exposure due to the differences in trocar trajectory. The TO approach is often noted to have a higher chance of exposure at the fornix because the vaginal skin is thinner at that location, predisposing the chance of buttonhole injury or a delayed extrusion. The TOMUS trial reported iatrogenic vaginal wall injury with trocar passage noted at time of surgery to occur 4.4% of the time with TO slings compared with 2.3% with RP slings. Rate of mesh exposure upon postoperative follow-up was more likely with TO slings (1.3%) compared with RP slings (0.7%).[20]

As noted above, vascular injury and subsequent bleeding and hematoma are not uncommon in sling placement. Vascularity is increased closer to the periurethral fascia, and deep dissection while creating vaginal tunnels may lead to bleeding and subsequent hematoma formation. Trocar passage through the endopelvic fascia may also disrupt vasculature and cause significant bleeding at the vaginal tunnels. Most bleeding is self-limited and will stop once the incision is closed. Vaginal packing may also be placed after closure of the incision. Closure should be performed with an interlocking suture to increase hemostasis along the incision. Recognition and response to bleeding are important because formation of a hematoma behind the vaginal mucosal closure may create pressure along the suture line and may contribute to dehiscence, tissue breakdown, and eventual mesh exposure.

POSTOPERATIVE CONSIDERATIONS FOR SYNTHETIC MESH MIDURETHRAL SLING SURGERY

The AUA guidelines for surgical treatment of female SUI recommend patients be seen and examined within 6 months of their surgery and that a physical examination, with attention to incisional sites and evaluation for healing, tenderness, mesh exposure, and other abnormalities, should be performed.[3] Although surgeon preference dictates follow-up further than 6 months after surgery, the authors believe the patient should be counseled and knowledgeable of common presentations for mesh complications so that they can return to the office for complete evaluation should any of these signs or symptoms occur.

PATIENT PRESENTATION WITH MESH EXPOSURE AND PERFORATION

Although there are many symptoms associated with vaginal mesh erosion, it is not uncommon that patients may be asymptomatic with a diagnosis made only upon physical examination. Regardless, a focused history should be obtained from the patient detailing the most common presenting symptoms of exposed mesh, including vaginal discharge or bleeding, dyspareunia, pelvic/groin pain, palpated mesh on self-examination, voiding dysfunction, and urinary tract infections as well as the timing/onset of any of these symptoms.

A retrospective review of patients who underwent surgical removal of a sling due to mesh-related complications revealed that vaginal pain was the most common reason for sling removal. Patients who underwent TO sling placement were more likely to complain of groin pain, whereas those who underwent RP sling reported suprapubic pain.[21] Partner pain during intercourse, also termed "hispareunia," may be present and may be an initial indication of sling exposure when the patient is otherwise asymptomatic.[21,22]

Wang and colleagues[23] also suggest that presenting symptoms of mesh complications evolve over time. Within their cohort of 278 patients, the mean number of presenting symptoms per patient was 3.8 ± 1.4 and increased significantly in relation to time since MUS placement. There was a higher rate of pain complaints in those presenting within 2 years of surgery and a higher rate of recurrent urinary tract infections and urinary incontinence in the later groups.

In addition to the symptoms noted above for vaginal mesh exposure, symptoms associated with mesh perforation into the bladder, urethra, or bowel/rectum vary and may include hematuria, recurrent urinary tract infections, dysuria, weak stream, urinary retention, irritative voiding, constant urinary or fecal drainage secondary to fistula, suprapubic pain, urethral pain, rectal pain, and fecal urgency or incontinence.[24] Therefore, it is imperative to always suspect and evaluate for a possible mesh exposure or complication when a patient presents with new symptoms, even if it is remote from their initial MUS procedure.

EVALUATION AND DIAGNOSIS OF MESH EXPOSURE AND PERFORATION

Previous operative reports should be requested before consultation or planned surgical intervention. Pelvic examination is performed with a half speculum and appropriate lighting. Inspection might reveal findings ranging from small areas of granular tissue to visible mesh through the vaginal skin (**Fig. 1**). Careful palpation should be used to try to identify the entire course of the sling. Vaginoscopy with a cystoscope should be considered if a patient cannot tolerate a thorough examination with a speculum due to pain, or in select cases if the sling cannot be visualized but is palpable. Based on patient presentation and history, a cystourethroscopy may also be performed, especially when a bladder or urethral perforation is suspected (**Figs. 2** and **3**).

Although sling exposure into the vagina is often easily assessed during physical examination, and sling perforation is typically visualized on cystourethroscopy, there are instances whereby the degree of mesh complication is more subtle. A synthetic MUS appears as an easily visualized echogenic structure on ultrasound, which can be imaged by transvaginal, translabial, or introital approaches. Recent literature suggests 2-dimensional and 3-dimensional imaging may be used to allow dynamic assessment of the sling and can help in diagnosis of sling failure, obstruction, sling exposure/perforation, or mesh-related pain. Perforated slings may become calcified, making them easily visible on ultrasound and configuration of sling arms, especially when multiple slings have been placed, can be identified to help with preoperative planning during sling removal.[25] Staack and colleagues[26] reviewed a series of women who underwent repeat surgery after sling placement and had clinical and intraoperative translabial ultrasound performed. The group was consistently able to identify whether a sling was TO or RP; however, identification of mesh exposure was less reliable given the variable thickness of vaginal tissue.[25]

The physician should have a high degree of suspicion for a mesh exposure or perforation

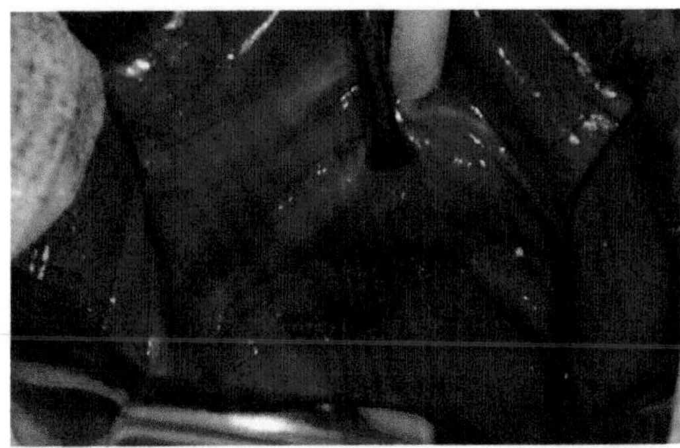

Fig. 1. Vaginal mesh exposure near midline.

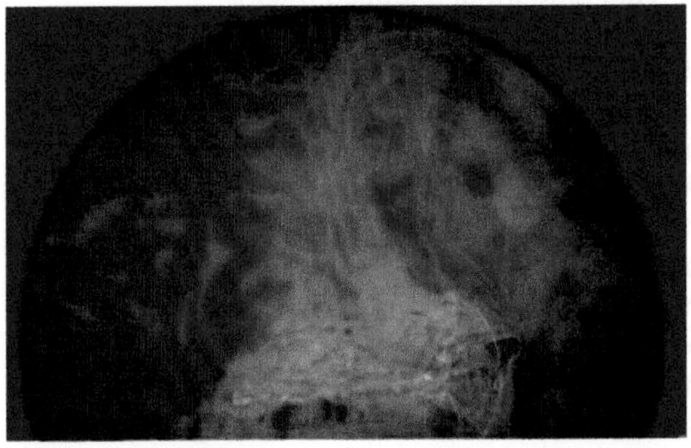

Fig. 2. Mesh perforation into base of bladder as visualized on cystoscopy.

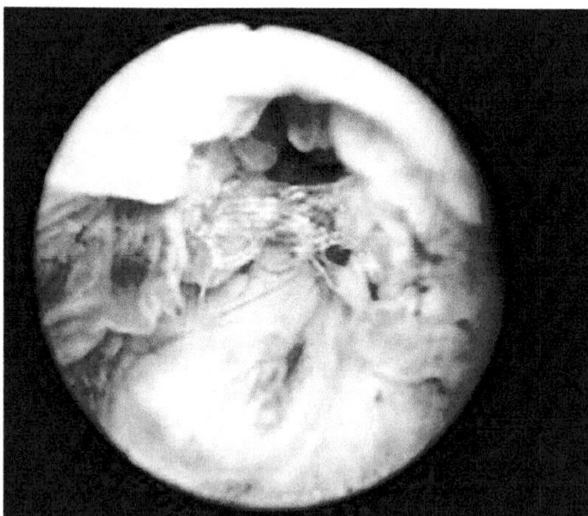

Fig. 3. Mesh perforation into the urethra as visualized on cystourethroscopy.

based on the patient's history before the physical examination. An accurate diagnosis based on physical examination findings will aid the physician in further conservative or surgical management.

MANAGEMENT OF MIDURETHRAL SLING MESH EXPOSURE

Once a mesh exposure has been identified, management depends on several factors. In terms of the patient's history, it is necessary to consider if the patient is symptomatic, is sexually active, and/or has pain. Based on the physical examination, the size and location of the exposure should be noted as well as the quality of vaginal tissue. Return to the operating room to excise exposed vaginal mesh is typically the most definitive treatment option, although it is not without risk of bleeding and possible injury to the urethra and lower urinary tract. For these reasons, less-invasive treatment options are often offered as initial management to patients who are asymptomatic, who are not sexually active, or who have a limited amount of exposed mesh.

Conservative management of mesh exposure includes observation, topical estrogen cream application, or local excision of the exposed mesh in the office setting. Expectant management is not unreasonable in an asymptomatic patient with exposure of type 1 mesh.[27] A retrospective review of women presenting to a tertiary care center with a mesh complication demonstrated that 51% of women were initially treated with conservative management, but of this 51%, 59.3% went on to a surgical intervention, including in office, operating room, and combination of both.[28]

Although there are minimal prospective data on the use of topical estrogen, the American College of Obstetricians and Gynecologists and AUGS Committee Opinion offers that there is little risk in offering a trial of hormonal cream for 6 to 12 weeks to improve or resolve the mesh exposure. It is recommended to reserve this management for exposures less than 0.5 cm.[29] Efficacious outcomes were noted by Kobashi and Govier[9] when they described 4 patients with MUS exposure, approximately 0.5 to 1.0 cm in length, all noted on physical examination at 6-week follow-up. With time alone, all exposures reepithelialized spontaneously without further complication. The authors have not had the same degree of success.

Local excision in the office is appropriate if the area of exposed mesh is small, easily visible, and accessible without significant retraction. Exposure of this sort is commonly at the incision site and/or is just an edge of distorted mesh. The surgeon should infiltrate the surrounding vaginal mucosa using lidocaine with epinephrine and excise the visible portion of the mesh with surgical scissors. Closure of the defect should be performed, if possible. Patients should be counseled that the in-office success rate of mesh trimming is not high. Abbott and colleagues[28] showed that 73.3% of women who underwent an in-office trimming of their exposed vaginal mesh went to the operating room for definitive treatment. To a large degree, the success rate depends on the size of the exposure.

For more extensive mesh exposure, treatment options include covering the exposed mesh with vaginal flaps or partial versus total sling excision. Covering the exposed mesh with vaginal skin flaps is a treatment option when the exposure is limited and a goal is to preserve urinary continence. Giri and colleagues[30] reviewed their series of 5 patients with vaginal mesh exposure who underwent primary reclosure of the vaginal skin over the mesh as a first-line treatment option. The margin of the vaginal skin and granulation tissue was trimmed; vaginal flaps were mobilized and closed with absorbable suture over the mesh with interrupted vertical mattress sutures in a single layer. Patients remained symptom free, without additional exposure or SUI recurrence at 12-month follow-up. In a slightly larger series, Kim and colleagues[31] described 8 mesh exposures treated by covering with vaginal flaps, of which 2 patients (25%) had recurrent exposure. Alternately, a series by Lee and colleagues[32] attempted to preserve mesh with vaginal flap coverage, but all 3 patients who underwent conservative management failed.

Although this approach may be successful in some patients, they must understand that the exposure can recur, necessitating further surgery.

If conservative measures fail, or more definitive treatment is sought for larger, symptomatic mesh exposures, partial or total mesh excision may be considered. During partial excision, dissection is begun at the tissue underlying the exposed mesh. Dissection is carried out at least 0.5 cm in either direction of the exposed portion. Hemostats or surgical clamps are placed at the part of mesh to be removed, and surgical scissors are used to cut out the exposed mesh. Vaginal mucosa is closed with absorbable suture.

In select circumstances, such as mesh-related pain or infection, total mesh excision may be performed. As noted previously, non–type 1 mesh is less porous and may not allow for adequate tissue ingrowth. The mesh may become encapsulated instead of scarred into place allowing mobility of the mesh. The mesh may become encapsulated instead of scarred into place allowing mobility of the mesh and for the sling to be removed more easily at the time of excision (**Fig. 4**). Although total mesh excision may help alleviate chronic pain from nerve or muscle compression or irritation, this is not always the case. Patients who present with pain should be carefully examined, and the surgeon should identify if the pain is overlying the area near the mesh exposure, or if the pain follows the trajectory of the sling arms to help determine if a partial versus total excision is necessary. The more mesh that is excised, the higher the likelihood of recurrent SUI. A retrospective review of 94 patients with no preoperative stress incontinence who underwent surgery for excision of MUS mesh exposure demonstrated that there was greater postoperative stress incontinence with complete versus partial removal of sling at short-term (42% vs 14%, P = .03) and long-term (59% vs 7%, P = .003) follow-up.[33] Patients must be counseled about the risks and benefits of total sling excision, including that their pain may not be improved or resolved with total excision, and that the chance of SUI with need for repeat SUI procedure is significant.

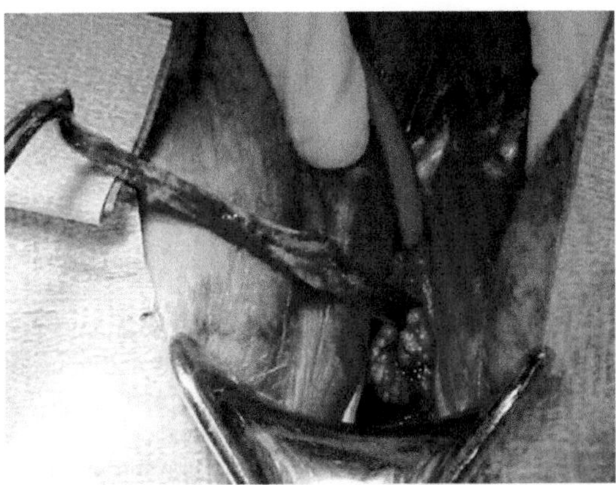

Fig. 4. Older, non–type 1 mesh. Because of less porous material and possible decreased tissue ingrowth, the sling may slide out with minimal dissection during surgical intervention.

MANAGEMENT OF MIDURETHRAL SLING MESH PERFORATION INTO THE URETHRA OR BLADDER

Sling perforation into the urinary tract, specifically the urethra, is uncommon with a <1% overall incidence. Risk factors for mesh perforation into the urethra include decreased vascularity due to excessive vaginal dissection or vaginal atrophy, excessive sling tensioning, or missed intraoperative perforation. As previously noted, careful intraoperative cystourethroscopy is essential to recognize injury at time of surgery. Once injury is acknowledged, synthetic sling placement is aborted. If the perforation is small, placing a urethral catheter to allow for healing may be sufficient, but if there is a significant laceration, primary repair of the urethra should be performed. Many patients who end up with a urethral perforation likely had the sling placed with excessive tension, and over time the sling eroded into the urethra. The authors have seen many patients with a history of postsling retention, prolonged catheterization, continued difficulty voiding, and ultimately, symptoms related to urethral perforation.

Treatment options include endoscopic management as well as transvaginal removal. The authors generally perform a transvaginal removal of the perforating mesh as well a few centimeters laterally in each direction.

Trocar perforation into the bladder is more common with incidence rates ranging from 0% to 24% in RP MUS series. Bladder perforation incidence with a TO approach is low, but higher with an outside-in than inside-out technique. Management options of perforated mesh into the lower urinary tract includes endoscopic intervention via Holmium laser ablation or resection with electrocautery, or excision via a transvaginal or abdominal (either open or laparoscopic) approach.

Endoscopic management is viewed as a less-invasive treatment option to avoid significant reconstruction of the urethra or bladder. Laser ablation of mesh perforating the urethra or bladder is meant to obliterate the exposed portion the synthetic sling, allow reepithelialization of the vaporized tissue, and potentially avoid more invasive reconstructive efforts. However, attempts at transurethral removal of mesh are often incomplete (**Fig. 5**). Residual mesh within the urethra might cause stone formation, recurrent urinary tract infections, or irritable voiding symptoms. A case series of 6 patients who underwent holmium transurethral removal of eroded mesh demonstrated that although intraoperatively they were able to achieve complete endoscopic removal and excision of the exposed mesh, 4 of the 6 patients represented with exposed fibers at repeat cystoscopy.[34] Transurethral endoscopic excision is another method proposed as a minimally invasive way to remove exposed mesh in the bladder. In a small case series of 14 patients, 13 had complete resolution at 18-month follow-up.[35] If one chooses one of these minimally invasive techniques, it is critical to resect/excise the mesh deep to the mucosal layer so that adequate healing without continued mesh exposure results.

Definitive management of eroded mesh into the bladder can be achieved via a transvaginal or suprapubic cystotomy. With the advent of minimally invasive techniques, many surgeons are comfortable performing the cystotomy either laparoscopically or robotically.[35] Misrai and colleagues[36] describe their extraperitoneal laparoscopic approach to the removal of RP mesh and demonstrated no major complications in their 30 patients at a mean follow-up of 38.4 months.[35] Similarly, Macedo and colleagues[37] describe their robotic approach to the removal of mesh eroded into the bladder and demonstrate that this technique is efficacious and may provide an alternative to an open cystotomy in the experienced surgeon's hands.

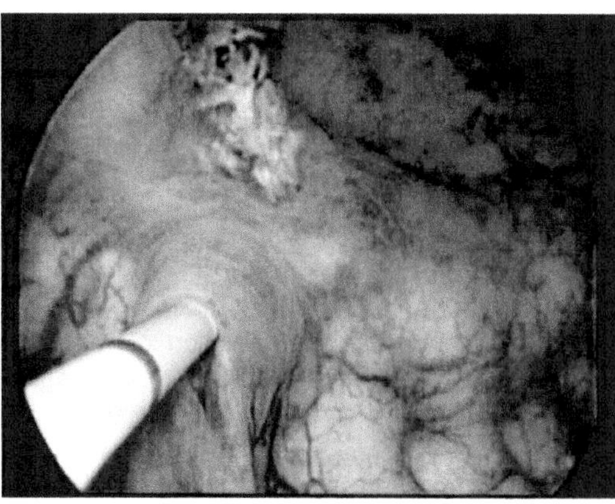

Fig. 5. Mesh perforation traversing bladder near ureteral orifice. Mesh arm appears transected secondary to prior laser ablation as attempted management.

SUMMARY

Mesh complications, including vaginal wall exposure and lower urinary tract perforation, after MUS surgery are not uncommon. Thorough preoperative evaluation and counseling should be provided to minimize risk and manage patient expectations of complications. Physicians should also have a high index of suspicion for mesh complications when a patient presents with bleeding, discharge, dyspareunia/hispareunia, recurrent urinary tract infections, pelvic/groin pain, or voiding dysfunction. Careful history taking and physical examination will lead to most diagnoses; however, additional diagnostics, such as cystourethroscopy, vaginoscopy, examination under anesthesia, or ultrasound, may be used. Treatment options for mesh exposure are patient and symptom dependent and include less-invasive management, such as observation, trial of topical estrogen cream, and local excision of mesh in the office setting, to more definitive procedures, such as covering mesh with vaginal flaps, and partial or total sling excision. Mesh perforation into the lower urinary tract requires more complex interventions. Minimally invasive techniques with transurethral resection or laser ablation can be attempted. More definitive treatments include transvaginal or abdominal (open or laparoscopic) surgery, or a combination of the 2.

REFERENCES

1. Luber KM. The definition, prevalence, and risk factors for stress urinary incontinence. Rev Urol 2004; 6(Suppl 3):S3–9.
2. Kobashi KC, Albo ME, Dmochowski RR, et al. Surgical treatment of female stress urinary incontinence: AUA/SUFU guideline. J Urol 2017;198(4):875–83.
3. Nager C, Tulikangas P, Miller D, et al. Position statement on mesh midurethral slings for stress urinary incontinence. Female Pelvic Med Reconstr Surg 2014;20(3):123–5.
4. Kenton K, Stoddard AM, Zyczynski H, et al. 5-year longitudinal follow-up after retropubic and transobturator midurethral slings. J Urol 2015;193(1):203.
5. Devices CF, Health R. Urogynecologic surgical mesh implants - considerations about surgical mesh for SUI. Available at: https://www.fda.gov/MedicalDevices/ProductsandMedicalProcedures/ImplantsandProsthetics/UroGynSurgicalMesh/ucm345219.htm. Accessed July 3, 2018.

6. Directorate-General for Health and Food Safety (European Commission). Opinion on the Safety of Surgical Meshes Used in Urogynecological Surgery. European Commission; 2015.
7. Haylen BT, Freeman RM, Swift SE, et al. An International Urogynecological Association (IUGA)/International Continence Society (ICS) joint terminology and classification of the complications related directly to the insertion of prostheses (meshes, implants, tapes) and grafts in female pelvic floor surgery. Neurourol Urodyn 2011;30(1):2–12.
8. Clemons JL, Weinstein M, Guess MK, et al. Impact of the 2011 FDA transvaginal mesh safety update on AUGS Members' use of synthetic mesh and biologic grafts in pelvic reconstructive surgery. Female Pelvic Med Reconstr Surg 2013;19(4): 191–8.
9. Kobashi KC, Govier FE. Management of vaginal erosion of polypropylene mesh slings. J Urol 2003; 169(6):2242–3.
10. Amid PK. Biomaterials and Abdominal Wall Hernia Surgery. Surg Laparosc Endosc Percutan Tech 1994;4(5):397.
11. Osborn DJ, Dmochowski RR, Harris CJ, et al. Analysis of patient and technical factors associated with midurethral sling mesh exposure and perforation. Int J Urol 2014;21(11):1167–70.
12. Ford AA, Rogerson L, Cody JD, et al. Mid-urethral sling operations for stress urinary incontinence in women. Cochrane Database Syst Rev 2017. https://doi.org/10.1002/14651858.cd006375.pub4.
13. Linder BJ, El-Nashar SA, Carranza Leon DA, et al. Predictors of vaginal mesh exposure after midurethral sling placement: a case-control study. Int Urogynecol J 2016;27(9):1321–6.
14. Kokanalı MK, Cavkaytar S, Kokanalı D, et al. A comperative study for short-term surgical outcomes of midurethral sling procedures in obese and nonobese women with stress urinary incontinence. J Obstet Gynaecol 2016;36(8):1080–5.
15. Krause M, Wheeler TL 2nd, Snyder TE, et al. Local effects of vaginally administered estrogen therapy: a review. J Pelvic Med Surg 2009;15(3):105–14.
16. Rahn DD, Ward RM, Sanses TV, et al. Vaginal estrogen use in postmenopausal women with pelvic floor disorders: systematic review and practice guidelines. Int Urogynecol J 2015;26(1):3–13.
17. Zambon JP, Matthews CA, Badlani GH. Midurethral slings. J Endourol 2018;32(S1):S - 105–10.
18. Gaines N, Gupta P, Sirls LT. Synthetic midurethral slings: exposure and perforation. In: H.G, editor. Complications of female incontinence and pelvic reconstructive surgery. Current clinical urology. Cham (Switzerland): Humana Press; 2017. p. 177–91.
19. Abbasy SA, Kenton K, Brubaker L, et al. Measurement of transurethral bladder neck displacement during tension-free vaginal tape procedure. Int Urogynecol J 2011;22(6):721–4.
20. Richter HE, Albo ME, Zyczynski HM, et al. Retropubic versus transobturator midurethral slings for stress incontinence. N Engl J Med 2010;362(22): 2066–76.
21. Chinthakanan O, Miklos JR, Moore RD, et al. The indication and surgical treatment of 286 midurethral synthetic sling complications: a multicenter study. Surg Technol Int 2016;29:167–71.
22. Petri E, Ashok K. Partner dyspareunia–a report of six cases. Int Urogynecol J 2012;23(1):127–9.
23. Wang C, Christie AL, Zimmern PE. Synthetic midurethral sling complications: evolution of presenting symptoms over time. Neurourol Urodyn 2018. https://doi.org/10.1002/nau.23534.
24. Cohen SA, Goldman HB. Mesh perforation into a viscus in the setting of pelvic floor surgery—presentation and management. Curr Urol Rep 2016;17(9). https://doi.org/10.1007/s11934-016-0621-3.
25. Chan L, Tse V. Pelvic floor ultrasound in the diagnosis of sling complications. World J Urol 2018; 36(5):753–9.
26. Staack A, Vitale J, Ragavendra N, et al. Translabial ultrasonography for evaluation of synthetic mesh in the vagina. Urology 2014;83(1):68–74.
27. Deffieux X, Thubert T, de Tayrac R, et al. Long-term follow-up of persistent vaginal polypropylene mesh exposure for transvaginally placed mesh procedures. Int Urogynecol J 2012;23(10):1387–90.
28. Abbott S, Unger CA, Evans JM, et al. Evaluation and management of complications from synthetic mesh after pelvic reconstructive surgery: a multicenter study. Am J Obstet Gynecol 2014;210(2): 163.e1-8.
29. Management of mesh and graft complications in gynecologic surgery. Female Pelvic Med Reconstr Surg 2017;23(3):171–6.
30. Giri SK, Sil D, Narasimhulu G, et al. Management of vaginal extrusion after tension-free vaginal tape procedure for urodynamic stress incontinence. Urology 2007;69(6):1077–80.
31. Kim SY, Park JY, Kim HK, et al. Vaginal mucosal flap as a sling preservation for the treatment of vaginal exposure of mesh. Korean J Urol 2010;51(6):416–9.
32. Lee T, Kim J-S, Jung J-K, et al. Surgical management of vaginal wound healing defects after tension-free vaginal tape placement. Int J Urol 2005; 12(7):699–701.
33. Jambusaria LH, Heft J, Stuart Reynolds W, et al. Incontinence rates after midurethral sling revision for vaginal exposure or pain. Am J Obstet Gynecol 2016;215(6):764.e1-5.
34. Doumouchtsis SK, Lee FYK, Bramwell D, et al. Evaluation of holmium laser for managing mesh/suture complications of continence surgery. BJU Int 2011; 108(9):1472–8.

35. Oh T-H, Ryu D-S. Transurethral resection of intravesical mesh after midurethral sling procedures. J Endourol 2009;23(8):1333–7.
36. Misrai V, Rouprêt M, Xylinas E, et al. Surgical resection for suburethral sling complications after treatment for stress urinary incontinence. J Urol 2009;181(5):2198–202 [discussion: 2203].
37. Macedo FIB, O'Connor J, Mittal VK, et al. Robotic removal of eroded vaginal mesh into the bladder. Int J Urol 2013;20(11):1144–6.

Surgery for Stress Urinary Incontinence

Autologous Fascial Sling

Jerry G. Blaivas, MD[a,*], Vannita Simma-Chiang, MD[b], Zeynep Gul, MD[b], Linda Dayan, BA[c,1], Senad Kalkan, MD[d,1], Melissa Daniel, MD[e]

KEYWORDS

• Pubovaginal sling • Fascial sling • Autologous pubovaginal sling • Synthetic midurethral sling • Stress urinary incontinence • Safety • Efficacy • Operative technique

KEY POINTS

- The autologous fascial pubovaginal sling (AFPVS) has been considered the gold standard treatment of both simple and complicated stress urinary incontinence in women since the late 1990s.
- The synthetic midurethral sling (SMUS) has gained popularity over the last decade because it is a minimally invasive operation associated with a quicker recovery and lower perioperative morbidity.
- Most studies show that cure rates for both procedures remain similar at 82%; 88% for objective success and 77% to 79% for subjective success.
- The safety profiles of AFPVS and SMUS are different; chronic pelvic pain, dyspareunia, and erosions are more common after SMUS while urethral obstruction and wound complications are more common after AFPVS.
- As longer-term outcomes of SMUS surgery come to light, the authors believe that the complication rate of SMUS will continue to increase, raising concerns about its long-term safety.
- The AFPVS remains a gold standard for the surgical treatment of stress urinary incontinence.

INTRODUCTION

For decades the autologous fascial pubovaginal sling (AFPVS) has been considered the gold standard for the treatment of stress urinary incontinence (SUI) in women. Although its safety and efficacy remain unchallenged, its popularity has waned dramatically over the last 15 years and, at present, it has been largely replaced by the synthetic midurethral slings (SMUS). In a recent poll of its membership, 99% of gynecologists and 87% of urologists consider SMUS as the treatment of choice for uncomplicated SUI.[1,2] The reason for this dramatic shift is not only the widespread belief among surgeons that the SMUS is as effective as, or more effective than, the AFPVS but also that its safety profile, ease of operation, and

Disclosure: Dr J.G. Blaivas receives paid expert testimony in mesh litigation cases. Dr V. Simma-Chiang has nothing to disclose. Dr Z. Gul has nothing to disclose. L. Dayan receives a salary from the Institute for Bladder and Prostate Research. Dr S. Kalkan has nothing to disclose. Dr M. Daniel has nothing to disclose.

[a] Department of Urology, Icahn School of Medicine at Mount Sinai, 1425 Madison Avenue, New York, NY 10029, USA; [b] Department of Urology, Icahn School of Medicine at Mount Sinai, 1425 Madison Avenue, New York, NY 10029, USA; [c] Institute for Bladder and Prostate Research, 445 East 77 Street, New York, NY 10075, USA; [d] Bezmialem Vakif University in Istanbul, Adnan Menderes Bulvarı Vatan Caddesi, 34093 Fatih/İstanbul, Turkey; [e] Department of Surgery, SUNY Downstate Medical Center, 450 Clarkson Avenue, Brooklyn, NY 11203, USA
[1] Present address: 445 East 77 Street, New York, NY 10075.
* Corresponding author. 445 East 77 Street, New York, NY 10075.
E-mail address: jerry.blaivas@mountsinai.org

Urol Clin N Am 46 (2019) 41–52
https://doi.org/10.1016/j.ucl.2018.08.014
0094-0143/19/© 2018 Elsevier Inc. All rights reserved.

perioperative morbidity are much better. However, the safety profile of SMUS has recently been challenged and it is our opinion that, when comparing the risks and benefits, the AFPVS outperforms the SMUS. Further, since the US Food and Drug Administration warning regarding transvaginal mesh, there has been an increase in AFPVS placement.[3] We believe this increase will continue as the full extent of the risks associated with SMUS come to light. This article reviews the surgical technique and long-term outcomes of the autologous rectus fascial sling in the treatment of women with SUI and compares outcomes after AFPVS and SMUS.

Operative Technique

Our operative technique has been described previously but has changed somewhat over the years and is discussed later. The patient is positioned in the dorsal lithotomy position. The vagina and abdomen are prepped to the level of the umbilicus and the patient is draped. To harvest rectus fascia, a 6-cm to 8-cm transverse incision is made just above the pubis (**Fig. 1**) and carried down to the rectus fascia. The incision can be extended as needed if the patient is obese. Starting about 2 cm above the pubis, in the midline, 2 parallel transverse incisions are made in the fascia approximately 2 cm apart (**Fig. 2**). The wound edges are retracted to allow these incisions to be extended toward the iliac crest. With proper wound retraction, final sling length is usually about 12 to 16 cm. The undersurface of the fascia is dissected off the rectus muscle and each end of fascia is secured with a running horizontal mattress, placed perpendicular to the direction of the fascial fibers, using a 2-0 permanent monofilament suture (**Fig. 3**). The fascia is then excised and placed in a basin of saline (**Fig. 4**). The wound is packed with saline-soaked sponges and attention is turned to the vagina.

A weighted speculum is placed into the vagina and a Foley catheter is inserted into the urethra. The labia are temporarily sutured to the drapes for retraction. Next, a gently curved horizontal incision is made over the bladder neck (**Fig. 5**). The

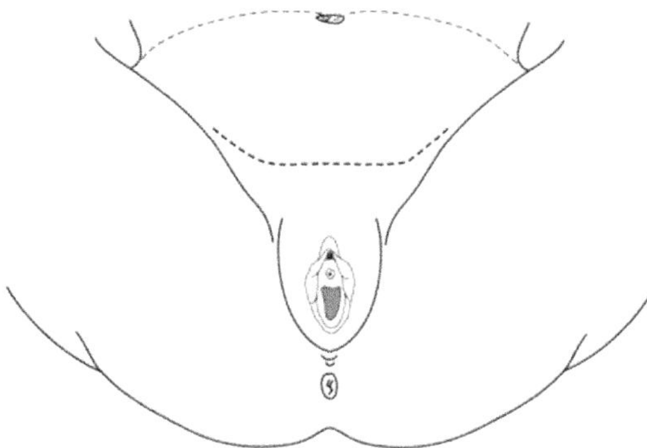

Fig. 1. Once the patient is positioned in dorsal lithotomy, a 6-cm to 8-cm incision is made just above the pubis. (*From* Blaivas JG, Chaikin DC. Pubovaginal fascial sling for the treatment of all types of stress urinary incontinence: surgical technique and long-term outcome. Urol Clin North Am 2011;38(1):8; with permission.)

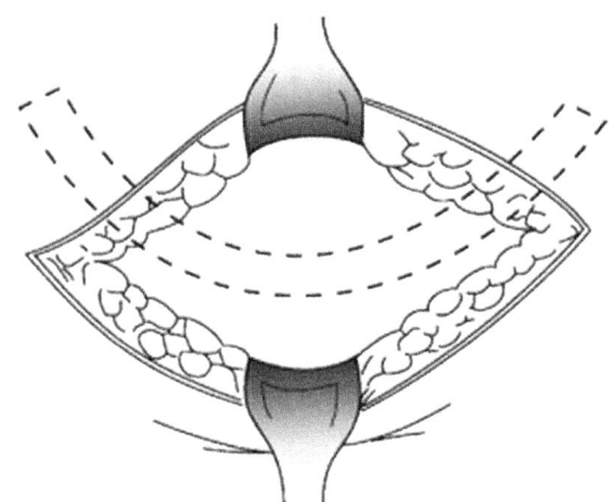

Fig. 2. To harvest the sling, 2 parallel transverse incisions (*dashed lines*) are made in the fascia 2 cm apart. The wound edges are retracted to maximize sling length. (*From* Blaivas JG, Chaikin DC. Pubovaginal fascial sling for the treatment of all types of stress urinary incontinence: surgical technique and long-term outcome. Urol Clin North Am 2011;38(1):8; with permission.)

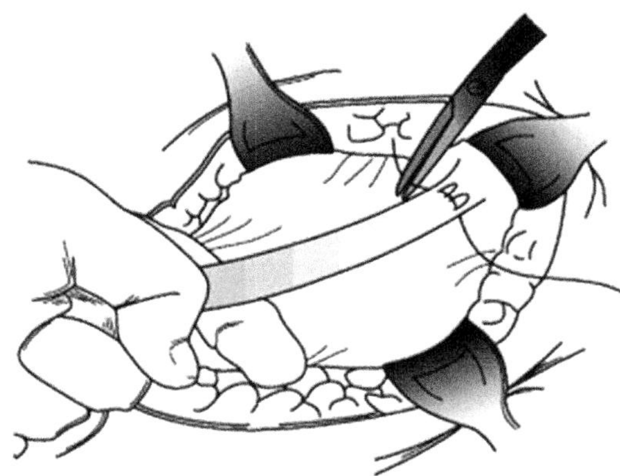

Fig. 3. A plane is created between the fascia and the muscle. The incision is extended at least until the point where the rectus divides to pass around the external oblique. Each end of fascia is secured with a running horizontal mattress, placed perpendicular to the direction of the fascial fibers, using a 2-0 permanent monofilament suture. (*From* Blaivas JG, Chaikin DC. Pubovaginal fascial sling for the treatment of all types of stress urinary incontinence: surgical technique and long-term outcome. Urol Clin North Am 2011;38(1):8; with permission.)

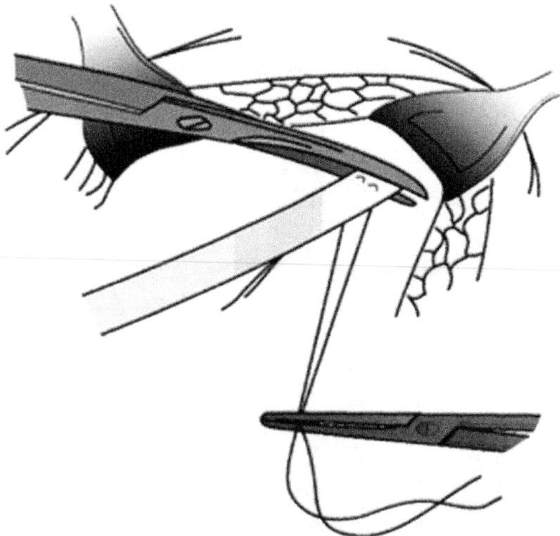

Fig. 4. After the mattress suture has been tied on either side, the fascial graft is transected bilaterally and placed in a basin of saline for later use as the sling. (*From* Blaivas JG, Chaikin DC. Pubovaginal fascial sling for the treatment of all types of stress urinary incontinence: surgical technique and long-term outcome. Urol Clin North Am 2011;38(1):9; with permission.)

incision should be about 2 cm proximal to the distal edge of the balloon and superficial to the pubocervical fascia. Identification of the bladder neck is facilitated by putting traction on the catheter and palpating the balloon. To avoid entering

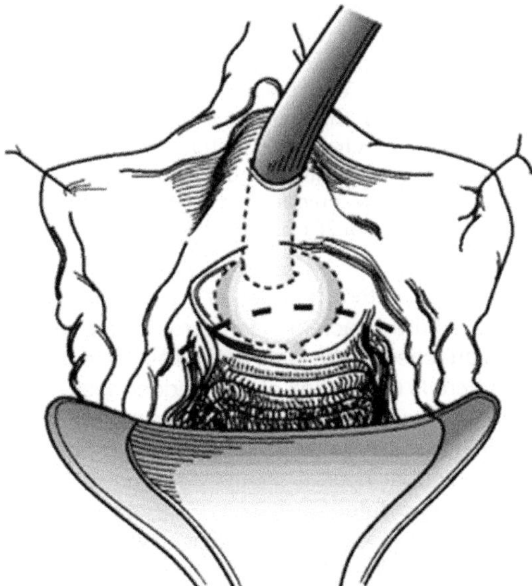

Fig. 5. A curved horizontal incision (*dashed line*) is made over the bladder neck, which should be about 2 cm proximal to the distal edge of the Foley balloon. (*From* Blaivas JG, Chaikin DC. Pubovaginal fascial sling for the treatment of all types of stress urinary incontinence: surgical technique and long-term outcome. Urol Clin North Am 2011;38(1):9; with permission.)

the wrong plane, an Allis clamp is placed on the cranial edge of the vaginal incision in the midline. The surgeon should then apply caudad traction with the Allis clamp with the nondominant hand while pushing upward with the index finger to help assess the depth of the dissection (**Fig. 6**). The plane is developed by careful dissection with Metzenbaum scissors, which should be held at a 60° to 90° angle to the undersurface of the vaginal incision. The correct plane is delineated by the characteristic shiny white appearance of the undersurface of the anterior vaginal wall (**Fig. 7**).

The dissection is then carried posterolaterally, to develop a tunnel for the sling, by retracting the

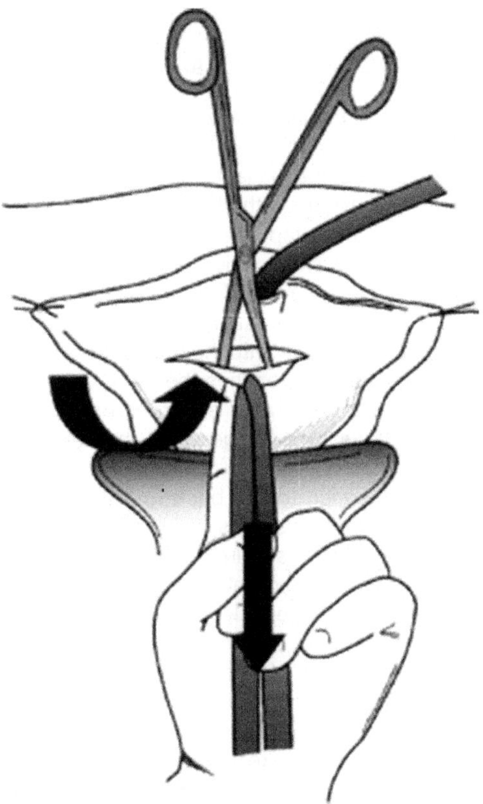

Fig. 6. The dissection should be superficial to the pubocervical fascia. To avoid entering the wrong plane, an Allis clamp is placed on the cranial edge of the vaginal incision in the midline. The surgeon should apply caudad traction with the Allis clamp while pushing upward with the index finger (curved arrow) to help assess the depth of the dissection. A vaginal flap is made for a distance of about 2 cm, just wide enough to accept the sling. The *black arrow* is illustrating the index finger pushing upward and pulling back on the flap. (*From* Blaivas JG, Chaikin DC. Pubovaginal fascial sling for the treatment of all types of stress urinary incontinence: surgical technique and long-term outcome. Urol Clin North Am 2011;38(1):9; with permission.)

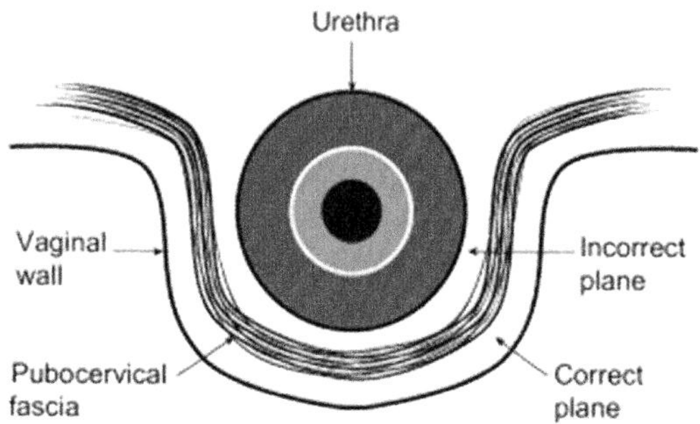

Fig. 7. The proper plane is superficial to the pubocervical fascia. If the incision is made too deep, the dissection proceeds underneath the urethra and bladder, exposing those structures to possible injury. (*From* Blaivas JG, Chaikin DC. Pubovaginal fascial sling for the treatment of all types of stress urinary incontinence: surgical technique and long-term outcome. Urol Clin North Am 2011;38(1):9; with permission.)

lateral edge of the incision with an Allis clamp and keeping the tips of the Metzenbaum scissors pointed toward the patient's ipsilateral shoulder (**Fig. 8**). To avoid urethral, bladder, or ureteral injury during this step, the dissection is kept as far lateral as possible, which is accomplished by orienting the concavity of the scissors laterally and applying constant lateral pressure against the vaginal epithelium with the tips of the scissors. Once the dissection reaches the pubis, the endopelvic fascia is perforated either with scissors or bluntly with an index finger and the retropubic space is entered (**Fig. 9**).

Attention is then turned back to the abdominal incision. A Kocher clamp is placed on the inferior edge of the rectus fascia in the midline. The fascia is lifted upward to facilitate passage of an index finger beneath the inferior leaf and along the undersurface of the pubis, until it meets the opposite index finger, which is placed in the vaginal incision (**Fig. 10**). While the index finger in the vaginal incision retracts the bladder and bladder neck medially, a long, curved clamp, like a DeBakey, is passed into the abdominal incision and follows the path created by the two index fingers (**Fig. 11**). Once the tip of the clamp is visible in the vaginal incision, one of the sutures attached to the fascial sling is passed into the clamp, and then pulled into the abdominal wound (**Fig. 12**). This procedure is then repeated on the opposite side.

Two small stab wounds are then made in the rectus fascia just above the pubis, and the sling is brought through them (**Fig. 13**). The sling is now in position, traversing from the abdominal wall, around the bladder neck, and back to the abdominal wall on the other side. Before securing the sutures, intravenous indigo carmine is given and a cystoscopy is performed to evaluate for

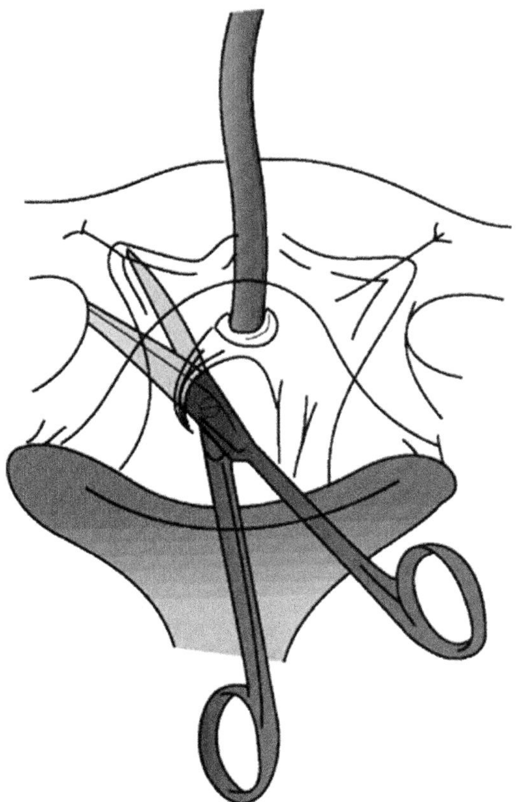

Fig. 8. The dissection is carried posterolaterally to develop a tunnel for the sling. To avoid urethral, bladder, or ureteral injury, the dissection is kept as far lateral as possible, which is accomplished by orienting the concavity of the scissors laterally and applying constant lateral pressure against the vaginal epithelium with the tips of the scissors. Once the dissection reaches the pubis, the endopelvic fascia is perforated. (*From* Blaivas JG, Chaikin DC. Pubovaginal fascial sling for the treatment of all types of stress urinary incontinence: surgical technique and long-term outcome. Urol Clin North Am 2011;38(1):10; with permission.)

injury to the urethra, bladder, or ureters. The cystoscope is pulled back to the midurethra and the sutures attached to the sling are pulled up to ensure that there is coaptation at the bladder neck. If the sling was inadvertently placed at the midurethra, it is left in place. However, if it was placed proximal to the bladder neck it should be removed and a new tunnel created.

The vaginal incision is then closed with a running 2-0 chromic. Then, the sutures on each end of the sling are pulled through the separate stab incisions in the fascia and the fascial defect is closed with continuous 2-0 delayed absorbable, monofilament sutures. The sutures that are attached to the ends of the graft are tied to one another in the midline to secure the sling in place, without any tension (**Fig. 14**).

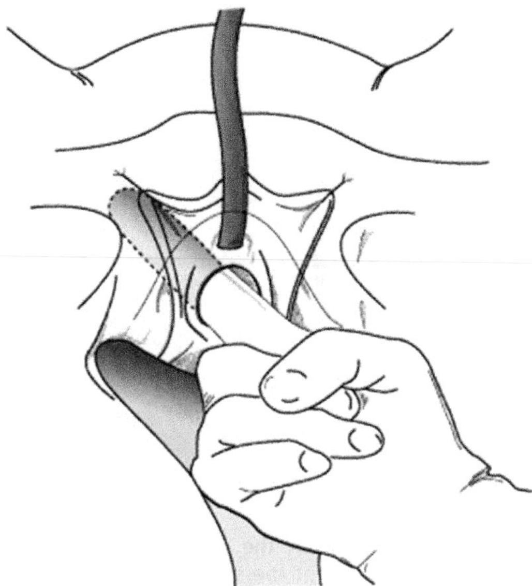

Fig. 9. The endopelvic fascia is perforated with scissors or with an index finger and the retropubic space is entered. (*From* Blaivas JG, Chaikin DC. Pubovaginal fascial sling for the treatment of all types of stress urinary incontinence: surgical technique and long-term outcome. Urol Clin North Am 2011;38(1):10; with permission.)

To avoid placing the sling on tension, the sutures on each end of the sling are pulled upward while downward pressure is applied to the cystoscope. This technique depresses the vesical neck and puts the sling on stretch. The sutures are then released and the cystoscope is removed. A well-lubricated Q-tip is placed in the urethra. If the urethral angle, as measured by the Q-tip, is negative, downward pressure is placed on the Q-tip until the angle is 0° or greater. The sutures can then be tied with confidence that the sling is not under excessive tension. It is usually possible to place 2 or 3 fingers comfortably between the sutures and the rectus fascia. A Foley catheter is left indwelling, but a vaginal pack is placed only if there is concern for bleeding. If used, it is soaked in sterile lubricating jelly to prevent vaginal pain or excoriation during its removal (**Fig. 15**).

Postoperative Management

If a vaginal pack was placed, it is removed before an active voiding trial, which is done once the patient is in the recovery room or, if the patient is admitted, on the first postoperative day. If the patient is still having significant discomfort, the catheter is left in longer. If the patient is unable to void before discharge, she is taught to do intermittent self-catheterization, which is continued until she is voiding satisfactorily (**Fig. 16**).

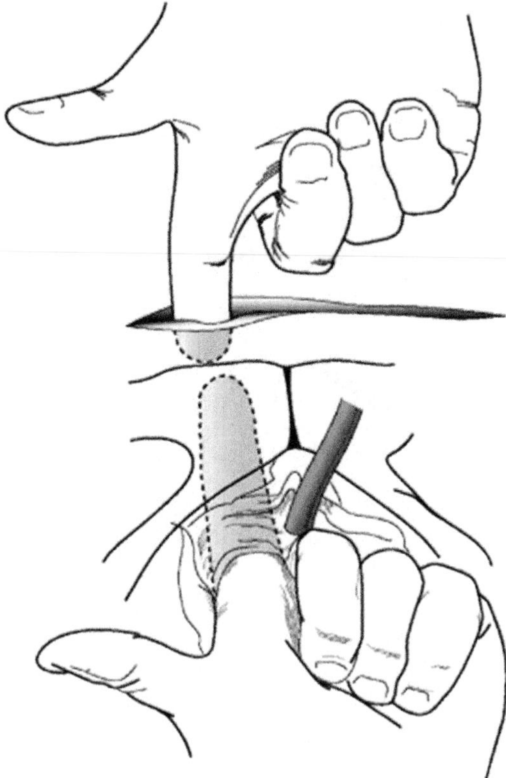

Fig. 10. An index finger is placed beneath the inferior leaf of rectus fascia and along the undersurface the pubis until it meets the opposite index finger, which is placed in the vaginal incision. (*From* Blaivas JG, Chaikin DC. Pubovaginal fascial sling for the treatment of all types of stress urinary incontinence: surgical technique and long-term outcome. Urol Clin North Am 2011;38(1):11; with permission.)

Fascia Lata Sling Harvest

In certain situations, such as if the patient is obese, has had prior abdominal surgery, or simply surgeon preference, a fascia lata graft may be taken for use as a sling. Typically, the patient is placed in the full lateral or the supine position with leg internally rotated at the hip. The thigh is prepped from below the knee to the anterior superior iliac spine. A 3-cm horizontal incision is then made approximately 2 cm above the patella and dissection is carried down to the level of the fascia lata, which can be identified by its characteristic shiny white appearance. Two parallel incisions are made 2 cm apart, perpendicular to the skin incision in the direction of the fascial fibers. The undersurface of the fascia is dissected off the muscle as far as possible (usually to 3–4 cm above the

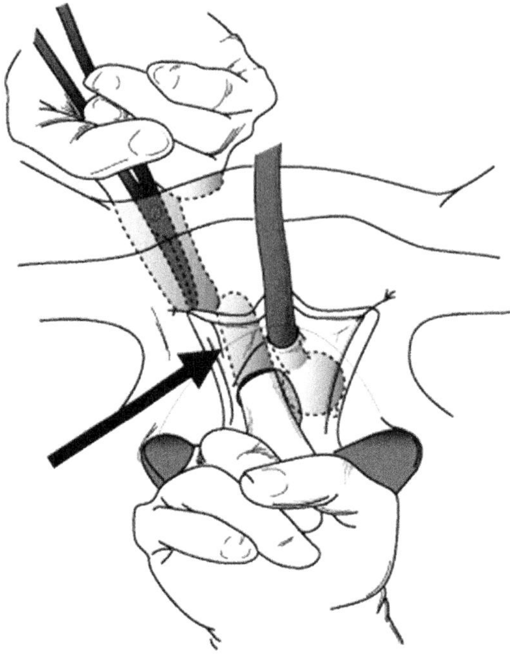

Fig. 11. While the index finger in the vaginal incision retracts the bladder and bladder neck medially, a long, curved clamp, such as a DeBakey, is passed into the abdominal incision and follows the path created by the two fingers. The *black arrow* illustrates the index finger retracting the bladder neck and urethra medially. (*From* Blaivas JG, Chaikin DC. Pubovaginal fascial sling for the treatment of all types of stress urinary incontinence: surgical technique and long-term outcome. Urol Clin North Am 2011;38(1):11; with permission.)

patella). The two parallel incisions are then connected, and this end of the graft is secured with a running horizontal mattress, placed perpendicular to the direction of the fascial fibers, using a 2-0 permanent monofilament suture. A thin malleable retractor is then placed superficially and deep to the planned fascial strip to free it from the subcutaneous fat and muscle, respectively. While placing gentle traction on the free end of the sling, the Crawford fascial stripper is used to extend the incision cephalad and divide it before removal. The other end of the graft is also secured with a 2-0 permanent monofilament suture in the same manner as before. The wound should be closed in 3 layers without closing the fascia lata. A compressive dressing is usually applied.[4,5]

RESULTS

The senior author's results with autologous rectus fascial pubovaginal slings have been reported in 4 reports over 15 years and have previously been summarized.[6–9] The largest series consisted of

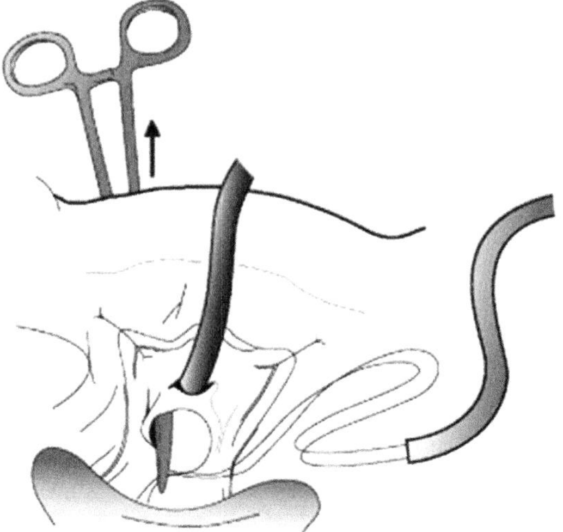

Fig. 12. Once the tip of the clamp is visible in the vaginal incision, one of the sutures attached to the fascial sling is passed into the clamp, and then pulled (*arrow*) into the abdominal wound. This step is then repeated on the opposite side. (*From* Blaivas JG, Chaikin DC. Pubovaginal fascial sling for the treatment of all types of stress urinary incontinence: surgical technique and long-term outcome. Urol Clin North Am 2011;38(1):11; with permission.)

251 women whose outcomes were assessed with the Simplified Urinary Incontinence Outcome Score (SUIOS).[6] The score is composed of 3 variables: a pad test, voiding diary, and questionnaire each graded on a 3-point scale. In this series, 75% of the women had complicated stress incontinence, which was defined as 1 or more of the following: mixed stress and urge incontinence, a so-called pipe-stem urethra, a urethral diverticulum, a vesicovaginal fistula, or a neurogenic bladder. Cure was defined as a dry pad test, no

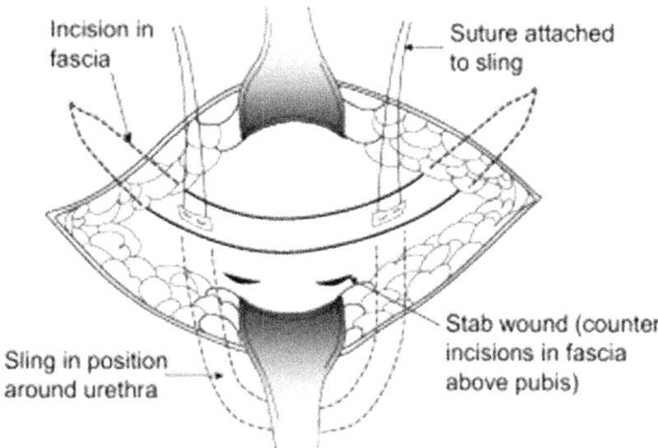

Fig. 13. Two stab wounds are then made in the rectus fascia just above the pubis. (*From* Blaivas JG, Chaikin DC. Pubovaginal fascial sling for the treatment of all types of stress urinary incontinence: surgical technique and long-term outcome. Urol Clin North Am 2011;38(1):12; with permission.)

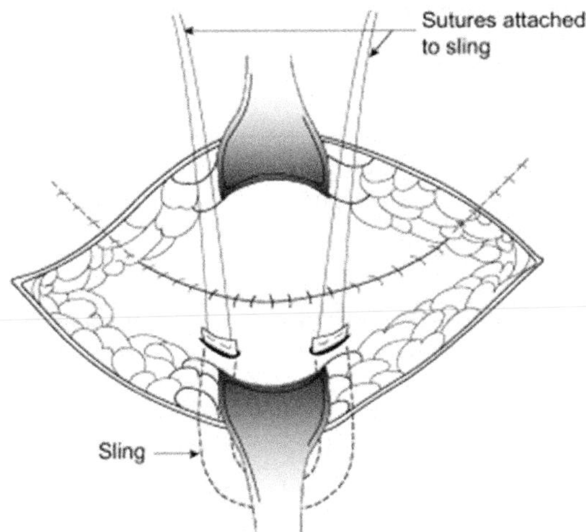

Fig. 14. The vaginal incision is closed. The sling is brought through the stab incisions. The rectus fascia is then closed. (*From* Blaivas JG, Chaikin DC. Pubovaginal fascial sling for the treatment of all types of stress urinary incontinence: surgical technique and long-term outcome. Urol Clin North Am 2011;38(1):12; with permission.)

reported episodes of incontinence, and patient-reported cure. Using the SUIOS, 45% of patients were cured, 41% had a good or fair response, and 15% had a poor response or failure. In a subsequent series of 67 women with simple stress incontinence (absence of complicated incontinence as defined earlier), the cure rate was 66% and all remaining patients experienced improvement; there were no failures. In a separate analysis of

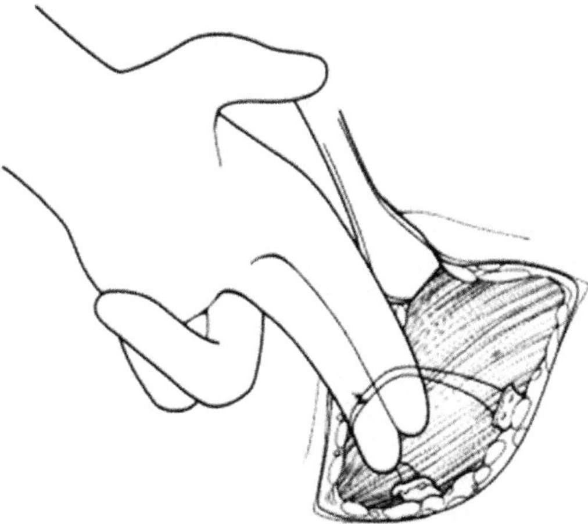

Fig. 15. The sutures attached to the sling are tied in the midline, without tension. See the text for tips on how to avoid tension. (*From* Blaivas JG, Chaikin DC. Pubovaginal fascial sling for the treatment of all types of stress urinary incontinence: surgical technique and long-term outcome. Urol Clin North Am 2011;38(1):12; with permission.)

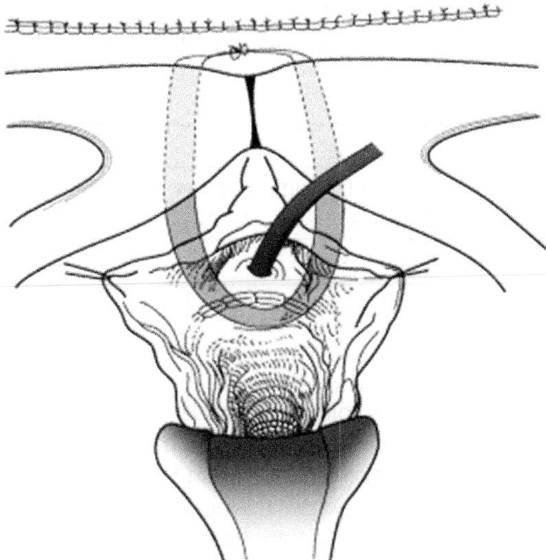

Fig. 16. The completed procedure. The sling is in place and each end is tied to each other over the rectus fascia. (*From* Blaivas JG, Chaikin DC. Pubovaginal fascial sling for the treatment of all types of stress urinary incontinence: surgical technique and long-term outcome. Urol Clin North Am 2011;38(1):12; with permission.)

98 women, we found no significant difference in the failure rates after AFPVS for patients with stress incontinence and mixed incontinence. However, when patients who were cured were compared with those who were not, patients who were not cured had more daily preoperative urgency episodes, more urge incontinence episodes, and voided more frequently.[7] Therefore, we deduce that the more severe the overactive bladder (OAB), the less likely the patient is to have a successful outcome.

Combining all of these series, most failures occurred within 6 months of surgery, and the most common cause of failure was persistent urge incontinence. De novo urge incontinence occurred in about 3% of cases. Overall complication rates were low. In more than 400 patients, wound infections, incisional hernias, and long-term urethral obstruction requiring surgery or catheterization each occurred in less than 1% of patients. The 2 causes of obstruction were grade 3 or 4 pelvic organ prolapse and placing the sling under too much tension. Adjusting tension comes with experience and can be optimized using the technique described earlier. All cases of urethral obstruction necessitating surgery or permanent intermittent catheterization occurred before 1988 in the senior author's experience.

In general, our success rates with autologous rectus fascial sling are similar to those reported in other large studies and meta-analyses and

Table 1
Efficacy of autologous fascial pubovaginal slings (AFPVS) versus synthetic midurethral slings (SMUS)

	AFPVS	SMUS	*P* value
Total size of cohort	n = 5733	n = 25,586	–
Mean follow-up (range), months	30 (12–67)	34 (12–204)	.21
Objective Success	82% (33–100)	88% (70–100)	.22
Subjective Success	79% (51–100)	77% (43%–99%)	.60

Data from Blaivas JG, Purohit RS, Benedon MS, et al. Safety considerations for synthetic sling surgery. Nat Rev Urol 2015;12(9):481–509.

are also comparable with SMUS (**Table 1**). For example, in a large randomized trial of 329 patients, Albo and colleagues[10] found that, at 2 years, patients randomized to undergo a pubovaginal sling had a 47% cure rate, which was defined as no incontinence episodes recorded in a 3-day voiding diary, no self-reported symptoms, an increase of less than 15 g during a 24-hour pad test, and no leakage during Valsalva and cough. Other small studies have reported similar cure rates ranging from 57% to 88%.[11–14]

Overall, the complication rates between AFPVS and SMUS are similar, except the SMUS has a higher rate of erosions, dyspareunia and chronic pain and the AFPVS has a higher rate of wound complications and urethral obstruction requiring surgery (**Table 2**).[14]

DISCUSSION

Long considered the gold standard for the treatment of stress incontinence in women, autologous fascial slings have lost popularity since the advent of SMUS, which gained popularity because of the ease of the procedure, shorter operative time, and reportedly reduced morbidity.[13,15–17] At present, SMUS is the most common procedure for stress urinary incontinence and several high-quality trials have shown that SMUS has comparable cure rates with the AFPVS as well as comparable (or lower) complication rates.[18,19]

Although the authors agree that success rates of the SMUS and AFPVS are similar, we believe the significant complication rate associated with synthetic midurethral slings are greater than those

Table 2
Nature and prevalence of complications due to autologous fascial pubovaginal slings (AFPVS) versus synthetic midurethral slings (SMUS)

	AFPVS (Prevalence %)	SMUS (Prevalence %)	Logistic Regression	Fisher's Exact Test
Total size of cohort	n = 5733	n = 25,586	–	–
Death	2/5733 (0.034)	2/7762 (0)	NA	0.48
Bladder perforation	50/3854 (1.3)	579/19,411 (3.0)	*<0.0001*	*<0.0001*
Bowel perforation	4/2936 (0.1)	4/3820 (0.1)	0.73	0.73
Wound complications	70/1982 (3.5)	NA	NA	NA
Urethral obstruction	358/4313 (8.3)	301/9375 (3.2)	*<0.0001*	*<0.0001*
Erosion surgery	8/2786 (0.28)	333/16,619 (2.0)	*<0.0001*	*<0.0001*
Vaginal	7/2786 (0.25)	235/13,705 (1.7)	*<0.0001*	*<0.0001*
Bladder	0/2786 (0)	29/13,393 (0.22)	NA	*0.004*
Urethral	1/2786 (0.04)	11/13,628 (0.08)	0.57	0.7
De novo OAB	320/2876 (11)	1512/14,765 (10)	0.16	0.16
Dyspareunia	4/454 (0.9)	24/324 (7.4)	*<0.0001*	*<0.0001*
Refractory pelvic pain	6/1004 (0.6)	247/7084 (3.5)	*<0.0001*	*<0.0001*

Data from Blaivas JG, Purohit RS, Benedon MS, et al. Safety considerations for synthetic sling surgery. Nat Rev Urol 2015;12(9):481–509.

associated with AFPVS. The conclusion that complication rates are similar comes from studies with limited follow-up; usually less than 5 years.[18,19] To better compare complication rates, the investigators performed a meta-analysis of complications after AFPVS and SMUS. Seventy-one studies were included in the analysis consisting of 5733 patients who underwent an AFPVS and 25,586 patients who underwent an SMUS. This analysis showed that sling erosion, refractory pelvic pain and dyspareunia were all more common after SMUS. Wound infection and urethral obstruction requiring surgery were more common between the two procedures and wound complications were more common after AFPVS.[5–8,10–17,20–81] In our judgment, what is lacking in almost all of the studies are certain lifestyle-altering complications that are practically unique to SMUS: refractory pelvic pain and dyspareunia and the cascade of symptoms and complications resulting from mesh revision surgeries.[82]

SUMMARY

Although, SMUSs have become more popular than pubovaginal slings, they are associated with severe complications that can be lifestyle altering for some patients. Pubovaginal slings are a safe and effective treatment of sphincter insufficiency. The authors believe that pubovaginal slings are still the gold standard for treatment of SUI. This study was funded by the Institute for Bladder and Prostate Research in New York, NY, USA.

REFERENCES

1. Nager C, Tulikangas P, Miller D, et al. Position Statement on Mesh Midurethral Slings for Stress Urinary Incontinence. Female Pelvic Med Reconstr Surg 2014;20(3):123–5.
2. Chughtai BI, Elterman DS, Vertosick E, et al. Midurethral sling is the dominant procedure for female stress urinary incontinence: analysis of case logs from certifying American urologists. Urology 2013; 82(6):1267–71.
3. Khan AA, Rosenblum N, Brucker B, et al. Changes in management of stress urinary incontinence following the 2011 FDA health notification. J Clin Urol 2017;10(5):440–8.
4. Dmochowski RR, Osborn DJ, Reynolds WS. Slings: autologous, biologic, synthetic, and midurethral. In: McDougal WS, Wein AJ, Kavoussi LR, Partin AW, Peters CA, editors. Campbell-Walsh urology. 11th edition; 2016. p. 1987–2038.
5. Latini JM, Lux MM, Kreder KJ. Efficacy and morbidity of autologous fascia lata sling cystourethropexy. J Urol 2004;171(3):1180–4.
6. Chaikin DC, Rosenthal J, Blaivas JG. Pubovaginal fascial sling for all types of stress urinary incontinence: long-term analysis. J Urol 1998;160(4):1312–6.
7. Chou EC-L, Flisser AJ, Panagopoulos G, et al. Effective treatment for mixed urinary incontinence with a pubovaginal sling. J Urol 2003;170(2 Pt 1):494–7.
8. Groutz A, Blaivas JG, Hyman MJ, et al. Pubovaginal sling surgery for simple stress urinary incontinence: analysis by an outcome score. J Urol 2001;165(5): 1597–600.
9. Blaivas JG, Chaikin DC. Pubovaginal fascial sling for the treatment of all types of stress urinary incontinence: surgical technique and long-term outcome. Urol Clin North Am 2011;38:7–15.
10. Albo ME, Richter HE, Brubaker L, et al. Burch colposuspension versus fascial sling to reduce urinary stress incontinence. N Engl J Med 2007;356(21): 2143–55.
11. Amaro JL, Yamamoto H, Kawano PR, et al. Clinical and quality-of-life outcomes after autologous fascial sling and tension-free vaginal tape: a prospective randomized trial. Int Braz J Urol 2009; 35(1):60–6.
12. Athanasopoulos A, Gyftopoulos K, McGuire EJ. Efficacy and preoperative prognostic factors of autologous fascia rectus sling for treatment of female stress urinary incontinence. Urology 2011;78(5): 1034–8.
13. Mock S, Angelle J, Reynolds WS, et al. Contemporary comparison between retropubic midurethral sling and autologous pubovaginal sling for stress urinary incontinence after the FDA advisory notification. Urology 2015;85(2):321–5.
14. Morgan TO, Westney OL, McGuire EJ. Pubovaginal sling: 4-year outcome analysis and quality of life assessment. J Urol 2000;163(6):1845–8.
15. Guerrero KL, Emery SJ, Wareham K, et al. A randomised controlled trial comparing TVT, Pelvicol and autologous fascial slings for the treatment of stress urinary incontinence in women. BJOG 2010;117(12):1493–502.
16. Morgan DM, Dunn RL, Fenner DE, et al. Comparative analysis of urinary incontinence severity after autologous fascia pubovaginal sling, pubovaginal sling and tension-free vaginal tape. J Urol 2007; 177(2):604–9.
17. Tubre RW, Padmanabhan P, Frilot CF, et al. Outcomes of three sling procedures at the time of abdominal sacral colpopexy. Neurourol Urodyn 2017;36(2):482–5.
18. Fusco F, Abdel-Fattah M, Chapple CR, et al. Updated systematic review and meta-analysis of the comparative data on colposuspensions, pubovaginal slings, and midurethral tapes in the surgical treatment of female stress urinary incontinence. Eur Urol 2017;72(4):567–91.

19. Ford AA, Rogerson L, Cody JD, et al. Mid-urethral sling operations for stress urinary incontinence in women. Cochrane Database Syst Rev 2017;(7): CD006375.
20. Aberger M, Gomelsky A, Padmanabhan P. Comparison of retropubic synthetic mid-urethral slings to fascia pubovaginal slings following failed sling surgery. Neurourol Urodyn 2016;35:851–4.
21. Al-Azzawi IS. The first Iraqi experience with the rectus fascia sling and transobturator tape for female stress incontinence: a randomised trial. Arab J Urol 2014;12(3):204–8.
22. Athanasopoulos A, Gyftopoulos K, McGuire EJ. Treating stress urinary incontinence in female patients with neuropathic bladder: the value of the autologous fascia rectus sling. Int Urol Nephrol 2012;44(5):1363–7.
23. Guan W, Bai J, Liu J, et al. Microwave ablation versus partial nephrectomy for small renal tumors: intermediate-term results. J Surg Oncol 2012; 106(3):316–21.
24. Barnes NM, Dmochowski RR, Park R, et al. Pubovaginal sling and pelvic prolapse repair in women with occult stress urinary incontinence: effect on postoperative emptying and voiding symptoms. Urology 2002;59(6):856–60.
25. Basok EK, Yildirim A, Atsu N, et al. Cadaveric fascia lata versus intravaginal slingplasty for the pubovaginal sling: Surgical outcome, overall success and patient satisfaction rates. Urol Int 2008;80(1):46–51.
26. Borup K, Nielsen JB. Results in 32 women operated for genuine stress incontinence with the pubovaginal sling procedure ad modum Ed McGuire. Scand J Urol Nephrol 2002;36(2):128–33.
27. Brito R, Ramos Carvalho C, Pedro Sérgio M, et al. Comparison of the efficacy and safety of surgical procedures utilizing autologous fascial and transobturator slings in patients with stress urinary incontinence. J Reprod Med 2013;58(1–2):19–24.
28. Brown SL, Govier FE, Morgan TO, et al. Cadaveric versus autologous fascia lata for the pubovaginal sling: surgical outcome and patient satisfaction. J Urol 2000;164(5):1633–7.
29. Brubaker L, Richter HE, Norton PA, et al. 5-year continence rates, satisfaction and adverse events of Burch urethropexy and fascial sling surgery for urinary incontinence. J Urol 2012;187(4):1324–30.
30. Beck RP, Nordstrom L, Nordstrom L. The fascia lata sling procedure for treating recurrent genuine stress incontinence of urine. Obstet Gynecol 1988;72(5): 699–703.
31. Blaivas JG, Jacobs BZ. Pubovaginal fascial sling for the treatment of complicated stress urinary incontinence. J Urol 1991;145(6):1214–8.
32. Brady CM, Ahmed I, Drumm J, et al. A prospective evaluation of the efficiency of early postoperative bladder emptying after the Stamey procedure or pubovaginal sling for stress urinary incontinence. J Urol 2001;165(5):1601–4.
33. Breen JM, Geer BE, May GE, et al. The fascia lata suburethral sling for treating recurrent urinary stress incontinence. Am J Obstet Gynecol 1997;177: 1363–6.
34. Carr LK, Walsh PJ, Victor E, et al. Favorable outcome of pubovaginal slings for geriatric women with stress incontinence. J Urol 1997;157(1):125–8.
35. Chan PTK, Fournier C, Corcos J. Short-term complications of pubovaginal sling procedure for genuine stress incontinence in women. Urology 2000;55(2): 207–11.
36. Chang Y-C, Fan Y-H, Lin A, et al. Which one stands longer? 20 years experience in retropubic suburethral sling surgery for female stress urinary incontinence: comparison between autologous fascia and prolene mesh. Eur Urol 2017;16(3):e1489–90.
37. Cross CA, Cespedes RD, McGuire EJ. Treatment results using pubovaginal slings in patients with large cystoceles and stress incontinence. J Urol 1997; 158(2):431–4.
38. Cross CA, Cespedes RD, McGuire EJ. Our experience with pubovaginal slings in patients with stress urinary incontinence. J Urol 1998;159(4):1195–8.
39. Demirci F, Yucel O. Comparison of pubovaginal sling and Burch colposuspension procedures in type I/II genuine stress incontinence. Arch Gynecol Obstet 2001;265(4):190–4.
40. El-Azab AS, El-Nashar SA. Midurethral slings versus the standard pubovaginal slings for women with neurogenic stress urinary incontinence. Int Urogynecol J 2015;26(3):427–32.
41. Enemchukwu E, Lai C, Reynolds WS, et al. Autologous pubovaginal sling for the treatment of concomitant female urethral diverticula and stress urinary incontinence. Urology 2015;85(6):1300–3.
42. Flynn BJ, Yap WT. Pubovaginal sling using allograft fascia lata versus autograft fascia for all types of stress urinary incontinence: 2-year minimum followup. J Urol 2002;167(2 Pt 1):608–12.
43. Frade AB, Frade CL, Leite TG, et al. Modified pubovaginal sling technique in the surgical management of female stress urinary incontinence. Rev Col Bras Cir 2015;42(6):377–81.
44. Fulford SCV, Flynn R, Barrington J, et al. An assessment of the surgical outcome and urodynamic effects of the pubovaginal sling for stress incontinence and the associated urge syndrome. J Urol 1999;162(1):135–7.
45. Govier FE, Gibbons RP, Correa RJ, et al. Pubovaginal slings using fascia lata for the treatment of intrinsic sphincter deficiency. J Urol 1997;157(1): 117–21.
46. Guerrero K, Watkins A, Emery S, et al. A randomised controlled trial comparing two autologous fascial sling techniques for the treatment

of stress urinary incontinence in women: short, medium and long-term follow-up. Int Urogynecol J 2007;18(11):1263–70.
47. Haab F, Trockman BA, Zimmern PE, et al. Results of pubovaginal sling for the treatment of intrinsic sphincteric deficiency determined by questionnaire analysis. J Urol 1997;158(5):1738–41.
48. Howden NS, Zyczynski HM, Moalli PA, et al. Comparison of autologous rectus fascia and cadaveric fascia in pubovaginal sling continence outcomes. Am J Obstet Gynecol 2006;194(5):1444–9.
49. Jeon MJ, Jung HJ, Chung SM, et al. Comparison of the treatment outcome of pubovaginal sling, tension-free vaginal tape, and transobturator tape for stress urinary incontinence with intrinsic sphincter deficiency. Am J Obstet Gynecol 2008;199(1). https://doi.org/10.1016/j.ajog.2007.11.060.
50. Khan ZA, Nambiar A, Morley R, et al. Long-term follow-up of a multicentre randomised controlled trial comparing tension-free vaginal tape, xenograft and autologous fascial slings for the treatment of stress urinary incontinence in women. BJU Int 2015; 115(6):968–77.
51. Kuo HC. Comparison of video urodynamic results after the pubovaginal sling procedure using rectus fascia and polypropylene mesh for stress urinary incontinence. J Urol 2001;165(1):163–8.
52. Kakizaki H, Shibata T, Shinno Y, et al. Fascial sling for the management of urinary incontinence due to sphincter incompetence. J Urol 1995;153(3):644–7.
53. Kaplan SA, Santarosa RP, Te AE. Comparison of fascial and vaginal wall slings in the management of intrinsic sphincter deficiency. Urology 1996; 47(6):885–9.
54. Kreder KJ, Austin JC. Treatment of stress urinary incontinence in women with urethral hypermobility and intrinsic sphincter deficiency. J Urol 1996;156(6): 1995–9.
55. Kwon E, Schulz JA, Flood CG. Success of pubovaginal sling in patients with stress urinary incontinence and efficacy of vaginal sling release in patients with post-sling voiding dysfunction. J Obstet Gynaecol Can 2006;28(6):519–25.
56. Lee D, Alhalabi F, Zimmern PE. Long-term outcomes of autologous fascia lata sling for stress incontinence secondary to intrinsic sphincter deficiency in women. Urol Sci 2017;28(3):135–8.
57. Luo DY, Wang KJ, Zhang HC, et al. Different sling procedures for stress urinary incontinence: a lesson from 453 patients. Kaohsiung J Med Sci 2014;30(3): 139–45.
58. Maccini M, Lhungay T, Doumaney T, et al. How to improve pubovaginal sling outcomes: comparison of two techniques for sling tensioning in 177 patients. Neurourol Urodyn 2017;36:S149.
59. Maher CF, O'Reilly BA, Dwyer PL, et al. Pubovaginal sling versus transurethral Macroplastique for stress urinary incontinence and intrinsic sphincter deficiency: a prospective randomised controlled trial. BJOG 2005;112(6):797–801.
60. Milose JC, Sharp KM, He C, et al. Success of autologous pubovaginal sling after failed synthetic mid urethral sling. J Urol 2015;193(3):916–20.
61. Mitsui T, Tanaka H, Moriya K, et al. Clinical and urodynamic outcomes of pubovaginal sling procedure with autologous rectus fascia for stress urinary incontinence. Int J Urol 2007;14(12):1076–9.
62. Malde S, Moore JA. Autologous mid-urethral sling for stress urinary incontinence: Preliminary results and description of a contemporary technique. J Clin Urol 2016;9(1):40–7.
63. Mason RC, Roach M. Modified pubovaginal sling for treatment of intrinsic sphincteric deficiency. J Urol 1996;156(6):1991–4.
64. McBride AW, Ellerkmann RM, Bent AE, et al. Comparison of long-term outcomes of autologous fascia lata slings with Suspend Tutoplast fascia lata allograft slings for stress incontinence. Am J Obstet Gynecol 2005;192(5 SPEC. ISS.):1677–81.
65. McCoy O, Vaughan T, Nickles SW, et al. Outcomes of autologous fascia pubovaginal sling for patients with transvaginal mesh related complications requiring mesh removal. J Urol 2016;196(2):484–9.
66. McGuire EJ, Lytton B. Pubovaginal sling procedure for stress incontinence. J Urol 1978;119(1):82–4.
67. Onur R, Singla A, Kobashi KC. Comparison of solvent-dehydrated allograft dermis and autograft rectus fascia for pubovaginal sling: questionnaire-based analysis. Int Urol Nephrol 2008;40(1):45–9.
68. Patel B, Kim J, Brook S, et al. Patients with complex stress urinary incontinence are satisfied with long-term outcomes following pressure regulating balloon gradient increase as. JURO 2013;189(4): e233.
69. Parker WP, Gomelsky A, Padmanabhan P. Autologous fascia pubovaginal slings after prior synthetic anti-incontinence procedures for recurrent incontinence: a multi-institutional prospective comparative analysis to de novo autologous slings assessing objective and subjective cure. Neurourol Urodyn 2016;35(5):604–8.
70. Petrou SP, Frank I. Complications and initial continence rates after a repeat pubovaginal sling procedure for recurrent stress urinary incontinence. J Urol 2001;165(6 Pt 1):1979–81.
71. Petrou SP, Davidiuk AJ, Rawal B, et al. Salvage autologous fascial sling after failed synthetic midurethral sling: greater than 3-year outcomes. Int J Urol 2016;23(2):178–81.
72. Sharifiaghdas F, Mortazavi N. Tension-free vaginal tape and autologous rectus fascia pubovaginal sling for the treatment of urinary stress incontinence: a medium-term follow-up. Med Princ Pract 2008; 17(3):209–14.

73. Sharifiaghdas F, Nasiri M, Mirzaei M, et al. Mini sling (Ophira) versus pubovaginal sling for treatment of stress urinary incontinence: a medium-term follow-up. Prague Med Rep 2015;116(3):210–8.
74. da Silva-Filho AL, Triginelli SA, Noviello MB, et al. Pubovaginal sling in the treatment of stress urinary incontinence for urethral hypermobility and intrinsic sphincteric deficiency. Int Braz J Urol 2003;29(6):540–4.
75. Simsiman AJ, Powell CR, Stratford RR, et al. Suburethral sling materials: best outcome with autologous tissue. Am J Obstet Gynecol 2005;193(6):2112–6.
76. Tcherniakovsky M, Fernandes CE, Bezerra CA, et al. Comparative results of two techniques to treat stress urinary incontinence: synthetic transobturator and aponeurotic slings. Int Urogynecol J 2009;20(8):961–6.
77. Trabuco EC, Klingele CJ, Weaver AL, et al. Medium-term comparison of continence rates after rectus fascia or midurethral sling placement. Am J Obstet Gynecol 2009;200(3):300.e1-e6.
78. Toledo LGM, Korkes F, Romero FR, et al. Bladder outlet obstruction after pubovaginal fascial sling. Int Urogynecol J 2009;20(2):201–5.
79. Wadie BS, Edwan A, Nabeeh AM. Autologous fascial sling vs polypropylene tape at short-term followup: a prospective randomized study. J Urol 2005;174(3):990–3.
80. Wadie BS, Mansour A, El-Hefnawy AS, et al. Minimum 2-year follow-up of mid-urethral slings, effect on quality of life, incontinence impact and sexual function. Int Urogynecol J 2010;21:1485–90.
81. Welk BK, Herschorn S. The autologous fascia pubovaginal sling for complicated female stress incontinence. Can Urol Assoc J 2012;6(1):36–40.
82. Dunn GE, Hansen BL, Egger MJ, et al. Changed women: the long-term impact of vaginal mesh complications. Female Pelvic Med Reconstr Surg 2014;20(3):131–6.

Burch Colposuspension

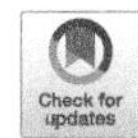

Ericka M. Sohlberg, MD[a], Christopher S. Elliott, MD, PhD[a,b,*]

KEYWORDS

• Burch • Colposuspension • Urethropexy

KEY POINTS

- Stress urinary incontinence is a prevalent condition for which surgical treatment continues to evolve.
- The Burch colposuspension has a 50-plus year history demonstrating strong long-term outcomes with few complications.
- Laparoscopic and open Burch colposuspension approaches have been shown to have equal efficacy.
- Other minimally invasive options, such as the mini-incisional Burch and robotic Burch, have less comparison data, although likely have similar outcomes.
- Although the use of the Burch colposuspension has waned in recent years secondary to a shift toward urethral sling operations, the Burch procedure still has an important role in the treatment of stress incontinence; specifically, a Burch should be considered when vaginal access is limited, intra-abdominal concurrent surgery is planned, or mesh is contraindicated.

INTRODUCTION

Stress urinary incontinence (SUI) is a prevalent condition affecting 25% to 35% of the US female population.[1–3] The current lifetime risk of surgery for SUI in the United States is approximately 13.5% with an estimated 200,000 women undergoing surgical repair annually.[4,5] These rates are predicted to increase in the coming years secondary to an aging population.[6]

SUI is generally attributable to urethral hypermobility as a result of diminished urethral support, although there can also be a component of urethral sphincter weakness. In women with incontinence secondary to urethral hypermobility, retropubic colposuspension surgery (or urethropexy) is a traditional repair that surgically elevates and reinforces periurethral tissue. Although once considered the "gold standard" in SUI treatment, the number of colposuspension procedures has waned since the turn of the twenty-first century following the introduction of the midurethral sling. In fact, over the past 2 decades, minimally invasive urethral sling procedures have become the dominant form of SUI treatment in the United States, accounting for nearly 90% of all surgical corrections in 2009.[7,8] However, following the 2011 Food and Drug Administration notification on serious complications associated with transvaginal mesh, the negative publicity associated with vaginal synthetic mesh products has extended to urethral slings.[9,10] Subsequently, the interest in colposuspension procedures has been rekindled as both women and practitioners alike seek alternative SUI treatment options. As a result, the Burch procedure continues to have a place in the operative armamentarium of the gynecologist and urologist.

THE COLPOSUSPENSION PROCEDURE: ORIGINS

The Burch procedure was first described by Dr John C. Burch in 1961.[11] Initially, he advocated for attaching the paravaginal fascia to the

Disclosure Statement: None.

[a] Department of Urology, Stanford University, 300 Pasteur Drive, Grant Building S285, Stanford, CA 94304, USA; [b] Division of Urology, Santa Clara Valley Medical Center, Valley Specialties Clinic, 751 South Bascom Avenue, 4th Floor, San Jose, CA 95128, USA

* Corresponding author. Valley Specialties Clinic, 751 South Bascom Avenue, 4th Floor, San Jose, CA 95128.
E-mail address: chrsuz@aol.com

Urol Clin N Am 46 (2019) 53–59
https://doi.org/10.1016/j.ucl.2018.08.002
0094-0143/19/© 2018 Elsevier Inc. All rights reserved.

tendinous arch of the fascia pelvis. This point of attachment was later changed to Cooper ligament in order to provide a more secure fixation. The procedure was further modified by Tanagho[12] in 1978 to its current state, where the paravaginal sutures are placed further lateral from the urethra, and a looser approximation of tissues is undertaken.

There are several other colposuspension variants, although none as commonly performed as the Burch procedure. One well-known urethropexy, the Marshall-Marchetti-Krantz (MMK) procedure, fixes the bladder neck to the periosteum of the symphysis pubis. The MMK historically has similar rates of short-term cure compared with the Burch procedure; however, it carries a risk of osteitis pubis (0.7%) that is not present with the Burch variant.[13] Because of the small but increased risk of potentially devastating infection, the International Consultation on Incontinence Committee determined in 2009 that there is no evidence for the continued use of the MMK cystourethropexy.[14,15]

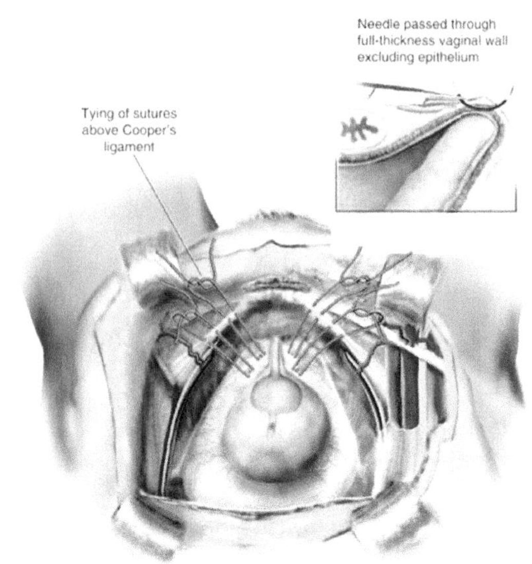

Fig. 1. Burch colposuspension suture placement. (*From* Karram MM. Retropubic urethropexy for stress incontinence. In: Baggish MS, Karram MM, editors. Atlas of pelvic anatomy and gynecology surgery. 3rd edition. St Louis (MO): Saunders; 2011. p. 406; with permission.)

BURCH MECHANISM OF ACTION

The Burch colposuspension procedure addresses SUI secondary to urethral hypermobility, but does not alleviate incontinence secondary to intrinsic sphincter deficiency. Interestingly, the precise mechanism of colposuspension surgery remains incompletely understood, although it is thought to restore anatomic support to the bladder neck and prevent urethral mobility with Valsalva.[16] This is borne out in imaging studies of women before and after Burch procedures, which demonstrate that postoperative cure rates are associated with a shorter distance between the bladder neck and levator ani muscle (**Fig. 1**).[17]

LONG-TERM EFFICACY AND PERIOPERATIVE COMPLICATIONS

Because of its use for 50-plus years, the Burch procedure has ample long-term outcomes data, with cure rates in small series up to 82% to 90% at 5- to 10-year follow-up.[18–20] Similarly, in a large review of 55 publications, the continence rates for open Burch procedures were noted to be 85% to 90% at 1 year postoperatively and approximately 70% at 5 years.[21]

As with any surgery, the Burch procedure carries its own set of complications. In a large review, the risk of significant bleeding resulting in postoperative hematoma or transfusion events was around 2%[22] and is consistent with small single-institution reports describing transfusion rates ranging from 0.7% to 3%.[23,24] Bleeding as a result of the Burch colposuspension occurs largely from injury to paravaginal veins when the surrounding fat pad is not fully cleared before suture placement. It is suggested that postoperative bleeding can be reduced with increased surgical exposure of the area.

Bladder injury may also occur at the time of Burch procedures, with an incidence of 0.4% to 9.6% (being more common in patients who have undergone prior pelvic surgery). Ureteral kinking or ureteral injury is even rarer, cited in 0.2% to 2%. Given the possibility of genitourinary harm, it is recommended that cystoscopy be performed at the end of a Burch procedure to ensure ureteral efflux and to rule out bladder injury. Among other postoperative complications, the rate of urinary tract infections ranges from 4% to 40% depending on the specific definition used and wound infections range from 4% to 10.8%.[22–24]

In addition to the above complications, immediate postoperative voiding dysfunction has been reported in up to 25% of patients following their Burch procedure.[22,25,26] The true profile of postoperative voiding symptoms is difficult to determine, however, because patients with frequency/urgency storage symptoms are often combined into the same category with those developing urinary retention. Furthermore, many publications define voiding dysfunction differently, making comparison difficult. Overall, the risk of urinary retention requiring long-term catheterization beyond 1 month is low, ranging from 0.7% to 7% (with most studies showing an incidence <3%). De novo detrusor instability may also occur (3%–8% of patients) and has been shown to be largely impacted by preoperative voiding function.[22,25–27] Interestingly, however, the Burch procedure may also improve bladder storage. Specifically, in a study of women undergoing preoperative urodynamics, a similar proportion of women had postoperative resolution of their detrusor overactivity compared with those who developed de novo detrusor overactivity (~8% each).[23]

Similar to other vaginal procedures, dyspareunia and pelvic pain may arise after Burch colposuspension. Long-term dyspareunia has been noted in 2% to 4% of women, whereas groin or suprapubic pain is reported by 2% to 6%.[26–30] Last, it has been theorized that by elevating the anterior vaginal wall, the Burch procedure may promote posterior vaginal wall weakness and resultant enterocele formation. This risk of developing a postoperative enterocele is reported to occur in 12% to 17% of women. It is noteworthy, however, that attempts to prevent enterocele formation with a concurrent culdoplasty have failed to decrease future enterocele rates.[27,31,32] As a result, it is not clear if the Burch colposuspension is the true cause of developing vaginal prolapse in certain compartments, or if it is simply the natural history of pelvic organ prolapse.

BURCH VERSUS SLING

As noted above, the urethral sling has largely taken the place of the Burch colposuspension as the current "gold standard" in female SUI surgery. The shift to sling based procedures is a result of several factors, which include but are not limited to decreased patient morbidity and increased rates of success in those undergoing sling procedures. In a recent meta-analysis comparing the results of 15,855 female patients enrolled in 28 randomized controlled trials, women who underwent sling placement had higher postoperative objective continence rates (based on a negative postoperative stress test) than those receiving a Burch colposuspension (79% vs 68%, respectively).[33] The superior cure rate for slings also holds true in the setting of concomitant surgery for pelvic organ prolapse. In a randomized controlled trial of women undergoing sacrocolpopexy randomized to Burch versus midurethral sling surgery, although the continence outcomes were similar at 6-month follow-up, those receiving a sling had superior continence rates at the 1- and 2-year follow-up timepoints.[34] In addition to increased continence outcomes, slings are also noted to have shorter operative times, shorter length of hospital stay, and decreased intraoperative blood loss as compared with open Burch urethropexy[35,36] (although similar rates of dyspareunia and pelvic pain occur with each).[37]

Despite the increased cure rates (both objective and subjective) provided by sling procedures, the improved efficacy may come at a cost. In the SISTeR trial, a randomized controlled trial comparing pubovaginal fascial slings to open Burch procedures, the higher success rates in the sling group were offset by increased rates of urinary tract infections, postoperative de novo urge incontinence, voiding dysfunction, and reoperation.[38] Specifically, more patients with a sling had urinary retention issues (defined as either the requirement for catheterization after 6 weeks or repeat surgery to facilitate bladder emptying) when compared with the Burch group (14% vs 2%), and treatment of postoperative urge incontinence was also increased in the sling group (27 vs 20%). The increased risk of adverse events in women undergoing sling surgery as compared with Burch colposuspension was further reiterated in a systematic review demonstrating colposuspension to have decreased risks of postoperative voiding dysfunction.[21] Taking these tradeoffs into account, Weber and Walters[39] published a decision analysis showing that the Burch procedure should be considered if the risk of urinary retention or detrusor instability is higher than 10% in women undergoing slings.

LAPAROSCOPIC BURCH COLPOSUSPENSION

The laparoscopic colposuspension was introduced in 1991 as a minimally invasive modification to the open Burch procedure.[40] Initial studies in the early 2000s showed that the laparoscopic colposuspension had a steep learning curve with a trend toward higher complication rates and longer operative times compared with the open approach. The increased learning curve and operative times were tempered, however, by similar objective cures rates, decreases in blood loss, improvements in postoperative pain, and shorter hospital stays using the laparoscopic approach.[41,42]

The early laparoscopic Burch series also described several modifications that affect postoperative continence. The first was the use of clips (rather than traditional sutures) to approximate Cooper ligament to the periurethral tissue. Although the clip technique made laparoscopy more accessible to many surgeons,[42] it was found over time to result in inferior postoperative continence outcomes compared with suture-based repairs.[43–45] Similarly, another means to decrease the surgery learning curve, stapled mesh as a fixation method, had objective cure rates that were inferior to that of suture-based repairs.[43–45] Likewise, the placement of only one laparoscopic suture per side was noted to be less effective than 2 sutures per side.[46]

As with most procedures, the outcomes of the laparoscopic Burch approach have improved with time. There have been 2 recent large randomized controlled trials comparing open and laparoscopic Burch surgeries. Carey and colleagues[47] evaluated a cohort of 200 women with SUI randomized to open or laparoscopic Burch and demonstrated that with up to 5 years of follow-up, there were no significant differences in either anatomic success or subjective perception of cure between the groups. In addition, it was noted that although the mean operating time was actually longer in the laparoscopic group, there was decreased blood loss and less postoperative pain in those undergoing laparoscopic surgery. Kitchener and colleagues[48] similarly evaluated 291 women randomized to a laparoscopic or open Burch procedure and found no difference in objective or subjective outcomes, although fewer patients in the laparoscopic group experienced significant pain (23 vs 60%, respectively). A systematic review of laparoscopic versus open approaches to the Burch colposuspension further supports the conclusion that there are no significant differences in postoperative continence rates between the approaches.[21] Given that the subjective and objective cure rates are equivalent between the laparoscopic and open methods, the consensus is that surgeons should undertake the approach with which they are most comfortable.[49,50]

ROBOTIC BURCH COLPOSUSPENSION

The robotic Burch urethropexy was first reported by Francis and colleagues[51] in 2015 and Bora and colleagues[52] in 2017. Their technique requires the use of 3 robotic ports and an assistant port. Although the cost of robotic surgery to perform a Burch colposuspension procedure alone is significant, the authors propose that a robotic approach to Burch colposuspension is particularly useful in patients undergoing other concurrent robotic surgeries.[52] In addition to the 2 case reports, there has since been a small study of 20 women randomized to robotic-assisted hysterectomy with robotic Burch versus open abdominal hysterectomy with open Burch. Although the concurrent hysterectomy is a potential confounding factor for several potential outcomes, the study demonstrated no difference in incontinence rates between the 2 groups and support the use of robotic Burch urethropexy at the time of a concurrent robotic surgery in the appropriate patient population with the appropriate surgeon.[53]

MINI-BURCH PROCEDURE

Another proposed minimally invasive variant of the Burch colposuspension is the "Mini-Incisional Burch." This procedure modification was proposed by Lind and colleagues[54] in 2004, with the goal of providing the same surgical correction through a smaller incision. The modified procedure was performed in 40 women under spinal anesthesia using a 1.5- to 2.5-cm horizontal skin incision above the pubic bone, as compared with the classic 5-cm open Burch incision. Using a suturing device that allows suture passage and retrieval in one motion, they were able to place sutures with a combination of visualization and proprioception via a hand in the vagina. The study authors reported a complete cure (cough stress test and questionnaire) in 97% of patients at short-term follow-up (9 months), and 85% of the procedures were performed on an outpatient basis.

OPERATIVE PEARLS

The critical aspects of the Burch procedure, regardless of surgical approach, are to obtain adequate exposure and to avoid reapproximating tissue under undue tension. The surgical goal is to loosely approximate the Cooper ligament to the periurethral tissue in order to allow postoperative adhesion formation that provides broad support for the urethra and bladder neck. To date, there are no randomized trials to suggest superiority of one suture type over another; however, most surgeons use absorbable suture. In addition, reviews have shown no difference in outcomes whether placing 2, 3, or 4 sutures per side, although as mentioned above it has been demonstrated that one suture per side is insufficient.[42] It is also critical to understand that although the Burch colposuspension does suspend the bladder neck and may repair small cystoceles, it is insufficient for repairing significant anterior pelvic organ prolapse. Hence, women with significant prolapse defects with concomitant SUI undergoing colposuspension should additionally have a dedicated cystocele repair.[55]

The following steps describe the open Burch colposuspension:

1. Either a pfannenstiel or straight midline subumbilical incision is made (at least 5 cm).
2. The retropubic space is exposed and peritoneum is swept superiorly. The periurethral fat is removed for adequate visualization of the anterolateral vaginal wall.

3. A Foley catheter is inserted per urethra, and the balloon is inflated. With an index finger in the vagina and gentle traction on the catheter, the bladder neck with the Foley balloon is palpable. With an assistant providing exposure by retracting the bladder medially and superiorly, the endopelvic and vaginal fascia are visible.
4. Two (or 3) absorbable stitches are then placed through the endopelvic and vaginal fascial complex, using the index finger to determine the appropriate depth (care should be taken to not violate the vaginal mucosa). The most cephalad suture is usually placed at the level of the bladder neck (2 cm lateral), and sutures are placed about 1 cm apart caudally.
5. The vaginal sutures are then placed through Cooper ligament and tied loosely (2- to 4-cm suture bridge between vagina and Cooper ligament) in a tension-free manner.
6. Cystoscopy is performed to rule out suture penetration into the bladder/urethra and also to confirm ureteral efflux. The placement of a drain in the retropubic space is usually unnecessary.
7. Many surgeons leave a catheter in place for several days postoperatively before a void trial; however, this may not be necessary.

Laparoscopic or robotic (intraperitoneal approach):

1. The surgeon starts with a 10-mm port at the umbilicus for the camera, with two 5-mm lower lateral working ports on either side of the abdomen (generally several fingerbreadths above and medial to the anterior superior iliac spine bilaterally)
2. The bladder is filled in a retrograde fashion through a Foley catheter to define its outline. The space of Retzius is then opened sharply in a semilunar fashion to access the bladder neck and periurethral tissue.
3. Suture placement and postoperative care are similar to the open procedure from this point on.

SUMMARY

Despite waning enthusiasm for the Burch procedure over the past 20 years by many surgeons, there remains an appropriate niche for the colposuspension in today's day and age. Given excellent long-term outcomes over the course of the last half-century, the Burch colposuspension should be considered an appropriate surgical treatment for any woman with SUI. Given excellent long-term outcomes over the course of the last half-century, the Burch colposuspension shuld be considered an appropriate surgical treatment for any woman with SUI, especially in settings where vaginal access is limited, where intra-abdominal surgery is already planned, or if mesh is contraindicated. As such, the Burch procedure has an ongoing role in the surgical repair of female SUI and should remain in the surgical repertoire of female pelvic medicine and reconstructive surgeons.

REFERENCES

1. Hampel C, Artibani W, Espuna Pons M, et al. Understanding the burden of stress urinary incontinence in Europe: a qualitative review of the literature. Eur Urol 2004;46(1):15–27.
2. Hampel C, Wienhold D, Benken N, et al. Definition of overactive bladder and epidemiology of urinary incontinence. Urology 1997;50:4–14.
3. Markland AD, Richter HE, Fwu CW, et al. Prevalence and Trends of Urinary incontinence in adults in the US 2001 to 2008. J Urol 2011;186(2):589–93.
4. Oliphant SS, Jones KA, Wang L, et al. Trends over time with commonly performed obstetric and gynecologic inpatient procedures. Obstet Gynecol 2010;116(4):926–31.
5. Wu JM, Matthews CA, Conover MM, et al. Lifetime risk of stress urinary incontinence or pelvic organ prolapse surgery. Obstet Gynecol 2014;123(6): 1201–6.
6. Nygaard I, Barber MD, Burgio KL, et al. Prevalence of symptomatic pelvic floor disorders in US women. JAMA 2008;300(11):1311–6.
7. Jonsson Funk M, Levin PJ, Wu JM. Trends in the surgical management of stress urinary incontinence. Obstet Gynecol 2012;119(4):845.
8. Rogo-Gupta L, Litwin M, Saigal C, et al. Trends in the surgical management of stress urinary incontinence among female medicare beneficiaries 2002-2007. Urology 2013;82(1):38–41.
9. Drain A, Khan A, Ohmann E, et al. Use of Concomitant Stress incontinence surgery at time of pelvic organ prolapse surgery since release of the 2011 notification on serious complications associated with transvaginal mesh. J Urol 2017; 197(4):1092–8.
10. Rac G, Younger A, Clemens J, et al. Stress urinary incontinence surgery trends in academic female pelvic medicine and reconstructive surgery urology practice in the setting of the food and drug administration public health notifications. Neurourol Urodyn 2017;36(4):1155–60.
11. Burch JC. Urethrovaginal fixation to Cooper's ligament for correction of stress incontinence, cystocele, and prolapse. Am J Obstet Gynecol 1961;81:281–90.
12. Tanagho EA. Colpocystourethropexy: the way we do it. J Urol 1978;116:751–3.

13. Kammerer-Doak DN, Cornella JL, Magrina JF, et al. Osteitis pubis after Marshall-Marchetti-Krantz urethropexy: a pubic osteomyelitis. Am J Obstet Gynecol 1998;179(3):586–90.
14. Smith AR, Chand D, Dmochowski R, et al. Committee 14. Surgery for urinary incontinence in women. In: Abrams P, Cardozo L, Khoury S, editors. Incontinence. Plymouth (United Kingdom): Health Publications; 2009. p. 1191–272.
15. Green J, Herschorn S. The contemporary role of Burch colposuspension. Curr Opin Urol 2005;15(4):250–5.
16. Burch JC. Cooper's ligament urethrovesical suspension for stress urinary incontinence: nine years' experience: results, complication, technique. Am J Obstet Gynecol 1968;100:764–74.
17. Digesu GA, Bombieri L, Hutchings A, et al. Effects of Burch colposuspension on the relative positions of the bladder neck to the levator ani muscle: an observational study that used magnetic resonance imaging. Am J Obstet Gynecol 2004;190:614–9.
18. Alcalay M, Monga A, Stanton S. Burch colposuspension: a 10-20 year follow up. Br J Obstet Gynaecol 1995;102:740–5.
19. Bergman A, Elia G. Three surgical procedures for genuine stress incontinence: five-year follow-up of a prospective randomized study. Am J Obstet Gynecol 1995;173:66–71.
20. Kjolhede P, Ryden G. Prognostic factors and long-term results of the Burch colposuspension. A retrospective study. Acta Obstet Gynecol Scand 1994;73:642–7.
21. Lapitan MCM, Cody JD, Mashayekhi A. Open retropubic colposuspension for urinary incontinence in women. Cochrane Database Syst Rev 2017;(7): CD002912.
22. Demirci F, Petri E. Perioperative complications of Burch colposuspension. Int Urogynecol J Pelvic Floor Dysfunct 2000;11(3):170–5.
23. Kenton K, Oldham L, Brubaker L, et al. Open Burch urethropexy has a low rate of perioperative complications. Am J Obstet Gynecol 2002;187(1):107–10.
24. Wee HY, Low C, Han HC. Burch colposuspension: review of perioperative complications at a women's and children's hospital in Singapore. Ann Acad Med Singap 2003;32(6):821–3.
25. Natale F, La Penna C, Saltari M, et al. Voiding dysfunction after anti-incontinence surgery. Minerva Ginecol 2009;61(2):167–72.
26. Demirci F, Yucel O, Eren S, et al. Long-term results of Burch colposuspension. Gynecol Obstet Invest 2001;51(4):243–7.
27. Eriksen BC, Hagen B, Eik-Nes SH, et al. Long-term effectiveness of the Burch colposuspension in female urinary stress incontinence. Acta Obstet Gynecol Scand 1990;69:45–50.
28. Galloway NTM, Davies N, Stephanson TP. The complications of colposuspension. Br J Urol 1987;60: 122–4.
29. Wang AC. Burch colposuspension vs. Stamey bladder neck suspension. A comparison of complications with special emphasis on detrusor instability and voiding dysfunction. J Reprod Med 1996;41:529–33.
30. Jorgensen L, Lose G, Mortensen SO, et al. The Burch colposuspension for urinary incontinence in patients with stable and unstable detrusor function. Neurourol Urodyn 1988;7:435–41.
31. Kjølhede P. Genital prolapse in women treated successfully and unsuccessfully by the Burch colposuspension. Acta Obstet Gynecol Scand 1998;77(4): 444–50.
32. Kiilholma P, Mäkinen J, Chancellor MB, et al. Modified Burch colposuspension for stress urinary incontinence in females. Surg Gynecol Obstet 1993; 176(2):111–5.
33. Fusco F, Abdel-Fattah M, Chapple CR, et al. Updated systematic review and meta-analysis of the comparative data on colposuspensions, pubovaginal slings, and midurethral tapes in the surgical treatment of female stress urinary incontinence. Eur Urol 2017;72(4):567–91.
34. Trabuco EC, Linder BJ, Klingele CJ, et al. Two-year results of burch compared with midurethral sling with sacrocolpopexy. Obstet Gynecol 2017; 131(1):31–8.
35. Sivaslioglu AA, Caliskan E, Dolen I, et al. A randomized comparison of transobturator tape and Burch colposuspension in the treatment of female stress urinary incontinence. Int Urogynecol J Pelvic Floor Dysfunct 2007;18(9):1015–9.
36. Asıcıoglu O, Gungorduk K, Besımoglu B, et al. A 5-year follow-up study comparing Burch colposuspension and transobturator tape for the surgical treatment of stress urinary incontinence. Int J Gynaecol Obstet 2014;125(1):73–7.
37. Demirci F, Yucel O. Comparison of pubovaginal sling and burch colposuspension procedures in type I/II genuine stress incontinence. Arch Gynecol Obstet 2001;265(4):190–4.
38. Albo ME, Richter HE, Brubaker L, et al. Burch colposuspension versus fascial sling to reduce urinary stress incontinence. N Engl J Med 2007;356: 2143–55.
39. Weber AM, Walters MD. Burch procedure compared with sling for stress urinary incontinence: a decision analysis. Obstet Gynecol 2000;96(6):867–73.
40. Vancaillie TG, Schuessler W. Laparoscopic bladder-neck suspension. J Laparoendosc Surg 1991;1: 169–73.
41. Moehrer B, Ellis G, Carey M, et al. Laparoscopic colposuspension for urinary incontinence in women. Cochrane Database Syst Rev 2002;(1): CD002239.
42. Dean NM, Ellis G, Wilson PD, et al. Laparoscopic colposuspension for urinary incontinence in women. Cochrane Database Syst Rev 2006;(3):CD002239.

43. Zullo F, Morelli M, Russo T, et al. Two techniques of laparoscopic retropubic urethropexy. J Am Assoc Gynecol Laparosc 2002;9(2):178–81.
44. Ross J. Two techniques of laparoscopic Burch repair for stress incontinence: a prospective, randomized study. J Am Assoc Gynaecologic Laparoscopists 1996;3(3):351–7.
45. Ankardal M, Milsom I, Stjerndahl JH, et al. A three-armed randomized trial comparing open Burch colposuspension using sutures with laparoscopic colposuspension using sutures and laparoscopic colposuspension using mesh and staples in women with stress urinary incontinence. Acta Obstet Gynecol Scand 2005;84(8):773–9.
46. Persson J, Wolner-Hanssen P. Laparoscopic Burch colposuspension for stress urinary incontinence: a randomized comparison of one or two sutures on each side of the urethra. Obstet Gynecol 2000;95(1):151–5.
47. Carey M, Goh JT, Rosamilia A, et al. Laparoscopic versus open Burch colposuspension: a randomized controlled trial. BJOG 2006;113:999–1006.
48. Kitchener HC, Dunn G, Lawton V, et al. Laparoscopic versus open colposuspension-results of a prospective randomized controlled trial. BJOG 2006;113:1007–13.
49. Jenkins TR, Liu CY. Laparoscopic Burch colposuspension. Curr Opin Obstet Gynecol 2007;19(4):314–8.
50. Reid F, Smith AR. Laparoscopic versus open colposuspension: which one should we choose? Curr Opin Obstet Gynecol 2007;19(4):345–9.
51. Francis S, Agrawal A, Azadi A, et al. Robotic Burch colposuspension : a surgical case and instructional video. Int Urogynecol J 2015;26(1):147–8.
52. Bora GS, Gupta VG, Mavuduru RS, et al. Robotic Burch colposuspension-modified technique. J Robot Surg 2017;11(3):381–2.
53. Ulubay M, Dede M, Öztürk M, et al. Comparison of robotic-assisted and abdominal hysterectomy with concomitant burch colposuspension: preluminary study. J Minim Invasive Gynecol 2015;22(6S):S242–3.
54. Lind LR, Gunn GC, Mattox TF, et al. Mini-incisional Burch urethropexy: a less invasive method to accomplish a time-tested procedure for treatment of genuine stress incontinence. Int Urogynecol J Pelvic Floor Dysfunct 2004;15(1):20–4.
55. Sekine H, Kohima S, Igarashi K, et al. Burch bladder neck suspension for cystocele repair: the necessity of combined vaginal procedures for severe cases. Int J Urol 1999;6(1):1–6.

Surgery for Anterior Compartment Prolapse

Surgery for Anterior Compartment Vaginal Prolapse: Suture-Based Repair

Katherine Amin, MD, Una Lee, MD*

KEYWORDS

• Anterior compartment • Vaginal prolapse • Native tissue

KEY POINTS

- Pelvic organ prolapse is a major health problem among parous women and anterior colporrhaphy is the most commonly performed prolapse repair procedure.
- In anterior prolapse, lack of bladder support is often caused by 3 types of abnormalities (or a combination thereof) including a central defect, a lateral (paravaginal) defect, and a transverse–proximal defect.
- A reconstruction of the anterior vaginal wall is performed by placing sutures that plicate and reduce the weakened tissues, and other native techniques have been introduced to further augment tissue and improve durability.
- Native tissue repair, although associated with a higher anatomic rate of prolapse recurrence compared with mesh-augmented repair, has been well-studied and using contemporary composite definitions of success is successful in relieving vaginal bulge symptoms and reducing prolapse within the vagina.

BACKGROUND

Anterior Vaginal Wall Pelvic Prolapse: Definition and Clinical Presentation

Pelvic organ prolapse (POP) is the downward decent of 1 or more components of the vaginal wall (anterior, posterior, and/or apical including the vaginal vault or posthysterectomy cuff).[1] It is a common finding on physical examination that has been reported in up to 50% of parous women; however, the prevalence of symptom-based POP may be as low as 3% to 6%.[2–4] Most women remain asymptomatic until the leading edge of the prolapse extends at least 0.5 cm beyond the hymenal ring[5]; however, symptom burden varies significantly among women with prolapse. The anterior compartment of the vagina is the most common site affected by prolapse and has a known and variable rate of recurrence after surgical repair. Women with anterior compartment prolapse (cystocele) may present with a wide range of pelvic floor symptoms, including the sensation of pelvic heaviness or vaginal bulge. Pertinent to cystocele, patients may report concomitant obstructive urinary symptoms such as poor urinary stream or urinary urgency. Other associated urinary bladder, bowel, or sexual dysfunction symptoms are common, including vaginal splinting to aid with urination, constipation, or dyspareunia.

Anterior Vaginal Wall Pelvic Prolapse: Treatment

The wide range of treatment options for anterior prolapse include conservative management, a pessary, or surgical repair. Conservative management is a viable option for women who are

Disclosure Statement: K. Amin has no disclosures to report. U. Lee is a preceptor surgeon for Medtronic.
Female Pelvic Medicine and Reconstructive Surgery, Section of Urology, Virginia Mason Medical Center, 1100 9th Avenue, C7-URO, Seattle, WA 98101, USA
* Corresponding author.
E-mail address: una.lee@virginiamason.org

Urol Clin N Am 46 (2019) 61–70
https://doi.org/10.1016/j.ucl.2018.08.008
0094-0143/19/© 2018 Elsevier Inc. All rights reserved.

minimally bothered by prolapse and find reassurance from education about prolapse and obtaining a diagnosis. Many women have intermittent and/or manageable symptoms, and opting for conservative treatment is reasonable. Management is often tailored based on the individual woman's general health, severity of symptoms, and surgeon preference and training. Currently, there is no standardized approach to the surgical repair of POP, and it is crucial to discuss the risks and benefits of each option during the decision-making process. The most common surgical procedure to treat the anterior compartment is the traditional anterior colporrhaphy, also called anterior repair or cystocele repair. The term "colporrhaphy" is etymologically derived from the Greek word *Kolpos* (a female bosom, womb, or vagina) and *raphe* (which means suture). The medical terminology of "–rrhaphy" is a suture-based repair; therefore, anterior colporrhaphy refers to a suture operation to repair lax and redundant vaginal tissue in cases of prolapse of the vaginal wall. Anterior colporrhaphy can be combined with other prolapse procedures or concomitant antistress urinary incontinence (SUI) surgery. Outcome-based measurements for this type of procedure have been historically controversial owing to the variability in reported definitions of success, which is further discussed elsewhere in this article. Outcome criteria have ranged from anatomic restoration to patient-perceived overall improvement of symptoms or quality of life. Overall, data show that the anterior compartment has the greatest risk of surgical failure.[6] Success rates for native tissue anterior compartment repair range from 30% to 97%,[7,8] compared with anatomic cure rates for native posterior[9,10] and apical compartment of 67% to 98%.[11,12] Given the high recurrence rate for native tissue repair, biologic grafts and synthetic mesh were introduced to further augment tissue during POP repair. Biologic graft augmentation in the anterior compartment has not been shown to be correlated with superior results, but also do not cause adverse complications.[13,14] In contrast, transvaginal mesh in the anterior compartment has demonstrated superior anatomic results, but a high rate of mesh-related complications. The significant morbidity and detrimental effects of transvaginal mesh complications led the US Food and Drug Administration to issue a notification of the rate of complications with transvaginal use.[6,15,16] Given the increased awareness and risk of complications associated with mesh-augmented cystocele repair, women are increasingly interested in the surgical treatment of prolapse without mesh augmentation. Pelvic floor surgeons are appropriately being judicious with the use of polypropylene transvaginal mesh, so there is a renewed interest in native tissue repairs. The goal of prolapse surgery is both relief of vaginal bulge symptoms and restoration of anatomy while avoiding detrimental complications. Native tissue cystocele repair can achieve symptom relief and restore anatomy to the leading edge within the hymen with a low risk of complications. The objective of this article is to discuss suture-based or native tissue repair for vaginal anterior compartment defects.

EPIDEMIOLOGY AND PREVALENCE

It is well-documented that the incidence of POP increases with age, with 1 study showing that 10% of women between 20 and 39 years of age are affected by POP, compared with 50% of octogenarians.[17] With new preventative health initiatives and an aging patient population, POP is expected to continue to be an important pelvic health problem among women. A study from the National Health and Nutritional Examination Survey predicts that by 2050, 9.2 million women will have vaginal prolapse.[18] Furthermore, older but still relevant landmark epidemiologic data by Olsen and colleagues[19] in 1997 has shown that women within the US health care system have an 11% lifetime risk of needing surgery for pelvic floor disorders and a 29% reoperation risk for incontinence and prolapse. Between 2005 and 2006, the treatment of POP was estimated to cost the US health care system approximately $300 million, reflecting the magnitude of the financial burden POP places on the health care system.[20] Anterior vaginal repair is the most commonly performed POP procedure, such that more than 80% of the POP surgeries performed in the United States correct the anterior compartment.[4] The etiology of anterior vaginal wall defects is multifactorial. Other risk factors besides age include pregnancy, mode of delivery during childbirth, connective tissue abnormalities, levator ani weakness, hysterectomy, and conditions related to increased intraabdominal pressure.[21,22]

ANATOMY

Support for the pelvic viscera is maintained through intimate relationships within the pelvis that include bony structures (pubis and ischium), fascial connective tissue (sacrospinous ligament, sacrotuberous ligament, obturator membrane, and pubocervical fascia), muscular attachments (levator ani, piriformis, and obturator muscles), nerves, and vessels. More specifically, supportive structures and connective tissue, such as the vaginalis muscularis and the condensation of tissues associated with the anterior vagina and bladder, are often in continuity with the organs that they support, rather than distinct anatomic structures. For example, the arcus tendineus fascia pelvis serves as a connective tissue that supports the vagina, bladder, and urethra to the lateral pelvic walls, then splits into the perivesical fascia or pubocervical fascia (vaginal side) and endopelvic fascia (abdominal side) at the level of the bladder.

A midline incision along the anterior vaginal wall, commonly performed in an anterior repair, exposes the pubocervical fascia and dissection toward the lateral pelvic wall exposes the arcus tendineus. In anterior prolapse, a lack of bladder support is often caused by 3 types of abnormalities (or a combination thereof), including a central defect, a lateral (paravaginal) defect, and/or a transverse–proximal defect. In central defects, the bladder herniates in the midline but lateral support is preserved, whereas in lateral defects the lateral pelvic wall attachments are weakened, which creates a sliding displacement of the bladder wall. Last, a transverse defect occurs when the bladder descends proximally owing to a separation between the pubocervical fascia and its attachment to the cervix.[23] Hypermobility of the urethra and bladder neck is also a common finding seen in anterior vaginal wall defects. Furthermore, the cardinal–uterosacral ligament complex anchors the cervix to the sacrum and deep pelvic fascia, providing support to the proximal third of the vagina and results in a posteriorly oriented vaginal access. Delancey[24] has reported that the association of apical descent is 3-fold more likely in anterior-predominant vaginal prolapse compared with posterior-predominant prolapse. This group has also described the role of dynamic and static MRI to assist with delineating anatomic structures in patients with POP.[25]

TECHNIQUE

Anterior Colporrhaphy

The classic approach for cystocele repair is the anterior colporrhaphy. Vaginal exposure is obtained and anatomic landmarks are noted including the bladder neck, urethra, and vaginal apex. A midline incision is made in the prolapsed anterior vaginal wall tissues. A dissection is performed bilaterally to expose the weakened prolapsed tissues of the anterior vaginal wall. The layer of tissue exposed is the vaginalis muscularis. A central defect is often encountered and the dissection is carried out laterally to the level of the arcus tendineous fascia pelvis. A reconstruction of the anterior vaginal wall is performed by placing sutures that plicate and reduce the weakened tissues. Sutures are placed that travel through the vaginalis muscularis and adventitial layers of the vaginal wall and the endopelvic fascia. Anterior colporrhaphy is traditionally performed with a synthetic braided absorbable sutures, such as polyglactin. These sutures are placed to imbricate the prolapsed tissues while creating additional support. The sutures can be placed in a Christmas tree configuration, U configuration, or purse string fashion to reduce the prolapse of the anterior vaginal wall and associated adventitial bladder tissues. The sutures are placed sequentially to provide support, while not placing deep sutures that obstruct the ureters. Cystocele repair can be performed in a single layer or additional layers can be used. Meticulous hemostasis is important before closure to prevent the formation of a hematoma. Cystoscopy is performed to demonstrate no injury to the urethra or bladder and to confirm ureteral patency. The anterior vaginal layer is then closed.

The Kelly plication, or placement of additional sutures at the urethra and bladder neck, can be performed in conjunction with a cystocele repair, but was more commonly performed before the introduction of the midurethral sling for SUI.[26] The Kelly plication was originally described as an anti-SUI procedure, but can offer additional support along the distal plate of the bladder wall. Kelly plication sutures can be associated with obstructive voiding so avoidance of obstructive suture placement near the bladder neck and urethra is essential to facilitate normal voiding and bladder emptying.

Anterior colporrhaphy, with or without Kelly plication, has considerable variability in reported outcomes. Suture type, technique of suture placement, and the presence or placement of vaginal or abdominal apical support may affect and/or improve success rates. A population-based longitudinal cohort study from Sweden showed that slow absorbable suture, such as PDS or Maxon, decreased the rate of recurrence as compared with rapidly absorbable suture (ie, Vicryl, Dexon, and Polysorb).[27] However, the use of PDS slow absorbable suture can also be associated with exposure of suture tails or knots vaginally that may or may not require further treatment. Additionally, Song and colleagues[28] reported a 98% success rate at 4 years with the use of 3 additional purse string sutures for reinforcement.

Durable native tissue repair of high-grade cystoceles remains challenging in pelvic floor reconstruction, likely owing to the innate pathophysiology and progression of pelvic prolapse as well as the limited tissue support anteriorly in some women. In an effort to improve outcomes, various surgical techniques have been described to augment the traditional native tissue anterior colporrhaphy. Performing a transvaginal needle suspension has been suggested to restore the anterior vaginal wall and offer support of the bladder base by repositioning the bladder neck in a high retropubic position.[29] In addition, the use of autologous rectus fascia or autologous fascia lata as a graft for cystocele augmentation has been shown to have upwards of a 97% success rate at a median of 5 years of follow-up.[30] As an alternative to transvaginal mesh and its associated mesh-specific complications, the use of interlocking permanent sutures can be used to construct a network of support along the anterior vaginal wall. This technique has been described by using a standard vertical incision from the bladder neck to the cuff followed by the development of bilateral tissue flaps. Then, 2-0 polypropylene sutures are used to incorporate the obturator and perivesical fascia on each side for lateral support. Lateral sutures are then interlocked with separate central sutures and finally tied to reduce the cystocele.[31] This technique, however, may be prone to exposed permanent sutures postoperatively because the anterior vaginal wall is associated with postmenopausal vaginal atrophy and hypoestrogenization over time.

Paravaginal Repair

Anterior compartment POP may be associated with defects of the lateral wall and, in such cases, concomitant paravaginal repair may improve outcomes. A paravaginal repair consists of the reattachment of lateral perivesical tissue to the arcus tendineus with multiple sutures. The transabdominal approach for paravaginal cystocele repair was initially described in 1976 via a Pfannenstiel incision, but a laparoscopic approach has grown in popularity because it offers improved visualization and a shorter recovery. Placement of the surgeon's fingers in the vagina can aid in placement of the sutures during the operation. Reported success rates of laparoscopic and open transabdominal paravaginal repair vary between 60% and 93%.[32,33] Additionally, transvaginal paravaginal repair has also been described by obtaining vaginal access to the retropubic space and incorporating the pubocervical fascia, arcus tendineous, and vaginal wall during the reconstruction.[34,35] To date, no randomized trials have evaluated the efficacy of paravaginal defect repair for anterior compartment prolapse. However, retrospective evidence has shown that an apical procedure alone (ie, sacrocolpopexy) was as effective as a combined apical and paravaginal repair.[36]

CONTROVERSIES IN SURGICAL OUTCOMES

Definition of Success in Pelvic Organ Prolapse Surgery

Defining success in POP surgery has been a controversial and important topic, and a standardized method has yet to be established. Research describing surgical outcomes has used various end-points including the POP quantification assessment, questionnaire responses (such as the Pelvic Floor Distress Inventory or Pelvic Floor Impact Questionnaire), retreatment or reoperation rates, and subjective patient-perceived ratings of overall treatment success and global improvement. Barber and colleagues[35] in collaboration with the Pelvic Floor Disorders Network, performed a secondary analysis of the Colpopexy and Urinary Reduction Efforts (CARE) trial, a randomized study assessing SUI in women without preoperative SUI who underwent abdominal sacrocolpopexy for POP with or without Burch colposuspension. Eighteen different definitions were applied for surgical success after surgery for grades 2 to 4 POP. Success rates varied greatly depending on the definition, ranging from 19.2% to 97.1%.[37,38] One of the most important findings was that subjective cure, or absence of vaginal bulge symptoms, was most strongly correlated with patient assessment of overall improvement and treatment success, and that anatomic definitions of success had weak correlation with patient perceptions of surgical outcome.[37]

Weber and colleagues[39] performed a prospective, randomized study of 114 patients who underwent 3 different types of anterior colporrhaphy including midline plication, ultrawide plication, or plication with polyglactin mesh graft overlay and reported an equivalent anatomic success rate (38%) among the 3 approaches at almost 2 years of follow-up. This study was then reanalyzed using a more contemporary definition of surgical success (ie, no prolapse beyond the hymen, no bulge symptoms, and no retreatment).[38] The results showed that, for patients who underwent traditional anterior colporrhaphy, the success rate was 89% at 1 year. Similarly, there was no difference in outcomes between the 3 contrasting surgical approaches.[7] Based on a recent Cochrane Database Systemic Review, native tissue repairs seem to be associated with higher rates of postoperative objective and subjective prolapse, but have similar and low reoperation rates when compared with synthetic mesh or biologic grafts (2%–9%).[6]

In summary, native tissue repair of anterior prolapse is associated with less anatomic success by strict definition, but with high rates of symptomatic success (**Table 1**). Using a more contemporary definition of surgical success (ie, a composite of no prolapse beyond the hymen, no bulge symptoms, and no retreatment), native tissue cystocele is associated with good surgical outcomes. These data are helpful for counseling patients on reasonable expectations and weighing the pros and cons of various surgical approaches for primary and recurrent anterior wall prolapse. The high rate of anatomic failure associated with anterior colporrhaphy is often the reason cited for the need for transvaginal mesh-augmented repair. However, the rate of success and failure depends on how success and failure are defined. In many cases, women have relief of bulge symptoms and are satisfied with their surgical outcome, so subjectively they experience success. Objectively, their examination may demonstrate descent of the anterior vaginal wall within the vagina that is associated with no or minimal symptoms.

Operative complications for native tissue repair of the anterior compartment are similar to other vaginal pelvic floor reconstructive procedures, including hemorrhage, urinary tract injury, infection, and de novo urinary incontinence. The rate of postoperative complications with native tissue cystocele repair are generally low and resolve with treatment. When compared with permanent mesh repair, native tissue repair was associated with reduced risk of de novo SUI, decreased bladder injury, and lower rates of repeat surgery for prolapse, SUI, and mesh exposure (combined outcome).[6] One distinct advantage of a native tissue cystocele repair is avoidance of the rare but potentially devastating morbidity of a serious complication uniquely associated with transvaginal mesh, including chronic pelvic pain, nerve injury, neuropathic pain, erosion of mesh into the bladder, and/or exposure of the mesh vaginally.

Mid- to Long-Term Recurrence and Reoperation Rates

Much of the literature to date reflects short- to mid-term outcomes for native tissue repair of the anterior compartment with 1 to 2 years of follow-up.[6] Additional mid- to long-term outcome data with contemporary follow-up is needed. Lavelle and colleagues[40] reported single-institution outcomes over an 18-year period with a mean follow-up of 5.8 years and defined failure as POP quantification assessment stage 2 or higher, or surgery for recurrent prolapse symptoms. They found a 7.4% rate of recurrent isolated anterior compartment prolapse, a 10.7% apical prolapse rate, a 8.3% posterior prolapse rate, and a 19% multiple compartment prolapse rate. Although 33% of patients with recurrent prolapse required a secondary procedure, only 3.3% of patients with isolated recurrent anterior compartment prolapse required a secondary procedure. However, a recent claims-based study reports promising results, with 5-year reoperation rates for POP surgery of less than 10% for women both younger and older than 65 years of age.[41]

Cystocele Alone Versus Concomitant Apical Repair

Providing anatomic apical restoration can correct anterior wall prolapse based on POP quantification assessment results in up to 63% of women with high-grade POP.[42] Greater prolapse recurrence rates have been demonstrated among women who do not undergo an apical repair.[6,43,44] Resuspension of the vaginal apex has been associated with a decrease in anterior compartment repair failure at either the time of hysterectomy or during a posthysterectomy prolapse repair. In a Medicare database study of almost 3000 women comparing isolated anterior repair versus combined anterior and apical repair, the 10-year reoperation rates were lower in the group who underwent a combination of anterior and apical repair (11.6% vs 20.2%).[45] Therefore, assessment of apical descent is crucial for preoperative planning in patients with POP. Addressing the vaginal apex and providing apical support at the time of cystoscele repair is a key component of providing a durable repair of anterior wall prolapse.

Uterine Preservation

Personal preference may motivate some patients to prefer uterine-sparing procedures while undergoing surgery for POP. A multicenter, noninferiority trial sought to compare uterus-preserving vaginal sacrospinous hysteropexy using permanent sutures with vaginal hysterectomy with suspension of the uterosacral ligaments in women with stage 2 or higher uterine prolapse.[46] The primary outcomes assessed were recurrent apical prolapse, bothersome bulge symptoms, or retreatment. Overall, this 2015 study concluded that sacrospinous hysteropexy is noninferior to vaginal hysterectomy with suspension of the uterosacral ligaments. Of note, however, 51 of 101 patients in the hysteropexy group and 44 of 100 in the hysterectomy group had recurrences. Of these patients, most were anterior wall recurrences (47 of 101 sacrospinous hysteropexy vs 33 of 99 vaginal hysterectomy) with no difference between

Table 1
Summary of AC success and outcomes

Author, Year	Type of Study	Single vs Multi Center	Apical Repair Performed if Indicated	No. of Patients Treated with AC	Mean Follow- up (mo)	Definition of Success	Success Rate	Other Reported Outcomes/ Complications
Gandhi et al,[13] 2005	RCT	Single center	Yes	78	12	<Stage II anterior vaginal wall prolapse (POP-Q) Resolution of pelvic pressure Resolution of vaginal bulge	71% 69% 89%	
Meschia et al,[47] 2007	RCT	Multicenter	No	103	12	Anatomic point Ba ≤-1 (POP-Q) Resolution of prolapse sensation	81% 87%	SUI: 13% OAB: 17% Dyspareunia: 10%
Guerette et al,[14] 2009	RCT	Multicenter	No	33	24	<Stage II anterior vaginal wall prolapse (POP-Q)	63%	Dyspareunia: 20%
Hviid et al,[48] 2010	RCT	Single center	No	31	12	<Stage II anterior vaginal wall prolapse (POP-Q)	85%	
Nieminen et al,[49] 2010	RCT	Multicenter	No	96	36	<Stage II anterior vaginal wall prolapse (POP-Q) Resolution of pelvic pressure	59% 72%	Reoperation rate: 10%
Altman et al,[50] 2011	RCT	Multicenter	No	186	12	(Composite) Stage 0 or I anterior vaginal wall prolapse (POP-Q) and subjective absence of vaginal bulge symptoms	35%	POP-Q Stage 0 or I:48% Bulge symptoms: 62% De novo SUI: 6% Bladder perforation: 0.5%

Vollebregt et al,[51] 2011	RCT	Multicenter	Yes	58	12	Rate of not having to undergo reoperation for anatomic failure	95%	Resolution of baseline dyspareunia: 80% De novo dyspareunia: 9%
Song et al,[28] 2012	Retrospective review	Single center	Yes	69	48	<Stage II anterior vaginal wall prolapse (POP-Q)	98%	Two patients had grade IV anterior vaginal wall prolapse and no recurrent of anterior prolapse
Lavelle et al,[40] 2016	Retrospective review	Single center	No	121	69	<Stage II anterior vaginal wall prolapse (POP-Q) OR no reoperation for symptomatic pelvic organ prolapse	54.6%	Intraoperative complication rate: 1.6% 30-d complication rate (Clavien I): 5.7% Rate of isolated recurrent anterior prolapse requiring secondary procedure: 3.3%

Abbreviations: AC, anterior colporrhaphy; OAB, overactive bladder; POP-Q, pelvic organ prolapse quantification system; RCT, randomized, controlled trial; SUI, stress urinary incontinence.

procedure groups, although posterior compartment recurrence was significantly higher in the hysterectomy group (14% vs 4%). This trial further supports the intimate relationship of apical and anterior compartment prolapse. More long-term data are needed on transvaginal (nonmesh), suture-based, uterine-sparing apical suspension at the time of anterior repair.

PATIENT COUNSELING

Patients should be counseled that prolapse does have a real risk of recurrence over one's lifetime, because the pathophysiology of prolapse continues as women age and a surgical repair does not stop this biologic process. Patients and surgeons alike desire a single procedure for prolapse that treats the prolapse, avoids complications, and does not recur. However, this expectation may or may not be reasonable based on many contributing factors, including individual connective tissue quality, increased intraabdominal pressures, wound healing factors, and progression of the disease. Shared decision making is important to discuss patient-centered goals and setting reasonable expectations on what can be achieved with a transvaginal cystocele repair, that is, a high likelihood of symptomatic relief with less than perfect anterior vaginal wall anatomy, but with the leading edge within the hymen. There is also a low but real risk of prolapse recurrence over time, with a possible need for future prolapse procedures. However, recurrence and the associated need for reoperation can occur with all surgical approaches for prolapse repair. Using modern definitions of success, the data show that native tissue cystocele repair does not perform as poorly as once thought, and therefore can be safely offered and used to treat symptomatic anterior wall prolapse.

Native Tissue Cystocele Repair in the Current Era of Knowledge Regarding Mesh Complications

In the last 15 years, transvaginal mesh for prolapse has been associated with an unacceptable rate of serious complications. Some complications are treatable, but some have caused serious injury and disability in women, even after the mesh is surgically removed. In the current era of knowledge after notification from the US Food and Drug Administration regarding transvaginal mesh complications, a thorough informed consent between surgeon and patient is essential to discuss the rare but real risk of complications associated with polypropylene mesh. Given the unique and distinct risks associated with transvaginal mesh, transvaginal native tissue repair remains a safe and viable surgical option for treatment of cystocele, ideally with concurrent apical support. Medical professionals adhere to principles of medical ethics. The well-known Latin phrase, *primum non nocere*, which translates to *first do no harm*, is an important concept. When we treat prolapse, we must first do no harm. Native tissue cystocele repair avoids the distinct risks associated with mesh placed in the vagina. Native tissue repair has its limitations as discussed elsewhere in this article, but remains an important surgery for primary or recurrent prolapse in women. The limitations of current surgical treatments highlight the need for further research into the pathophysiology of pelvic prolapse to develop therapies that target the mechanisms of the female pelvic floor and treat women in a safe durable manner, thus improving women's health and quality of life.

SUMMARY

Native tissue anterior compartment prolapse repair, whether performed solely or concomitantly with other prolapse surgery, is the most common POP procedure and remains an important surgical procedure for pelvic prolapse. Native tissue repair has been well-studied and using contemporary composite definitions of success, is successful in relieving vaginal bulge symptoms and reducing prolapse within the vagina. Native tissue repair may be associated with a higher anatomic rate of prolapse recurrence compared with mesh-augmented repair, but depends on the definition of anatomic success used. Additionally, the key role of apical support in contributing to the durability of anterior prolapse surgery has been established. Native tissue cystocele repair has been performed safely since the advent of modern vaginal surgery for prolapse. Reoperation rates for cystocele repair are low but not negligible. Native tissue cystocele repair is safe, effective, and addresses symptom relief for women, and for these reasons should continue to be a part of pelvic floor reconstructive surgery.

REFERENCES

1. Haylen BT, de Ridder D, Freeman RM, et al. An International Urogynecological Association (IUGA)/International Continence Society (ICS) joint report on the terminology for female pelvic floor dysfunction. Neurourol Urodyn 2010;29(1):4–20.
2. Handa VL, Garrett E, Hendrix S, et al. Progression and remission of pelvic organ prolapse: a longitudinal study of menopausal women. Am J Obstet Gynecol 2004;190(1):27–32.

3. Hendrix SL, Clark A, Nygaard I, et al. Pelvic organ prolapse in the Women's Health Initiative: gravity and gravidity. Am J Obstet Gynecol 2002;186(6):1160–6.
4. Barber MD, Maher C. Epidemiology and outcome assessment of pelvic organ prolapse. Int Urogynecol J 2013;24(11):1783–90.
5. Gutman RE, Ford DE, Quiroz LH, et al. Is there a pelvic organ prolapse threshold that predicts pelvic floor symptoms? Am J Obstet Gynecol 2008;199(6):683.e1-7.
6. Maher C, Feiner B, Baessler K, et al. Surgery for women with anterior compartment prolapse. Cochrane Database Syst Rev 2016;(11):CD004014.
7. Chmielewski L, Walters MD, Weber AM, et al. Reanalysis of a randomized trial of 3 techniques of anterior colporrhaphy using clinically relevant definitions of success. Am J Obstet Gynecol 2011;205(1):69.e1-8.
8. Gotthart PT, Aigmueller T, Lang PFJ, et al. Reoperation for pelvic organ prolapse within 10 years of primary surgery for prolapse. Int Urogynecol J 2012;23(9):1221–4.
9. Madsen LD, Nüssler E, Kesmodel US, et al. Native-tissue repair of isolated primary rectocele compared with nonabsorbable mesh: patient-reported outcomes. Int Urogynecol J 2017;28(1):49–57.
10. Nieminen K, Hiltunen K-M, Laitinen J, et al. Transanal or vaginal approach to rectocele repair: a prospective, randomized pilot study. Dis Colon Rectum 2004;47(10):1636–42.
11. Margulies RU, Rogers MAM, Morgan DM. Outcomes of transvaginal uterosacral ligament suspension: systematic review and metaanalysis. Am J Obstet Gynecol 2010;202(2):124–34.
12. Mothes AR, Wanzke L, Radosa MP, et al. Bilateral minimal tension sacrospinous fixation in pelvic organ prolapse: an observational study. Eur J Obstet Gynecol Reprod Biol 2015;188(1–5).
13. Gandhi S, Goldberg RP, Kwon C, et al. A prospective randomized trial using solvent dehydrated fascia lata for the prevention of recurrent anterior vaginal wall prolapse. Am J Obstet Gynecol 2005;192(5):1649–54.
14. Guerette NL, Peterson TV, Aguirre OA, et al. Anterior repair with or without collagen matrix reinforcement: a randomized controlled trial. Obstet Gynecol 2009;114(1):59–65.
15. "FDA Public Health Notification. Serious complications associated with transvaginal placement of surgical mesh in repair of pelvic organ prolapse and stress urinary incontinence. 2008. Available at: http://www.fda.gov/cdrh/safety/102008-surgicalmesh.html". Accessed June 15, 2018.
16. FDA Safety Communication. UPDATE on serious complications associated with transvaginal placement of surgical mesh for pelvic organ prolapse", 2011. Available at: https://www.fda.gov/MedicalDevices/ProductsandMedicalProcedures/ImplantsandProsthetics/UroGynSurgicalMesh/ucm345201.html. Accessed June 15, 2018.
17. Nygaard I, Barber MD, Burgio KL, et al. Prevalence of symptomatic pelvic floor disorders in US women. JAMA 2008;300(11):1311–6.
18. Wu JM, Hundley AF, Fulton RG, et al. Forecasting the prevalence of pelvic floor disorders in U.S. Women: 2010 to 2050. Obstet Gynecol 2009;114(6):1278–83.
19. Olsen A, Smith V, Bergstrom J, et al. Epidemiology of surgically managed pelvic organ prolapse and urinary incontinence. Obstet Gynecol 1997;89(4):501–6.
20. Sung VW, Washington B, Raker CA. Costs of ambulatory care related to female pelvic floor disorders in the United States. Am J Obstet Gynecol 2010;202(5):483.e1-4.
21. DeLancey JO, Morgan DM, Fenner DE, et al. Comparison of levator ani muscle defects and function in women with and without pelvic organ prolapse. Obstet Gynecol 2007;109(2 Pt 1):295–302.
22. Jelovsek JE, Chagin K, Gyhagen M, et al. Predicting risk of pelvic floor disorders 12 and 20 years after delivery. Am J Obstet Gynecol 2018;218(2):222.e1–19.
23. Raz S. Atlas of vaginal reconstructive surgery. New York: Springer; 2015.
24. Berger MB, Kolenic GE, Fenner DE, et al. Structural, functional, and symptomatic differences between women with rectocele versus cystocele and normal support. Am J Obstet Gynecol 2018;218(5):510.e1–8.
25. DeLancey JOL. "What's new in the functional anatomy of pelvic organ prolapse? Curr Opin Obstet Gynecol 2016;28(5):420–9.
26. Kelly HA, Dumm WM. Urinary incontinence in women, without manifest injury to the bladder. 1914. Int Urogynecol J Pelvic Floor Dysfunct 1998;9(3):158–64.
27. Bergman I, Söderberg MW, Kjaeldgaard A, et al. Does the choice of suture material matter in anterior and posterior colporrhaphy? Int Urogynecol J 2016;27(9):1357–65.
28. Song H-S, Choo GY, Jin L-H, et al. Transvaginal cystocele repair by purse-string technique reinforced with three simple sutures: surgical technique and results. Int Neurourol J 2012;16(3):144.
29. Raz S, Klutke CG, Golomb J. Four-corner bladder and urethral suspension for moderate cystocele. J Urol 1989;142(3):712–5.
30. Cormio L, Mancini V, Liuzzi G, et al. Cystocele repair by autologous rectus fascia graft: the pubovaginal cystocele sling. J Urol 2015;194(3):721–7.
31. Lee U, Raz S. Emerging concepts for pelvic organ prolapse surgery: what is cure? Curr Urol Rep 2011;12(1):62–7.
32. Demirci F, Ozdemir I, Somunkiran A, et al. Abdominal paravaginal defect repair in the treatment of paravaginal defect and urodynamic stress incontinence. J Obstet Gynaecol 2007;27(6):601–4.

33. Chinthakanan O, Miklos JR, Moore RD. Laparoscopic paravaginal defect repair: surgical technique and a literature review. Surg Technol Int 2015;27: 173–83.
34. Mallipeddi P, Kohli N, Steele AC, et al. Vaginal paravaginal repair in the surgical treatment of anterior vaginal wall prolapse. Prim Care Update Ob Gyns 1998;5(4):199–200.
35. Young SB, Daman JJ, Bony LG. Vaginal paravaginal repair: one-year outcomes. Am J Obstet Gynecol 2001;185(6):1360–6 [discussion: 1366–7].
36. Shippey SH, Quiroz LH, Sanses TVD, et al. Anatomic outcomes of abdominal sacrocolpopexy with or without paravaginal repair. Int Urogynecol J 2010; 21(3):279–83.
37. Barber MD, Brubaker L, Nygaard I, et al. Defining success after surgery for pelvic organ prolapse. Obstet Gynecol 2009;114(3):600–9.
38. Lee U, Raz S. Words of wisdom. Re: defining success after surgery for pelvic organ prolapse. Eur Urol 2010;58(4):633–4.
39. Weber AM, Walters MD, Piedmonte MR, et al. Anterior colporrhaphy: a randomized trial of three surgical techniques. Am J Obstet Gynecol 2001;185(6): 1299–304 [discussion: 1304–6].
40. Lavelle RS, Christie AL, Alhalabi F, et al. Risk of prolapse recurrence after native tissue anterior vaginal suspension procedure with intermediate to long-term followup. J Urol 2016;195(4 Pt 1):1014–20.
41. Wu JM, Dieter AA, Pate V, et al. Cumulative incidence of a subsequent surgery after stress urinary incontinence and pelvic organ prolapse procedure. Obstet Gynecol 2017;129(6):1124–30.
42. Lowder JL, Park AJ, Ellison R, et al. The role of apical vaginal support in the appearance of anterior and posterior vaginal prolapse. Obstet Gynecol 2008;111(1):152–7.
43. Summers A, Winkel LA, Hussain HK, et al. The relationship between anterior and apical compartment support. Am J Obstet Gynecol 2006;194(5): 1438–43.
44. Siff LN, Barber MD. Native tissue prolapse repairs: comparative effectiveness trials. Obstet Gynecol Clin North Am 2016;43(1):69–81.
45. Eilber KS, Alperin M, Khan A, et al. Outcomes of vaginal prolapse surgery among female Medicare beneficiaries: the role of apical support. Obstet Gynecol 2013;122(5):981–7.
46. Detollenaere RJ, den Boon J, Stekelenburg J, et al. Sacrospinous hysteropexy versus vaginal hysterectomy with suspension of the uterosacral ligaments in women with uterine prolapse stage 2 or higher: multicentre randomised non-inferiority trial. BMJ 2015;351:h3717.
47. Meschia M, Pifarotti P, Bernasconi F, et al. Porcine skin collagen implants to prevent anterior vaginal wall prolapse recurrence: a multicenter, randomized study. J Urol 2007;177(1):192–5.
48. Hviid U, Hviid TVF, Rudnicki M. Porcine skin collagen implants for anterior vaginal wall prolapse: a randomised prospective controlled study. Int Urogynecol J 2010;21(5):529–34.
49. Nieminen K, Hiltunen R, Takala T, et al. Outcomes after anterior vaginal wall repair with mesh: a randomized, controlled trial with a 3 year follow-up. Am J Obstet Gynecol 2010;203(3):235.e1-8.
50. Altman D, Väyrynen T, Engh ME, et al, Nordic Transvaginal Mesh Group. Anterior colporrhaphy versus transvaginal mesh for pelvic-organ prolapse. N Engl J Med 2011;364(19):1826–36.
51. Vollebregt A, Fischer K, Gietelink D, et al. Primary surgical repair of anterior vaginal prolapse: a randomised trial comparing anatomical and functional outcome between anterior colporrhaphy and trocar-guided transobturator anterior mesh. BJOG 2011;118(12):1518–27.

Surgery for Anterior Compartment Prolapse Synthetic Graft-Augmented Repair

Osnat Israeli, MD[a,b], Adi Y. Weintraub, MD[a,b,*]

KEYWORDS

• Pelvic organ prolapse • Anterior colporrhaphy • Native tissue • Polypropylene mesh

KEY POINTS

Anterior colporrhaphy can be performed using either native tissue or synthetic materials such as polypropylene mesh:

- There seems to be superiority in efficacy and durability in anterior prolapse repair with synthetic mesh.
- High rates of reported complications and accompanied litigation steer surgeons away from using synthetic materials for prolapse repair.
- No uniform consensus exists regarding the optimal surgical technique and mesh kits used, identifying the finest implanted materials and tools for assessing success.
- Accurate estimations of the true benefits and actual rates of adverse effects remain uncertain.

INTRODUCTION

Pelvic organ prolapse (POP) is the descent of 1 or more of the vaginal walls, cervix, or vaginal cuff following hysterectomy. POP is a common condition that affects many women worldwide.[1] Its prevalence is currently estimated to be approximately 40% in women aged 45 to 85 years and about 30% of these women are symptomatic.[2] Symptoms include complains of urinary, bowel, or sexual dysfunction, as well as symptoms of vaginal pressure, heaviness or pain,[3] greatly impacting patients' well-being and quality of life.[4]

The efficacy of conservative treatment such as pelvic floor exercise or a pessary is limited. It is estimated that about 11% of all women will undergo surgery for POP repair during their lifetime, and 30% of these will need reoperation because of prolapse recurrence within 4 years after the initial surgery.[5]

In the United States, the most common surgery for correction of POP is anterior colporrhaphy for the prolapse of the anterior wall, and the results of this surgery are generally poor with an anatomic recurrence rate of greater than 40%.[6] Anterior colporrhaphy can be performed using either native tissue or with synthetic materials such as a polypropylene mesh.

Transvaginal mesh kits represent a newer technique that differs from the traditional colporrhaphy. Instead of individual sutures used to plicate the anterior endopelvic connective tissue, trocars are used to insert and fasten a standardized mesh to augment support to the pelvic structures and overlay the anterior vaginal wall central defect. These standardized kits represent a departure from an individualized assessment of the patient's anatomy to a more standardized approach. Another major difference between the techniques is that a permanent mesh is used instead of delayed absorbable sutures.[7]

Disclosure: The author has nothing to disclose.

[a] Department of Obstetrics and Gynecology, Soroka University Medical Center, Rager Boulevard, PO Box 151, Beer Sheva 85025, Israel; [b] Department of Obstetrics and Gynecology, Soroka University Medical Center, Faculty of Health Sciences, Ben-Gurion University of the Negev, Beer Sheva, Israel
* Soroka University Medical Center, Rager Boulevard, PO Box 151, Beer Sheva 85025, Israel.
E-mail address: adiyehud@bgu.ac.il

Urol Clin N Am 46 (2019) 71–78
https://doi.org/10.1016/j.ucl.2018.08.009
0094-0143/19/© 2018 Elsevier Inc. All rights reserved.

The rational for using mesh involves avoiding the use of the structurally deficient native tissue that was present during the initial disease presentation.[8]

Abundant literature exists showing the superiority of synthetic implants in reducing recurrence of POP, which is reviewed elsewhere in this article. However, inserting foreign materials into the body carries with it an increased risk of complications. These complications are also reviewed elsewhere in this article.

The use of synthetic materials in general and specifically of mesh for the repair of POP has been the issue of controversy in the past few years. Warnings about the abundance of complications have steered surgeons away from preforming mesh repairs, ignoring the advantages that this technique carries with it. As with many clinical issues, professional opinions have a tendency of swaying from one extremity to the other, until, finally a wide consensus is reached.

In this article, we look back at the history of POP mesh repair, examine its efficacy and advantages, assess common complications, review current opinions, and look to the future for ways in which improved use of mesh can lead to better results and fewer complications. Because there is an abundance of literature, the most updated trails and reviews were chosen.

HISTORY BACKGROUND AND CLINICAL PROGRESSION

Surgical mesh has been used for internal repairs since the 1950s and was originally developed to support the abdominal wall in the repair of hernias. By the 1970s, gynecologists began to believe that mesh may be used in the repair of POP, and by the 1990s, surgical mesh was being used to do transvaginal repairs of POP and to treat stress urinary incontinence (SUI).[7]

Kits for vaginal repair have been used in the United States since 2005 to augment repair with native tissue. Instead of using individual sutures, the use of trocars was presented for a simpler, faster, and more standardized approach.[6] Mesh kits were introduced and aggressively marketed, faster than data were collected and before sufficient information on short- and long-term safety concerns were available.[9] With time, clinical use became more common and with it increasing reports of postoperative complications.

In 2008 2 big reviews were published. The first by Sung and colleagues[10] reviewed studies comparing mesh repair with native tissue, totaling 16 comparative studies and 37 noncomparative studies. These investigators found limited efficacy or safety evidence and called for further randomized, controlled trails with adequate power. In the second publication, Feiner and colleagues[11] reviewed all trails that used transvaginal mesh to assess success and complication rates. Thirty studies were included, reporting on 2653 women. Both anatomic and subjective outcomes were reviewed, and these researchers concluded that apical augmentation with mesh products resulted in successful outcomes, but mesh erosion and dyspareunia were well-known complications. In the same year, the US Food and Drug Administration (FDA) issued the first publication regarding serious complications of using mesh for treatment of prolapse.[12] A review published in 2009 by Bako and Shar[13] further emphasized mesh-related complications, reporting mesh erosion rates of 2% to 25% and infection rates of up to 8%. They also discussed reasons for complications, including mesh misplacement, dissection plane problems, and excessive mesh tension. In 2011, an additional safety communication was issued owing to increasing reports of complications.[3] After the FDA safety update in 2011, the use of synthetic mesh in transvaginal POP surgery decreased. Haya and colleagues[14] investigated the rates and types of POP surgery in the OECD countries, and reported that the greatest decrease was seen in the United States. In that same year, Altman and colleagues[6] published a multicenter, parallel group, randomized, controlled trail showing that mesh repair had higher short-term rates of success compared with native tissue repairs. However, this trial also showed higher rates of complications.

In 2014, the FDA demanded premarket studies to evaluate safety and effectiveness of vaginal mesh implants[4] and finally in 2016 reclassified them as class III high-risk devices.[15]

A systematic review published in 2016 reviewed new literature and compared it with the Sung and colleagues[10] review from 2008 and another large review from the same year published by Murphy.[16] This review included relatively more randomized, controlled trails and a better strength of evidence. In the reviewed studies, the use of mesh consistently resulted in improved anatomic outcomes compared with native tissue repair. Superior relief of subjective bulge symptoms was also shown. However, there was no difference in quality of life or urinary and sexual function.[17]

In 2016, the PROSPECT trial—a large, randomized, controlled trail—included 865 women and showed that a primary transvaginal anterior or posterior prolapse repair with nonabsorbable synthetic mesh confers no symptomatic or anatomic benefits to women in the short term (follow-up of $\leq$2 years). More than 1 woman in 10 had mesh complications, but most were asymptomatic and there was no difference in other adverse effects.[18] With that, concerns exist addressing the methodology of this study, mainly owing to a lack of unity between surgical techniques and surgent experience.

To date, there is no consensus as to the use of mesh for anterior POP repair. In the past few years, several position statements and committee opinions were published on this topic around the world.

The American College of Obstetricians and Gynecologists and the American Urogynecologist Society published a committee opinion in 2011 offering recommendations for the safe and effective use of vaginal mesh for POP repair. Among their recommendations were using both subjective and objective measures of success, patient selection (mainly patients with a high risk for recurrence), an emphasis on surgeon training, demanding specific research for every new kit released, and stressing the importance of informed consent and the need for additional randomized, controlled trails on the subject.[19]

In 2017, the European Urology Association and the European Urogynecology Association published a consensus statement reaching the conclusion that mesh should only be used in the repair of POP in complex cases, with recurrent prolapse, and restricted to those surgeons with appropriate training who are working in multidisciplinary referral centers. They also emphasized that patients should be adequately informed regarding the potential success rates and mesh-related adverse effects.[20]

The Canadian Urologic Association's position statement published in 2017 went even further, concluding that it is not recommended to use mesh for repair of POP owing to the relatively small advantages and the increased rate of adverse effects. If, however, mesh repair is offered to a patient it is important to state and explain advantages and disadvantages of the procedure. It is also important that the surgeon be able to diagnose and treat possible complications if they occur.

ADVANTAGES OF MESH AUGMENTATION PELVIC ORGAN PROLAPSE REPAIR

The main argument for using a synthetic graft repair in the anterior compartment would be its superior efficacy and durability in treating the signs and symptoms of prolapse, compared with native tissue repair, with fewer recurrences and reoperations.[21]

In a Cochrane report published in 2016, 25 randomized, controlled trials comparing native tissue repair with permanent mesh in woman having anterior or multicompartment prolapse, the superiority of mesh repair was clearly demonstrated. Of patients with native repair, 19% had an awareness of prolapse after native tissue surgery as compared with 10% to 15% after mesh repair. The rate of recurrence (38% vs 11%–20%) and the rate of reoperation (3% vs 1%–3%) for prolapse was lower in the mesh group.[22]

High anatomic success rates, standing at about 90%, have been reported in literature since the 1990s[23–25] and these are still true in recent publications.[26,27] In addition, there seems to be superiority of mesh repair in improving prolapse symptoms.[6,28] There are additional reports of increased both subjective and objective success rates and lower rates of reoperation than were reported previously.[29]

COMPLICATIONS OF MESH AUGMENTATION PELVIC ORGAN PROLAPSE REPAIR

As the use of mesh kits for vaginal repair increased throughout the years and their use became exceedingly widespread, reports and awareness of complications also increased, obligating the surgeon to take them into consideration when contemplating and counseling regarding what surgical technique to use.

The FDA monitors medical device performance to detect potential device-related safety issues, according to MAUDE (Manufacture and User Facility Device Experience). Mesh related complications of POP surgery include (in order of decreasing incidence): erosion/mesh exposure, pain, infection, bleeding, dyspareunia, organ perforation, urinary problems, vaginal scaring/shrinkage, neuromuscular problems, and prolapse recurrence.[30]

The main complication is mesh exposure, a complication obviously unique to mesh augmentation surgery. In a metanalysis published in 2016, 14 randomized, controlled trials were included, comparing complications after transvaginal mesh repairs with native tissue repairs. Mesh exposure was shown in more than 10% of women undergoing mesh surgery. Of these women, 7.7% had to undergo an additional surgery for mesh exposure.[22] A small mesh exposure may be asymptomatic and usually does not require additional surgery for mesh excision.[31]

Another complication noted with mesh repair is postoperative pain, including pelvic pain, groin pain, leg pain, and dyspareunia. Rates of pain after mesh repair are variable. In a Cochrane report, the rate was relatively low; only 0.5% of women underwent mesh removal for this reason. However, 38.6% of complaints to the FDA included vaginal pain and/or dyspareunia.[32] The etiology of this complication is thought to be mesh shrinkage owing to the inflammatory reaction of the body to foreign material and it is thought to be associated with the inherent properties of the selected material of the synthetic mesh.

De novo SUI is an additional reported complication. Twelve randomized trials have reported this complaint more common in mesh repairs in comparison to native tissue repairs (133 vs 96–1000 women).[22] These findings are duplicated and emphasized in controlled trials with a longer follow-up of 3 years,[26] showing a higher rate of de novo SUI in women undergoing mesh repair.

Intraoperative bladder injury has also been reported at increased rates. Luckily, this complication is uncommon and the reported rates are low (0.8%–1.8%)[33,34] Other less common complications include neuromuscular problems, vaginal scarring or shrinkage, and urethral injuries.[9,35,36]

PARAMETERS FOR THE EVALUATION OF TREATMENT SUCCESS

Assessing the rate of success for a specific repair can be measured either anatomically (objective success) or subjectively, according to the individual evaluation of the patient as to symptoms and quality of life. Success rates differ according to definitions and the assessment tool used. Anatomic success of the surgery is made using the POP-Q system, a relatively detailed and objective anatomic assessment of the degree of prolapse, carried out for each compartment separately.[37] Subjective success is based on quality of life questionnaires, for example, the Pelvic Organ Prolapse Symptom Score, a validated patient self-completed tool that has been shown to be sensitive to change after treatment,[38] the Pelvic floor Impact Questioner, the Pelvic Floor Distress Inventory short form, or the Pelvic Organ Prolapse/Urinary Incontinence Sexual Questioner, as well as many other questionnaires. It is likely that using different questioners in different trails leads to a variable definition of success; using different outcomes may have considerable impact on the results even of a single study.[39] It should be noted that there is no direct and predictable relationship between objective anatomic cure and subjective improvement of prolapse symptoms or patient subjective satisfaction.[40] The varying definitions of cure and success pose a limitation when analyzing literature in published reviews and metanalyses and may give inaccurate results.

WHAT DOES THE FUTURE HOLD?

Reviewing the past literature, official statements, and recent randomized, controlled trails, there is still no consensus on the issue of mesh repair for anterior POP. There seems to be some added value for synthetic graft repair in comparison to native tissue repair, especially in cases with increased risk for recurrence. However, according to the body of evidence so far it seems that the toll of adverse effects remains high, perhaps beyond what is reasonable for choice of action.

As to now, after FDA warnings and published reviews, many surgeons have migrated away from using this technique, withholding possible advantages from women suffering from POP. Poor publicity and litigation against doctors and device companies has led many doctors and patients to no longer use these products, and several large companies have withdrawn from the field of female pelvic floor surgery devices either partly or completely.[41] However, in our opinion it is too soon to part just yet with this modality of treatment all together, in accordance with personal experience.

In 2015, a study that examined the efficacy and safety of a skeletonized mesh performed on 103 patients evaluated the short-term (6 weeks) and long-term (6 months and 12 months) outcomes of surgery. Intraoperative complications included 2 cases (2%) of cystotomy that were corrected vaginally. The immediate postoperative complications included 1 patient (1%) with a urinary tract infection, 4 cases (3.9%) of self-resolved hematomas, and 6 cases (5.8%) of bladder outlet obstruction. At 12 months, a high success rate and low complication rate was noted. Recurrence of prolapse was reported by 7 patients (6.6%). However, only 4 (3.8%) underwent a repeat procedure. Two patients developed de novo SUI and 6 patients (5.7%) reported dyspareunia. No cases of mesh erosion/extrusion were noted. This study showed excellent anatomic and quality of life results in patients with advanced POP treated with a skeletonized and reduced mesh system. No mesh exposure was recorded within the first year after surgery. The reason for such low adverse outcomes may be due to the unique structure and properties of the mesh used and to the highly skilled surgeons who performed the procedures.[42]

Another study published in 2015 assessed subjective success in 79 women with a postoperative follow-up of 79 to 104 months. The recurrence of prolapse symptoms was reported by 11 patients (13.9%), mostly in the posterior compartment. Only 6 needed a corrective procedure. One patient had her mesh removed owing to dyspareunia. Eleven patients (13.9%) reported lower urinary tract symptoms other than prolapse, as follows: SUI,[1] overactive bladder,[8] and dyspareunia.[2] In this study, low rates of adverse outcomes were found and the same surgical technique and implanted materials were used, implying that in other studies other factors may contribute to higher rates of complications.[43]

The obvious limitation of these studies is their small sample size. However, it seems that the lack of unity in the methodology used in different trials, the different surgical kits used, varying surgeons' experience, research protocols, patient selection, and methods for assessing success limit the accuracy of existing data.

Additionally, in almost all the committee opinions and clinical statements there seems to be suggestions and recommendations for improving the clinical practice surrounding these procedures, such as meticulous patient selection and improved surgical training. It is, therefore, of great importance to develop strategies for decreasing complications, allowing transvaginal mesh repair to be an acceptable option of treatment. With improved research, increased attention to surgical technique, and meticulous patient selection there might still be hope for mesh repair, with its greater efficacy and expectable rates of adverse effects.

STRATEGIES FOR IMPROVING SUCCESS RATES AND DECREASING COMPLICATIONS

Patient Selection

Because there are reasons for and against the use of mesh repair, the decision to use it should be made on an individual basis. When there is a greater risk for prolapse recurrence, it becomes more reasonable to choose this surgical approach. Stage 3 or 4 (POP-Q) prolapse, age less than 60 years, diabetes mellitus, and recurrent prolapse are all risk factors for increased failure rates of native tissue repair[44] and may be a basis for considering synthetic graft repair.

Meticulous patient selection is paramount in decreasing the rate of mesh erosions. Several studies have demonstrated an increased risk of mesh exposure and wound infection with increasing body mass index, poorly controlled diabetes, and smoking,[30,45,46] younger, sexually active women are also at higher risk.[47,48] In addition, concurrent hysterectomy seems to increase the risk for this complication.[49,50]

Anatomic Considerations

A wide variety of kits were made available within a relatively short period of time, each with technical variations and different designs. These variations may have hindered surgeons' ability to become familiar with a specific procedure and its associated surgical anatomy. Moreover, this condition has likely contributed to the complexity of mesh excision procedures. In article study by Corton[51] published in 2013, a detailed review of the pelvic floor anatomy is provided along with specific information regarding the relevant anatomic structures with different kits for mesh repair.[52] Both the American College of Obstetricians and Gynecologists and the American Urogynecologist Society declare that the safe and effective use of vaginal mesh for the repair of POP requires that surgeons placing vaginal mesh should undergo appropriate training specific to each device and must have a thorough understanding of pelvic anatomy and experience with reconstructive procedures.[20]

Surgeon's Training

In a retrospective study of 198 cases, Achtari and colleagues[53] reported that the surgeons who were experienced with the surgical technique had less erosions than less experienced surgeons. Other studies have also shown a higher exposure risk for trainees in comparison with consultants (25.9% vs 13.5%).[8] Owing to the relatively high rate of complications and the delicate nature of these procedures, use of mesh should be performed only by pelvic floor surgeons with appropriate training and experience.

Patient Education

Nowadays, informed consent is a requirement before carrying out any surgical procedure. Owing to the complexity of choosing mesh for vaginal POP repair, the importance of informed consent is further emphasized. It is imperative to review the pros and cons of this approach and to include the patient in selecting the surgical pathway. In addition, coordination of patients' expectations is of great importance. Urodynamic studies can help to determine preoperative urinary continence and voiding function and whether a patient could benefit from concurrent surgery for SUI. POP surgery is frequently blamed for stress incontinence symptoms even when SUI was present before surgery.

Mesh Material Properties

Research in biomaterials (including the structure and properties of the actual mesh and the addition of coating materials) have recently emerged worldwide because of an urgent need for more appropriate options for reconstructive medicine and treatment of soft tissue disorders. Composite or coated meshes intending to get an antiadhesive profile, protection against infection, or to elicit less pronounced foreign body reactions have been tested. Although significant basic science information has been produced, there remain conflicting results. Also, tissue-engineering techniques have shown only limited evidence to date. Because life expectancy is advancing quickly, demands in biomaterials research must be reached to offer long-lasting therapeutic options for reconstructive surgery.[54]

SUMMARY

To date, no uniform consensus exists regarding the use of synthetic meshes for POP repair. Although there seems to be superiority in efficacy and durability, high rates of reported complications and accompanied litigation steers surgeons away from this technique. Unfortunately, even though much was published on this topic, a lack of unity regarding the optimal surgical technique and mesh kits used, identifying the finest implanted materials and tools for assessing success. All these conditions hinder accurate estimations of the true benefits and actual rates of adverse effects.

Further research, using unified techniques and outcome measures, is needed. Until then, careful patient selection and surgical education as well as thoughtful surgical protocols are in place for increasing efficacy and reducing complications.

REFERENCES

1. Olsen AL, Smith VJ, Bergstrom JO, et al. Epidemiology of surgically managed pelvic organ prolapse and urinary incontinence. Obstet Gynecol 1997;89:501–6.
2. Slieker-Ten Hove MCP, Pool-Goudzwaard AL, Eijkemans MJC, et al. Prediction model and prognostic index to estimate clinically relevant pelvic organ prolapse in a general female population. Int Urogynecol J Pelvic Floor Dysfunct 2009;20(9):1013–21.
3. Younger A, Rac G, Quentin C, et al. Pelvic organ prolapse surgery in academic female pelvic medicine and reconstructive surgery urology practice in the setting of the Food and Drug Administration public health notifications. Urology 2016;91:46–50.
4. Abdel-Fattah M, Familusi A, Fielding S, et al. Primary and repeat surgical treatment for female pelvic organ prolapse and incontinence in parous women in the UK: a register linkage study. BMJ Open 2011;1(2):e000206.
5. Wu JM, Matthews CA, Conover MM, et al. Lifetime risk of stress urinary incontinence or pelvic organ prolapse surgery. Obstet Gynecol 2014;123(6):1201–6.
6. Altman D, Vayrynen T, Engh ME, et al, Nordic Transvaginal Mesh Group. Anterior colporrhaphy versus transvaginal mesh for pelvic organ prolapse. N Engl J Med 2011;364(19):1826–36.
7. Iyer S, Bortos SM. Transvaginal mesh: a historical review and update of the current state of affairs in the United States. Int Urogynecol J 2017;28:527–35.
8. MacDonald S, Terlecki R, Constatini E, et al. Complications of transvaginal mesh for pelvic organ prolapse and stress urinary incontinence: tips for prevention, recognition, and management. Eur Urol Focus 2016;2:20–267.
9. Committee on Gynecologic Practice. Committee Opinion no. 513: vaginal placement of synthetic mesh for pelvic organ prolapse. Obstet Gynecol 2011;118:1459–64.
10. Sung VW, Rogers RG, Schaffer JI, et al. Graft use in transvaginal pelvic organ prolapse repair: a systematic review. Obstet Gynecol 2008;112(5):1131–42.
11. Feiner B, Jelovesk JE, Maher C. Efficacy and safety of transvaginal mesh kits in the treatment of prolapse in the vaginal apex: a systematic review. Br J Obstet Gynaecol 2009;116:15–24.
12. Food and Drug Administration. FDA public health notification: serious complications associated with transvaginal placement of surgical mesh in repair of pelvic organ prolapse and stress urinary incontinence. Silver Spring (MD): FDA; 2008.
13. Bako A, Dhar R. Review of synthetic mesh-related complications in pelvic floor reconstructive surgery. Int Urogynecol J 2009;20:103–11.
14. Haya N, Baessler K, Christmann-Schmid C, et al. Prolapse and continence surgery in countries of the organization for economic cooperation and development in 2012. Am J Obstet Gynecol 2015;212(6):755.e1–27.
15. FDA. Urogynecology surgical mesh implants. Available at: http://www.fda.gov/medicaldevices/productsandmedicalprocedures/implantsandprosthetics/urogynsurgicalmesh/. Accessed September 20, 2017.
16. Murphy M, Society of Gynecologic Surgeons Systematic Review Group. Clinical practice guidelines on vaginal graft use from the society of gynecologic surgeons. Obstet Gynecol 2008;112:1123–30.
17. Shhimpf M, Abed H, Sanses T, et al, for the Society of Gynecological Surgeons Systematic, Review group. Graft and mesh use in transvaginal prolapse repair: a systematic review. Obstet Gynecol 2016;128:81–91.
18. Glazer CMA, Breeman S, Elders A, et al. Mesh, graft, or standard repair for women having primary transvaginal anterior or posterior compartment prolapse surgery: two parallel-group, multicenter, randomized, controlled trials (PROSPECT). Lancet 2017;389:381–92.
19. ACOG Committee Opinion No.513. Vaginal placement of synthetic mesh for pelvic organ prolapse. 2011.
20. Chapple CR, Cruz F, Deffieux X, et al. Consensus statement of the European Urology Association

and the European Urogynecological Association on the use of implanted materials for treating pelvic organ prolapse and stress urinary incontinence. Eur Urol 2017;77:424–31.
21. Kontogiaanis S, Gooulimi E, Giannitas K. Reasons for and against use of non-absorbable, synthetic mesh during pelvic organ prolapse repair, according to the prolapsed compartment. Adv Ther 2016;33:2139–49.
22. Maher C, Feiner B, Baessler K, et al. Transvaginal mesh or grafts compared with native tissue repair for vaginal prolapse. Cochrane Database Syst Rev 2016;(2):CD012079.
23. Nicita G. A new operation for genitourinary prolapse. J Urol 1998;160(3 Pt 1):741–5.
24. Flood CG, Drutz HP, Waja L. Anterior colporrhaphy reinforced with Marlex mesh for the treatment of cystoceles. Int Urogynecol J Pelvic Floor Dysfunct 1998; 9(4):200–4.
25. Migliari R, De Angelis M, Madeddu G, et al. Tension-free vaginal mesh repair for anterior vaginal wall prolapse. Eur Urol 2000;38(2):151–5.
26. Rudnicki M, Laurikainen E, Pogosean R, et al. A 3-year follow-up after anterior colporrhaphy compared with collagen-coated transvaginal mesh for anterior vaginal wall prolapse: a randomized controlled trial. BJOG 2016;123(1):136–42.
27. Dias MM, De AC, Bortolini MAT, et al. Two-years results of native tissue versus vaginal mesh repair in the treatment of anterior prolapse according to different success criteria: a randomized controlled trial. Neurourol Urodyn 2016;35(4):509–14.
28. De Tayrac R, Cornille A, Eglin G, et al. Comparison between trans-obturator trans-vaginal mesh and traditional anterior colporrhaphy in the treatment of anterior vaginal wall prolapse: results of a French RCT. Int Urogynecol J 2013;24(10):1651–61.
29. Nieminen K, Hiltunen R, Takala T, et al. Outcomes after anterior vaginal wall repair with mesh: a randomized, controlled trial with a 3 year follow-up. Am J Obstet Gynecol 2010;203(3):235.e1-8.
30. Brill AI. The hoopla over mesh: what it means for practice. Obstetrics and Gynecology News 2012;14–5.
31. American Urological Association. Choosing wisely: ten things physicians and patients should question. 2016. Available at: http://www.choosingwisely.org/societies/american-urological-association/. Accessed September 20, 2017.
32. Maher CM, Feiner B, Baessler K, et al. Surgical management of pelvic organ prolapse in women: the updated summary version Cochrane review. Int Urogynecol J 2011;22(11):1445–57.
33. Bjelic-Radisic V, Aigmueller T, Preyer O, et al. Vaginal prolapse surgery with transvaginal mesh: results of the Austrian registry. Int Urogynecol J 2014; 25:1047–52.
34. Frankman EA, Alperin M, Sutkin G, et al. Mesh exposure and associated risk factors in women undergoing transvaginal prolapse repair with mesh. Obstet Gynecol Int 2013;2013:926313.
35. Derpapas A, Digesu AG, Pananayi D. A persistent bladder erosion with ureteric involvement following mesh augmented repair of cystocele. Am J Obstet Gynecol 2010;202:e5–7.
36. Heisler CA, Casiano ER, Klingele CJ. Ureteral injury during vaginal mesh excision: role of prevention and treatment options. Am J Obstet Gynecol 2012;207: e3–4.
37. Bump RC, Mattiasson A, Bø K, et al. The standardization of terminology of female pelvic organ prolapse and pelvic floor dysfunction. Am J Obstet Gynecol 1996;175(1):10–7.
38. Hagen S, Glazener C, Sinclair L, et al. Psychometric properties of the pelvic organ prolapse symptom score. BJOG 2009;116:25–31.
39. Barber MD, Brubaker L, Nygaard I, et al. Defining success after surgery for pelvic organ prolapse. Obstet Gynecol 2009;114(3):600–9.
40. Teleman P, Laurikainen E, Kinne I, et al. Relationship between the Pelvic Organ Prolapse Quantification system (POP-Q), the Pelvic Floor Impact Questionnaire (PFIQ-7), and the Pelvic Floor Distress Inventory (PFDI-20) before and after anterior vaginal wall prolapse surgery. Int Urogynecol J 2015;26(2): 195–200.
41. Karmaker D, Dwyer PL. Failure of expectations in vaginal surgery: lack pf appropriate consent, goals and expectations of surgery. Curr Urol Rep 2016; 17:87.
42. Weintraub AY, Neuman M, Reuven Y, et al. Efficacy and safety of skeletonized mesh implants for advanced pelvic organ prolapse: 12-month follow-up. World J Urol 2016;34:1491–8.
43. Weintraub AY, Friedman T, Baumfeld Y, et al. Long term subjective cure rate, urinary tract symptoms and dyspareunia following mesh augmented anterior vaginal repair. Int J Surg 2015;24(Pt A):33–8.
44. Whiteside JL, Weber AM, Meyn LA, et al. Risk factors for prolapse recurrence after vaginal repair. Am J Obstet Gynecol 2004;191(5):1533–8.
45. Araco F, Gravante G, Sorge R, et al. The influence of BMI, smoking, and age on vaginal erosions after synthetic mesh repair of pelvic organ prolapses. A multicenter study. Acta Obstet Gynecol Scand 2009;88(7):772–80.
46. Collinet P, Belot F, Debodinance P, et al. Transvaginal mesh technique for pelvic organ prolapse repair: mesh exposure management and risk factors. Int Urogynecol J 2006;17:315.
47. Kokanali MK, Doğanay M, Aksakal O, et al. Risk factors for mesh erosion after vaginal sling procedures for urinary incontinence. Eur J Obstet Gynecol Reprod Biol 2014;177:146–50.
48. Kaufman Y, Singh SS, Alturki H, et al. Age and sexual activity are risk factors for mesh exposure

following transvaginal mesh repair. Int Urogynecol J 2011;22:307–13.
49. Kasyan G, Abramyan K, Popov AA, et al. Meshrelated and intraoperative complications of pelvic organ prolapse repair. Cent European J Urol 2014; 67:296–301.
50. Bensinger G, Lind L, Lesser M, et al. Abdominal sacral suspensions: analysis of complications using permanent mesh. Am J Obstet Gynecol 2005;193: 2094–8.
51. Corton MM. Critical anatomical concepts for safe surgical mesh. Clin Obstet Gynecol 2013;56(2): 247–56.
52. American College of Obstetricians and Gynecologists ACOG Committee Opinion No. 513: vaginal.
53. Achtari C, Hiscock R, O'Reilly BA, et al. Risk factors for mesh erosion after transvaginal surgery using polypropylene (Atrium) or composite polypropylene/polyglactin 910 (Vypro II) mesh. Int Urogynecol J Pelvic Floor Dysfunct 2005;16(5): 389–94.
54. Goulart Fernandes Dias F, Goulart Fernandes Dias PH, Prudente A, et al. New strategies to improve results of mesh surgeries for vaginal prolapse repair – an update. Int Braz J Urol 2015; 41(4):623–34.

Surgery for Posterior Compartment Prolapse

Posterior Vaginal Wall Prolapse: Suture-Based Repair

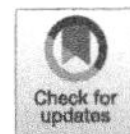

Juan M. Guzman-Negron, MD*, Michele Fascelli, MD, Sandip P. Vasavada, MD

KEYWORDS

• Rectocele • Posterior compartment prolapse • Posterior colporrhaphy

KEY POINTS

- Posterior vaginal wall prolapse is a herniation of the anterior rectal wall producing a vaginal bulge and is often associated with a wide range of clinical symptoms, including pain, constipation, and splinting to achieve defecation.
- Managing patient expectations is of utmost importance when considering any rectocele repair intervention and will make an impact on the postoperative perception of satisfaction and improvement of the patient.
- Randomized studies have shown no benefit to the use of synthetic or biological graft compared with suture-based posterior compartment repairs.
- Recurrence rates after posterior colporrhaphy are lower when compared with transanal approaches.
- Transvaginal techniques should be considered first choice when managing posterior compartment prolapse.

INTRODUCTION

Pelvic organ prolapse is estimated to be identified in nearly 40% to 60% of aging parous women, although approximately 3% of those women report symptoms.[1–3] The specific incidence of posterior compartment prolapse, or rectocele, is less well-reported. Posterior vaginal wall prolapse is a herniation of the anterior rectal wall that produces a posterior vaginal bulge. This is often associated with a wide range of clinical symptoms, including pain, constipation, and splinting to achieve defecation. Some patients are asymptomatic. It is often challenging to correlate anatomic findings and clinical symptoms, making prolapse repair a challenge. Data suggest that pelvic organ prolapse progresses until menopause and the number of women who suffer from this problem is expected to increase to nearly 5 million by 2050.[4]

Medical management with stool bulking agents, laxatives, and softeners can benefit some symptoms but not the resolution of a vaginal bulge or defecatory dysfunction. The use of vaginal pessary also has been shown to not be efficacious in helping manage the symptoms of posterior vaginal wall prolapse. Surgery, accordingly, has become the mainstay of therapy for symptomatic rectoceles. Though several surgical techniques have been described to repair a rectocele, no clear indications for type of repair have emerged in the literature. Defects in the posterior compartment mirror those found in the anterior compartment. Central and lateral defects have traditionally been repaired with plication of rectovaginal fascia in the midline (posterior colporrhaphy). Site-specific posterior repair attempts to correct rents in the rectovaginal fascia and may be performed as an alternative.[5] Perineal weakness may require reapproximating the perineal body (perineorrhaphy). Loss of proximal support may be associated with concomitant anterior prolapse and require more extensive surgical planning.

Glickman Urological and Kidney Institute, Lerner College of Medicine, Cleveland Clinic, 9500 Euclid Avenue, Cleveland, OH 44195, USA
* Corresponding author. 9500 Euclid Avenue, Cleveland, OH 44195.
E-mail address: guzmanj3@ccf.org

Urol Clin N Am 46 (2019) 79–85
https://doi.org/10.1016/j.ucl.2018.08.007
0094-0143/19/© 2018 Elsevier Inc. All rights reserved.

The objective of this article is to review the management strategies of posterior compartment prolapse while drawing conclusions about suture-based and site-specific techniques.

ANATOMY AND SUPPORT

The posterior vaginal wall is supported by the so-called rectovaginal fascia, also known as Denonvilliers fascia. Histologic studies performed to evaluate the presence of this fascia during posterior colporrhaphies have shown it is composed of moderately dense connective tissue with smooth muscle.[6] This rectovaginal fascia of the midvagina has been categorized by DeLancey[7] as level II support, along with the fascia of the levator ani muscles. Proximally, in the upper vagina, level I support is composed of the cardinal-uterosacral ligament complex. Distally, level III support is composed of the perineal body and the rectovaginal septum. The perineal body works as a point of fixation for the vaginal muscularis and pelvic floor muscles, thus providing distal support to the posterior vaginal wall.

PATHOPHYSIOLOGY

Within the posterior vaginal compartment, different organs may prolapse, depending on loss of level of support. Loss of level II support and/or attenuation of the rectovaginal fascia in the midvagina results in a herniation of the rectum, better known as a rectocele. If the defect extends to the proximal posterior vaginal wall, prolapse could manifest in the form of a herniation of small bowel or an enterocele. Loss of level I support affects the cardinal-uterosacral ligament complex, resulting as an enterocele or a high rectocele in the posterior vaginal wall. Loss of level III support in the posterior vaginal wall will manifest as a perineal body defect or a low rectocele. These pelvic floor defects result from weakening of the pelvic floor muscles and endopelvic connective tissues supporting the pelvic floor organs. Difficulty with defecation can also cause increase rectal pressure and predispose women to rectocele formation.

POSTERIOR COMPARTMENT SUTURE-BASED REPAIR

Rectocele suture-based repairs can be performed through a transvaginal, transanal, and transperineal route. The decision to undergo any of these repairs should be based on the degree of bothersome symptoms the patient is experiencing and the impact these have on quality of life. The main targets when repairing rectoceles are to alleviate prolapse symptoms, improve anatomic support, and restore bowel and sexual function. Realizing and managing these expectations is of utmost importance when considering any of these procedures, and will have an impact on the perceived satisfaction and improvement of the patient. The authors reviewed the literature on these approaches.

TRANSVAGINAL RECTOCELE REPAIR

Transvaginal rectocele native tissue repairs are subdivided into midline plication and site-specific defect repairs. Patients are placed in dorsal lithotomy and sequential compression devices are placed in the lower extremities. A midline plication repair consists of opening the vaginal epithelium, typically in the midline, and dissecting the posterior vaginal wall bilaterally with exposure of the vaginal muscularis tissue. The vaginal muscularis is plicated and brought over to the midline with interrupted transverse or vertical absorbable sutures, providing a shelf over the rectum (**Fig. 1**). The levator muscles can be plicated in the midline, depending on the widening of the vaginal hiatus, and carries an increased risk of postoperative pain and/or dyspareunia. The vaginal epithelium is then trimmed, if needed, and closed with running absorbable suture. A perineorrhaphy is performed if there is presence of rectovaginal septum detachment from the perineal body. The bulbocavernosus and transverse perineal muscles are brought together in the midline of the perineal body with absorbable sutures, making sure to keep continuity with the distal rectocele repair and to avoid ridges that may cause dyspareunia (**Fig. 2**). Site-specific defect repairs were originally developed to minimize posterior colporrhaphy complications, specifically dyspareunia. For these repairs, the vaginal epithelium is opened in the midline and dissection of the muscularis from the epithelium is performed bilaterally. Then, the index finger of the nondominant hand is placed in the rectum to identify areas of weakness and defects in the muscularis (**Fig. 3**). These defects are closed with interrupted absorbable suture in a vertical or transverse fashion (**Fig. 4**). The epithelium is then trimmed, if needed, and closed with running absorbable suture.

Most of the data looking at rectocele repair success rates are limited to 12-month to 24-month follow-up. The PROlapse Surgery: Pragmatic Evaluation and randomised Controlled Trials (PROSPECT) trial was a recent multicenter randomized trial that sought to compare outcomes of prolapse repair involving either synthetic mesh or biological grafts against standard suture-based repair in women.[8] Subjects were assigned to 1 of 2 trials: comparing standard (native tissue)

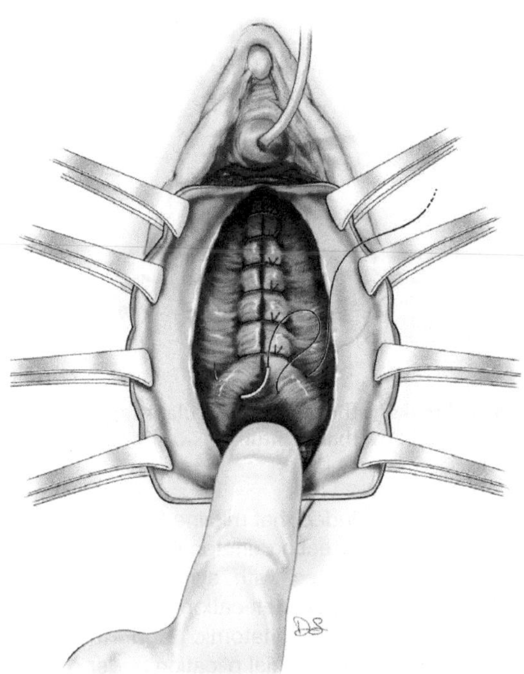

Fig. 1. Midline plication of the vaginal muscularis with interrupted absorbable sutures creating a shelf over the rectum. (*Courtesy of* Cleveland Clinic, Center for Medical Art & Photography © 2014–2018; with permission. All rights reserved.)

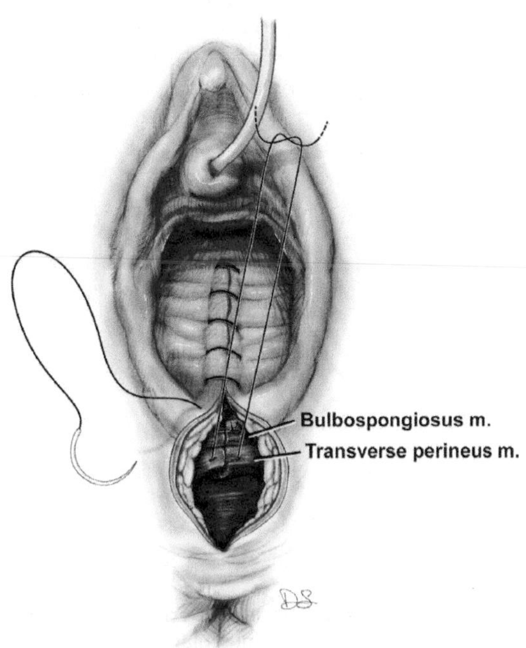

Fig. 2. Bulbocavernosus and transverse perineal muscles plicated in the midline in a perineorrhaphy with absorbable sutures keeping continuity with the distal rectocele repair. (*Courtesy of* Cleveland Clinic, Center for Medical Art & Photography © 2014–2018; with permission. All rights reserved.)

repair alone with standard repair augmented with either synthetic mesh or biological graft. The study included both anterior and posterior prolapse compartment repair subjects and surgeons were free to choose their preferred technique for transvaginal mesh, graft, and standard native tissue repairs. After 2-year follow-up, this study showed that augmenting a primary transvaginal anterior or posterior prolapse repair with nonabsorbable synthetic mesh or biological graft does not provide any short-term symptomatic or anatomic benefit compared with standard suture-based repair yet exposes the patient to the risk of mesh complications. A randomized trial by Paraiso and colleagues[9] compared anatomic and functional outcomes of 3 different approaches: posterior colporrhaphy (midline plication), site-specific repair, and graft-augmented site-specific repair. They had 106 subjects enrolled for the study with stage II or greater posterior vaginal wall prolapse and 98 had a mean follow-up of 17.5 plus or minus 7 months. Concomitant perineorrhaphy was performed if subjects reported splinting to defecate and/or a perineal defect was noted at the time of surgery. After 1 year of surgery, they reported 86% (24/28) of the subjects in the posterior colporrhaphy group and 78% (21/27) subjects in the site-specific group had an anatomic cure of their posterior vaginal wall prolapse, compared with 54% (14/26) of those subjects who received rectocele repair with graft augmentation (P = .02). Reoperation rates for prolapse during the study period were 3% (1/33) in the posterior colporrhaphy group, 5% (2/37) in the site-specific repair group, and 10% (3/29) in the graft augmentation group. All groups had significant improvements in the prolapse, colorectal, and urinary scales of their validated questionnaires, and defecatory dysfunction decreased significantly with no difference between groups. Postoperatively, they did not find a significant difference between groups in the global index of improvement. The investigators concluded posterior colporrhaphy and site-specific rectocele repairs resulted in similar anatomic and functional outcomes as graft-augmented rectocele repairs, and all 3 methods resulted in significant improvements in symptoms, quality of life, and sexual function.

Another randomized trial by Sung and colleagues[10] compared subjective and anatomic outcomes between native tissue repairs and porcine small intestinal submucosal graft augmentation. For the native tissue repair procedures, they

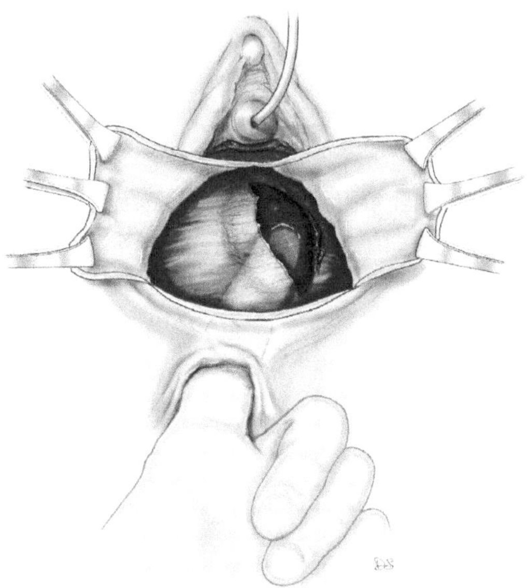

Fig. 3. Site-specific defect repair technique exposing weaknesses in the vaginal muscularis with the index finger of the nondominant hand. (*Courtesy of* Cleveland Clinic, Center for Medical Art & Photography © 2014–2018; with permission. All rights reserved.)

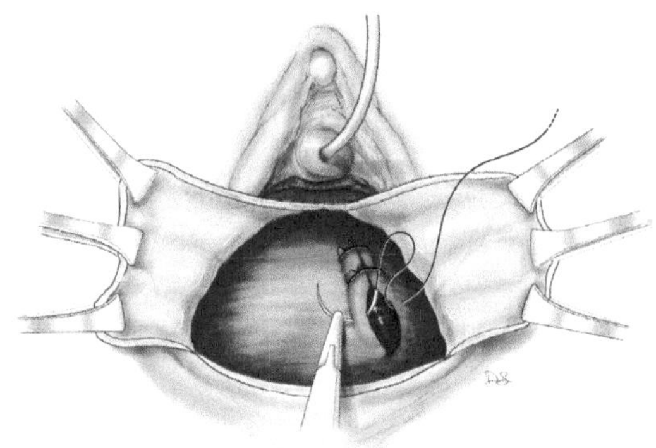

Fig. 4. Breaks in the vaginal muscularis repaired with interrupted absorbable sutures.

included subjects with midline plication or site-specific repair. They enrolled 160 subjects, of which 137 had 12-month anatomic follow-up. They included women with at least stage II symptomatic rectoceles and defined anatomic failure as points Ap or Bp −1 or greater on pelvic organ prolapse quantification system (POP-Q). They found no difference in anatomic failure (12% vs 9%, *P* = .5), vaginal bulge symptom failure (3% vs 7%, *P* = .4), or defecatory symptom failure (44% vs 45%, *P* = .9) for graft compared with native tissue repairs, and concluded that graft rectocele repairs are not superior to native tissue suture-based repairs.

Maher and colleagues[11] prospectively evaluated the efficacy of midline fascial plication of the posterior vaginal wall in women with rectoceles and obstructed defecation. They recruited 38 consecutive women with symptomatic rectoceles (stage II or greater) and obstructed defecation. With a median follow-up of 12.5 months, their subjective success rates after rectocele repair were 97% (95% CI 0.83–1.00) at 12 months and 89% (95% CI 0.55%–0.98%) at 24 months. The objective success rates were 87% (95% CI 0.64–0.96) at 12 months and 79% (95% CI 0.51–0.92) at 24 months. Functional outcomes were also improved, with 87% of women in this cohort no longer experiencing obstructed defecation, and a significant reduction in postoperative straining to defecate, hard stools, and dyspareunia (*P*<.001). Thus, they concluded that midline fascial plication is effective in correcting anatomic and functional outcomes associated with symptomatic rectoceles and obstructed defecation. Milani and colleagues[12] reported anatomic and functional outcome of midline fascial plication under continuous digital transrectal control. They prospectively recruited 233 subjects with posterior vaginal wall prolapse stage II or more with a median follow-up of 14 months (12–35 months). Anatomic success rates were 80.3% (95% CI 75–86) with independent predictors for failure being posterior prolapse stage greater than or equal to III (odds ratio [OR] 8.7, 95% CI 2.7–28.1) and prior history of colposuspension (OR 5.6, 95% CI 1.1–27.8). Obstructed defecation was relieved after midline fascial plication rectocele repair in 63% of affected subjects.

Site-specific rectocele repair has also been evaluated and reported on in the scientific literature. Cundiff and colleagues[5] operated on 69 women undergoing repairs limited to reapproximation of discrete defects in the rectovaginal fascia, without levator plication or perineorrhaphy, in a population with median preoperative stage II prolapse. They reported at 6 weeks of follow-up that POP-Q stage improved in all but 2 women and, by 12 months of follow-up, they had a rectocele recurrence rate of 18% (8/43). Recurrence was defined as no change in or worsening of the preoperative posterior wall prolapse stage. Interestingly, they reported a mean decrease in genital hiatus of 1.9 cm (SD 1.6 cm, range 3.5–5 cm, *P*<.001) even though they did not perform a levator plication or perineorrhaphy in any of the subjects. Bowel symptoms such as tenesmus, splinting, and fecal incontinence had statistically significant improvements after site-specific repairs. Kenton and colleagues[13] assessed rectocele repairs by using a fascial defect approach and reattaching the rectovaginal fascia to the perineal body with a series of vertically placed delayed absorbable sutures. Perineal body repairs were done if deficient. Sixty-six consecutive women underwent rectocele repairs after an anatomic rectocele was confirmed by fluoroscopy, with symptoms of posterior vaginal wall prolapse or difficult defecation attributable to distal stool trapping. Using their technique, they reported posterior vaginal wall topography was restored to a value of −2 or −3 cm in 77% of subjects (34/44) at 1-year follow-up. Postoperative symptom resolution was as follows: protrusion, 90% (35/39; *P*<.0005); difficult defecation, 54% (14/24; *P*<.0005); constipation, 43% (9/21; *P* = .02); dyspareunia, 92% (11/12; *P* = .01); and manual evacuation, 36% (4/11; *P* = .125).

In a retrospective observational study of 125 subjects, Porter and colleagues[14] sought to evaluate the anatomic, functional, and quality of life effects of site-specific repairs in the surgical management of rectocele. Surgical correction was found to have been achieved in 82% of eligible subjects (73/89) with a mean follow-up of 18 months (range 6–36 months). All daily aspects of living improved (*P*<.05), and reports of dyspareunia improved (*P*<.04) or were cured after the operation in 73% of subjects (19/26), worsened in 19% of subjects (5/26), and arose de novo in 3 subjects. Bowel symptoms showed significant improvement postoperatively with the following cure rates: stooling difficulties, 55%; pelvic pain or pressure, 73%; vaginal mass, 74%; and splinting, 65%. Constipation did not significantly change, with 60% (43/72) reporting symptoms before the operation and 50% (36/72) reporting symptoms after the operation (*P*<.07).

Finally, Abramov and colleagues[15] retrospectively reviewed 124 consecutive subjects following site-specific rectocele repair and 183 consecutive subjects following standard posterior colporrhaphy without levator ani plication to compare the anatomic and functional outcomes of these approaches. Women were offered surgical repair when they had symptomatic posterior vaginal wall prolapse, including a symptomatic bulge or constipation. Mean follow-up for both groups was approximately 12 months. Rectocele was defined as greater than or equal to second degree by the modified Baden-Walker halfway system. With no significant differences in baseline characteristics between groups, they found recurrence of rectocele beyond the midvaginal plane (33% vs 14%, *P* = .001) and beyond the hymenal ring (11% vs 4%, *P* = .02), bulge recurrence (11% vs 4%, *P* = .02), and postoperative Bp point (−2.2 vs −2.7 cm, *P* = .001) were significantly higher after the site-specific rectocele repair. Both approaches had similar rates of postoperative dyspareunia and bowel symptoms.

TRANSANAL AND TRANSPERINEAL RECTOCELE REPAIRS

Transanal and transperineal approaches are also performed for the management of rectocele repairs, especially by colorectal and general surgeons. Transanal repairs typically involve the patient being placed in a jackknife position, making an incision at the level of the dentate line, dissecting the anterior rectal mucosa proximal to the dentate line, and then plicating the rectal wall with absorbable sutures, either horizontally or vertically, following stripping of the anterior rectal mucosa.[16] Transperineal repairs consist of making a transverse incision in the perineum above the subcutaneous anal sphincter, identifying the rectovaginal septum, dissecting between the rectum and the vagina, and then suturing the rectal submucosa with absorbable sutures.[17]

In a randomized trial, Farid and colleagues[17] evaluated the functional outcomes of transperineal repair with and without levatorplasty versus transanal repair of rectocele in obstructed defecation. They had a total of 48 subjects with a rectocele larger than 2 cm with 1 or more of the following symptoms: need for digital manipulation during defecation, sense of incomplete evacuation, excessive straining, or sexual dyspareunia. At 6-month follow-up, they found transperineal repair of rectocele was superior to transanal repair in both structural and functional outcomes. Constipation improved significantly in both groups with transperineal repair but not in the group with transanal repair. Functional scores measured with a modified obstructed defecation syndrome questionnaire improved significantly in the transperineal groups (with levatorplasty, *P*<.001; without levatorplasty, *P*<.01) but not in the transanal group (*P* = .142). They concluded transperineal repair of rectocele was superior to transanal repair in both structural and functional outcomes. Nieminen and colleagues[18] did a prospective, randomized study comparing outcomes after transanal and vaginal techniques for rectocele repair. They randomized 30 subjects with a symptomatic rectocele to either a posterior colporrhaphy or a transanal rectoceleplasty. Transvaginal surgery was performed by a gynecologist and transanal surgeries were performed by colorectal surgeons. At 12-month follow-up, 14 (93%) subjects in the vaginal group and 11 (73%) in the transanal group reported improvement in symptoms (*P* = .08). Recurrence rates of rectocele were 1 (7%) in the transvaginal group compared with 6 (40%) in the transanal group ($P = .04$). Recurrence of enteroceles were 0 versus 4 ($P = .05$), respectively. In the transvaginal group, defecography showed a significant decrease in rectocele depth, whereas the difference did not reach statistical significance in the transanal group. They concluded both techniques were associated with statistically significant improvement in symptoms; however, the transanal technique was associated with more clinically diagnosed recurrences of rectocele and/or enterocele. Another randomized study by Kahn and colleagues[19] sought to evaluate the effectiveness between transanal rectocele repair technique performed by a colorectal surgeon and transvaginal rectocele repair technique performed by a gynecologist. They found a higher incidence of postoperative enteroceles in the transanal repair group and concluded that transanal repairs are not adequate because they do not address the presence of an enterocele and may contribute to their development and need for further surgery.

A Cochrane review from 2013 mentions these 2 studies[18,19] and states transvaginal rectocele repairs performed better than the transanal repair of rectocele in terms of a significantly lower recurrence of posterior vaginal wall prolapse, despite a higher blood loss and greater use of pain medication.[20] More women had difficulties in bowel evacuation after transanal operation but this did not reach statistical significance.

LEVATORPLASTY

Studies have shown good anatomic and functional outcomes can be achieved performing transvaginal rectocele repairs without the need of levator plication.[5,11,15] It has also been a common belief that levatorplasty increases the risk of postoperative pain and dyspareunia, although rates of dyspareunia have been seen even when a levatorplasty is not performed during posterior colporrhaphy.[21] After performing posterior colporrhaphies with levatorplasty, Kahn and Stanton[22] reported on these complications and found higher postoperative rates of bowel symptoms and sexual dysfunction. Considering there have been good anatomic and functional outcomes with posterior colporrhaphy without levator plication, it is the authors' practice to generally perform these repairs without performing a levatorplasty, especially in sexually active individuals. The most recent evidence-based surgical pathway for pelvic organ prolapse supports this recommendation against levatorplasty due to concerns for higher rates of dyspareunia.[23]

COMPLICATIONS

Early postoperative complications after rectocele repairs may include pain and constipation. Hematoma, surgical-site infection, and rectal injury resulting in rectovaginal fistula are infrequently seen after rectocele repairs. Long-term complications are usually related to sexual dysfunction or dyspareunia and defecatory dysfunction. An analysis of midline plication posterior colporrhaphy studies showed a mean postoperative dyspareunia rate of 18% (range 5%–45%) and a mean defecatory dysfunction rate of 17% (8%–36%).[24] A similar analysis on site-specific repair studies showed the same mean postoperative rates of dyspareunia and defecatory dysfunction.[24] A recent long-term study analyzing sexual function and quality of life in 151 subjects after posterior colporrhaphy found at a median 64-month follow-up that dyspareunia rates decreased after treatment, even after perineorrhaphy.[25]

SUMMARY

Suture-based rectocele repairs can be performed through transvaginal, transperineal, and transanal approaches. With the current scientific evidence limited to single-center trials, the best choice to perform a rectocele repair is the transvaginal approach, which gives excellent anatomic and functional outcomes while providing the lowest rate of anatomic recurrence. Randomized trials have shown excellent anatomic and functional outcomes with suture-based native tissue rectocele repairs compared with graft-augmented repairs.[9,10] When considering suture-based repairs, it is the opinion of the authors that a midline plication repair conveys objective results superior to site-specific defect repair. Whether this translates to superior improvement in functional outcomes needs further assessment. Most other studies looking at suture-based rectocele repairs are limited by their retrospective nature and short-term follow-up. As previously mentioned, understanding patient expectations before any surgical intervention and managing them are key to achieving successful outcomes after any pelvic organ prolapse repair. With rectocele repairs, surgeons should strive to improve anatomic support and improve prolapse symptoms while minimizing complications, such as dyspareunia and defecatory dysfunction. Moving forward, studies to assess the effectiveness of rectocele repairs should move toward composite outcomes that combine subjective and objective measurements to improve our understanding of a successful outcome in this challenging population.

REFERENCES

1. Handa VL, Garrett E, Hendrix S, et al. Progression and remission of pelvic organ prolapse: a longitudinal study of menopausal women. Am J Obstet Gynecol 2004;190(1):27–32.
2. Hendrix SL, Clark A, Nygaard I, et al. Pelvic organ prolapse in the Women's Health Initiative: gravity and gravidity. Am J Obstet Gynecol 2002;186(6):1160–6. Available at: http://www.ncbi.nlm.nih.gov/pubmed/12066091.
3. Wu JM, Vaughan CP, Goode PS, et al. Prevalence and trends of symptomatic pelvic floor disorders in U.S. women. Obstet Gynecol 2014;123(1):141–8.
4. Wu JM, Hundley AF, Fulton RG, et al. Forecasting the prevalence of pelvic floor disorders in U.S. Women: 2010 to 2050. Obstet Gynecol 2009;114(6):1278–83.
5. Cundiff GW, Weidner AC, Visco AG, et al. An anatomic and functional assessment of the discrete defect rectocele repair. Am J Obstet Gynecol 1998;179(6 Pt 1):1451–6 [discussion: 1456–7]. Available at: http://www.ncbi.nlm.nih.gov/pubmed/9855580.
6. Farrell SA, Dempsey T, Geldenhuys L. Histologic examination of "fascia" used in colporrhaphy. Obstet Gynecol 2001;98(5):794–8.
7. DeLancey JOL. Structural anatomy of the posterior pelvic compartment as it relates to rectocele. Am J Obstet Gynecol 1999;180(4):815–23.
8. Glazener CM, Breeman S, Elders A, et al. Mesh, graft, or standard repair for women having primary transvaginal anterior or posterior compartment prolapse surgery: two parallel-group, multicentre, randomised, controlled trials (PROSPECT). Lancet 2017;389(10067):381–92.
9. Paraiso MF, Barber MD, Muir TW, et al. Rectocele repair: a randomized trial of three surgical techniques including graft augmentation. Am J Obstet Gynecol 2006;195(6):1762–71.
10. Sung VW, Rardin CR, Raker CA, et al. Porcine subintestinal submucosal graft augmentation for rectocele repair: a randomized controlled trial. Obstet Gynecol 2012;119(1):125–33.
11. Maher CF, Qatawneh AM, Baessler K, et al. Midline rectovaginal fascial plication for repair of rectocele and obstructed defecation. Obstet Gynecol 2004;104(4):685–9.
12. Milani AL, Withagen MIJ, Schweitzer KJ, et al. Midline fascial plication under continuous digital transrectal control: which factors determine anatomic outcome? Int Urogynecol J 2010;21(6):623–30.
13. Kenton K, Shott S, Brubaker L. Outcome after rectovaginal fascia reattachment for rectocele repair. Am J Obstet Gynecol 1999;181(6):1360–4.
14. Porter WE, Steele A, Walsh P, et al. The anatomic and functional outcomes of defect-specific rectocele repairs. Am J Obstet Gynecol 1999;181(6):1353–9.
15. Abramov Y, Gandhi S, Goldberg RP, et al. Site-specific rectocele repair compared with standard posterior colporrhaphy. Obstet Gynecol 2005;105(2):314–8.
16. Kahn MA, Stanton SL. Techniques of rectocele repair and their effects on bowel function. Int Urogynecol J 1998;9(1):37–47.
17. Farid M, Madbouly KM, Hussein A, et al. Randomized controlled trial between perineal and anal repairs of rectocele in obstructed defecation. World J Surg 2010;34(4):822–9.
18. Nieminen K, Hiltunen KM, Laitinen J, et al. Transanal or vaginal approach to rectocele repair: a prospective, randomized pilot study. Dis Colon Rectum 2004;47(10):1636–42.
19. Kahn MA, Stanton SL, Kumar DFS. Posterior colporrhaphy is superior to the transanal repair for treatment of posterior vaginal wall prolapse. Neurourol Urodyn 1999;18(4):329–30.
20. Maher C, Baessler K. Surgical management of pelvic organ prolapse in women. Cochrane Database Syst Rev 2010;(4):CD004014.
21. Weber AM, Walters MD, Piedmonte MR. Sexual function and vaginal anatomy in women before and after surgery for pelvic organ prolapse and urinary incontinence. Am J Obstet Gynecol 2000;182(6):1610–5.
22. Kahn MA, Stanton SL. Posterior colporrhaphy: its effects on bowel and sexual function. Br J Obstet Gynaecol 1997;104(1):82–6.
23. Maher CF, Baessler KK, Barber MD, et al. Summary: 2017 International consultation on incontinence evidence-based surgical pathway for pelvic organ prolapse. Female Pelvic Med Reconstr Surg 2018. https://doi.org/10.1097/SPV.0000000000000591.
24. Karram M, Maher C. Surgery for posterior vaginal wall prolapse. Int Urogynecol J 2013;24(11):1835–41.
25. Schiavi MC, D'Oria O, Faiano P, et al. Vaginal native tissue repair for posterior compartment prolapse: long-term analysis of sexual function and quality of life in 151 patients. Female Pelvic Med Reconstr Surg 2017;19(4):210–3.

Surgery for Posterior Compartment Vaginal Prolapse: Graft Augmented Repair

Sunchin Kim, MD, Grant R. Pollock, MD,
Christian O. Twiss, MD, FACS, Joel T. Funk, MD, FACS*

KEYWORDS

• Rectocele • Posterior compartment prolapse • Graft augment • Mesh augment

KEY POINTS

- Posterior compartment vaginal prolapse can be approached with multiple surgical techniques, including transvaginally, transperineally, and transanally, repaired with either native tissue or with the addition of an augment.
- Augment material for posterior compartment prolapse includes biologic graft (dermal, porcine submucosal), absorbable mesh (Vicryl polyglactin), or nonabsorbable synthetic mesh (polypropylene).
- Anatomic success rates for posterior compartment repair with augment has ranged from 54% to 92%.
- Augmented posterior compartment repair has not been shown to have superior outcome to native tissue repair.

INTRODUCTION

Pelvic organ prolapse refers to descent of vaginal tissue into the vaginal canal.[1] The pelvic organ support system consists of anterior, apical, and posterior compartments,[2] and prolapse of these compartments are commonly seen variations in the office of any urologist.

An estimated 166,000 women underwent surgery for pelvic organ prolapse in 2010 in the United States,[3] with 52% of these women having a posterior compartment repair component as part of their surgery for prolapse.[4] The overall prevalence of posterior compartment prolapse alone is difficult to ascertain, as it tends to occur concurrently with anterior and apical prolapse. In addition, up to 80% of rectoceles can be asymptomatic,[5] leading to possible underestimation of its prevalence because not all patients with rectocele require surgical treatment. Treatment of posterior compartment prolapse is typically pursued when the patient becomes symptomatic, classically presenting with some defecatory dysfunction including rectal pain, constipation, tenesmus, splinting, and fecal incontinence.[6] There are multiple methods described in literature for the surgical management of posterior compartment prolapse. It can be approached either transvaginally, transperineally, or transanally, and can be repaired with native tissue or with an augment using mesh or graft material. The focus of this article is on the transvaginal approach comparing native tissue repair with a graft or mesh augmented repair.

Overall prolapse recurrence and reoperation rates has ranged greatly between 4.7% and

Disclosure Statements: None.

Department of Surgery, Division of Urology, University of Arizona, 1501 North Campbell Avenue, Box 245077, Tucson, AZ 84724, USA
* Corresponding author.
E-mail address: jfunk@surgery.arizona.edu

Urol Clin N Am 46 (2019) 87–95
https://doi.org/10.1016/j.ucl.2018.08.015
0094-0143/19/© 2018 Elsevier Inc. All rights reserved.

41.1%[7,8] within a 5-year follow-up. Løwenstein and colleagues[9] found that up to 12.1% of rectocele repairs had reoperation within 20 years of follow-up. A variety of graft and mesh materials have been introduced in the recent past for the purpose of strengthening the prolapse repair, and improving the anatomic success rate by reducing the risk of a rectocele recurrence. With an augment, a second layer of support is created using a rectangular piece of mesh or graft placed over the defect-directed repair. This acts as a collagen scaffold for fibroblast infiltration and scar formation, and can potentially replace the fascia as a permanent barrier to prolapse recurrence.[10] The ideal material used for an augment should have a very low rejection rate, be relatively inexpensive, decrease recurrence rates, and cause no harm with respect to bowel and sexual function.[10] Augment materials are categorized into 3 major types: biological graft, synthetic absorbable mesh, and synthetic nonabsorbable mesh.

ANATOMY OF POSTERIOR VAGINAL PROLAPSE

Posterior pelvic organ prolapse is characterized primarily by 3 independent defects: rectocele, enterocele, and perineal body defects.[1] The key anatomic structures involved are the peritoneum of the cul-de-sac (also known as the rectouterine pouch, or "pouch of Douglas"), the rectum, and the perineum.[1] The perineum is the most inferior part of the pelvis.[11] The vagina is a fibromuscular potential space lined by vaginal epithelium.[12] This potential space requires significant support to remain suspended in the pelvis. In 1992, DeLancey described the anatomy of vaginal support[12,13] by performing cross-sectional dissections of nulliparous and multiparous cadavers. He confirmed that the support of the vagina and the posterior compartment is maintained by complex interactions of connective tissue and striated muscle.[14]

The vagina and its support system is divided into 3 different levels (**Fig. 1**). The upper one-fourth of

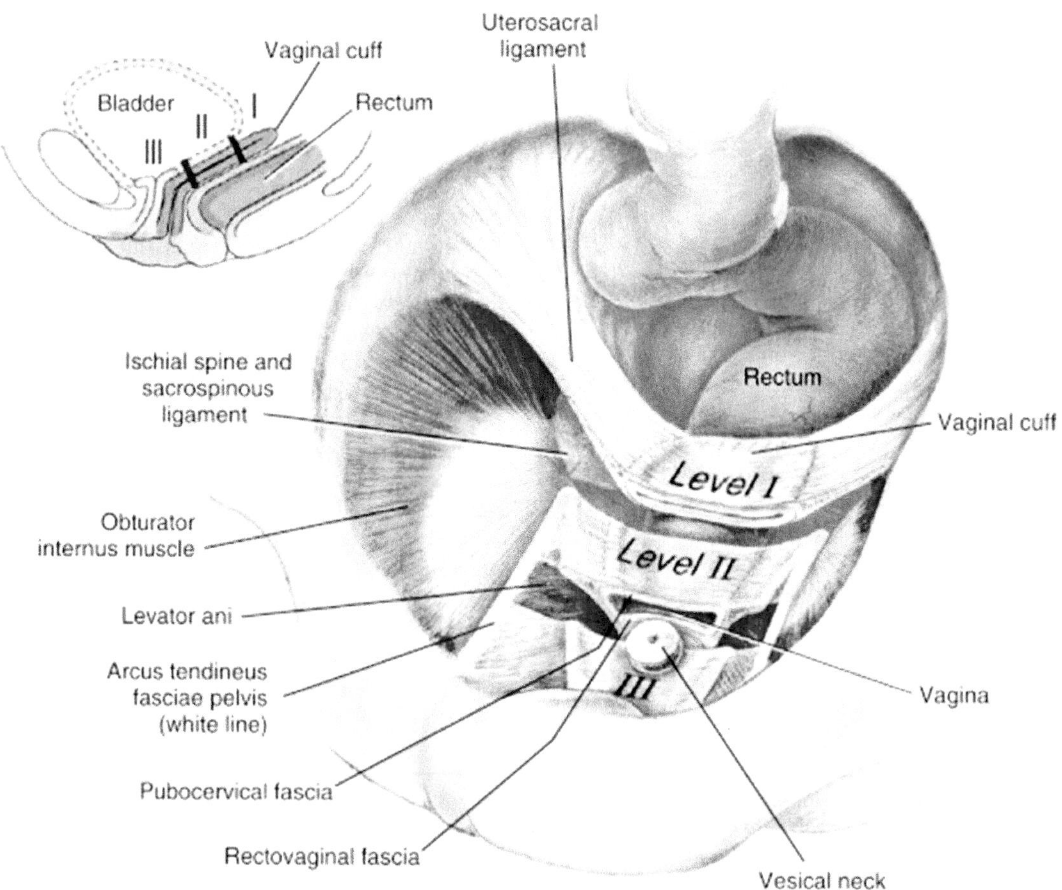

Fig. 1. DeLancey's 3 levels of vaginal support. (*From* DeLancey JOI. Anatomic aspects of vaginal eversion after hysterectomy. Am J Obstet Gynecol. 1992; 166:1717; with permission.)

the vagina is suspended by the cardinal/uterosacral ligament complex, designated as DeLancey Level I. The middle one-half of the vagina is maintained by endopelvic fascia connections to the arcus tendinous fascia pelvis, which attaches the vagina to the aponeurosis of the levator ani (DeLancey Level II). The lower one-fourth of the vagina is maintained by the fusion of the lower vagina to the urogenital diaphragm and the perineal body. Any bulge into the vagina represents a break in the continuity of one of these layers of support.[12,13]

In male individuals, a dense fascial tissue layer separating the rectum from the prostate and seminal vesicles was discovered by the French anatomist Denonvillier in 1839.[15] Likewise, female individuals have fascial layers around the vagina. The pubocervical fascia lines the anterior wall of the vagina and maintains the integrity and support of the anterior wall. In 1993, Richardson[15] performed gross dissections to characterize what many up to that point had called "Denonvilliers' fascia in the female." The strength and integrity of the posterior wall of the vagina is supplied by this fascia, also known as the rectovaginal septum or rectovaginal fascia.[12] This fascial layer separates the rectal and genital compartments of the lower pelvis and lies immediately below the vaginal mucosa. It courses from the perineal body to the cul-de-sac, where it merges with fibers of the uterosacral ligaments as well as the posterior cervix. Additionally, the rectovaginal fascia is associated with all of DeLancey's 3 levels of support. It merges with the lateral fibers of the cardinal/uterosacral complex at Level I. It merges with the parietal fascia covering the iliococcygeus and pubococcygeus at Level II. And last, it merges with the perineal body at the level of the UG diaphragm at Level III.[12] After years of studying the rectovaginal fascia in the autopsy suite and the operating room, Richardson[15] believed the rectovaginal fascia was the most important structure in terms of maintaining the integrity of the posterior compartment, and posterior compartment prolapse almost always was found to involve a break in some aspect of the rectovaginal fascia.

Significant posterior vaginal wall prolapse is most often the result of 3 anatomic deficiencies: loss of fascial support overlying the rectum, laxity and separation of the muscular levator plate with resultant widening of the levator hiatus, and tearing and separation of the perineal musculature.[16] The rectocele and the enterocele are the primary defects of posterior pelvic organ prolapse. Both rectoceles and enteroceles present as a bulge in the posterior vaginal wall. A rectocele occurs when bowel muscularis comes in contact with vaginal mucosa with no intervening fascia. The rectovaginal fascia that normally separates the vagina from the rectum has broken in some way allowing the rectal wall to push upward onto the vaginal mucosa.[12] The rectovaginal fascia can break in a variety of different manners. The most common fascial break is described by Richardson[15] as a transverse separation of the rectovaginal fascia immediately above its attachment to the perineal body. This type of tear yields a "low rectocele," or a bulge that begins just inside the introitus.[15] A transverse tear could extend up the lateral aspect of the posterior vaginal wall, leading to a "hockey stick" defect. If the break is high, it could extend down both lateral walls, leading to a "U-shaped" defect.[12]

Enteroceles occur when the peritoneum comes in contact with vaginal mucosa with no intervening fascia. Enteroceles can be classified into 3 groups based on the location of fascial tissue break: anterior, apical, and posterior. As with the rest of this article, we focus primarily on posterior enteroceles. The posterior enterocele is the most common type of enterocele with the uterus in place, and other defects like uterine prolapse or concomitant rectoceles are often present.[12] In enteroceles, the break in the fascia usually occurs somewhere in the upper or dorsal portion of the fascia where it adheres to the cul-de-sac peritoneum and merges with the cardinal/uterosacral fibers.[15] Breaks associated with enteroceles, however, are highly variable.[15]

A complete posterior repair can be a challenging case for even for an experienced pelvic surgeon because it involves evaluating and treating 3 separate structures. First, it is important to evaluate the integrity of the rectovaginal fascia, and repair it by closing any defects. Next, it is important to evaluate the size of the levator hiatus, and to bring the medial margins of the pubococcygeus together in the midline to narrow it if the hiatus is deemed to be too wide. Finally, the intrinsic muscles of the perineal body must be reconstructed if they are separated (which often is secondary to old obstetric injuries).[12] If an enterocele is present, repair also requires the completion of 3 tasks: the reconstruction of the vaginal fibrous tissue, reestablishing the suspension and lateral attachments of the reconstructed vagina, and excision of redundant peritoneum and vaginal mucosa.[12]

SURGICAL TECHNIQUE

There is considerable variation within the technical details, but here we describe a general approach to the augmented repair of posterior compartment prolapse. A longitudinal incision is made at the posterior wall of the vagina starting at the hymenal ring and extended toward the vaginal apex. The rectovaginal fascia is then dissected off the mucosa until the puborectalis muscles are located. The defects in the fascia are then corrected with a central plication of the fascia with delayed absorbable sutures. A wedge excision of the vaginal epithelium may be performed, along with plication of the levator ani muscles. The augment (absorbable, biologic, or synthetic), usually a rectangular piece with variable sizes depending on the degree of the prolapse, is then placed overlying the fascial repair and anchored to the sacrospinous ligaments (**Fig. 2**). Perineal defects are then repaired with deep sutures into the perineal muscles, after which the overlying vaginal and perineal skin is then closed.

ABSORBABLE MESH VERSUS NATIVE TISSUE

There is an overall paucity of literature regarding repair of posterior compartment prolapse using just absorbable mesh. As is the case with most studies regarding pelvic organ prolapse, the literature for absorbable mesh repair is confounded by combining multicompartment prolapse repair results,[17] repair for stress urinary incontinence, and the variability in surgeon technique that results due to the number of defects present. In addition, the mesh used in other studies also had variability, such as Vypro 2, which has both absorbable Vicryl and nonabsorbable Prolene incorporated into their mesh,[18,19] or a composite Monocryl-Prolene.[20]

One randomized study (**Table 1**) was performed with an absorbable mesh using Vicryl polyglactin 910 in the surgical repair of rectoceles. The mesh itself dissolves by hydrolysis and acts as a lattice for the formation of dense granulation tissue with

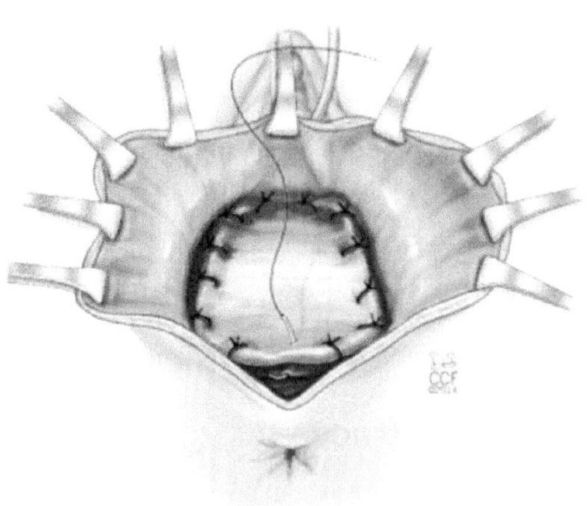

Fig. 2. Posterior graft augment. (*Reprinted with permission*, Cleveland Clinic, Center for Medical Art & Photography © 2014–2018. All Rights Reserved.)

minimal inflammatory response. Sand and colleagues[21] performed a prospective, randomized, controlled trial with 161 women with vaginal prolapse managed surgically, with either a native tissue or an absorbable mesh augmented repair, and were evaluated at 2, 6, 12, and 52 weeks postoperatively. All the women had cystoceles, and 132 had concurrent rectoceles; 80 of 161 patients received mesh. For patients selected to receive the mesh, a 6 × 6-inch piece of mesh was divided into 3 pieces, one underneath the trigone, one just anterior to the vaginal cuff, and the third for the posterior colporrhaphy placed just cephalad to the deep transverse perineal muscles.

At 1 year postoperatively, 119 (90%) of 132 patients with rectocele did not have recurrence. Of the 13 patients with recurrence, 7 had been treated surgically with native tissue repair, and 6 had been treated with absorbable mesh augmentation. This study is limited by the already low incidence of recurrent rectocele, making it difficult to detect a difference between the 2 study groups. With the given results, there is no significant difference between native tissue repair and absorbable mesh augmented repair regarding rectocele recurrence.

BIOLOGICAL GRAFT VERSUS NATIVE TISSUE

Oster and Astrup[22] were the first to report use of a dermal autograft for the repair of posterior compartment prolapse. Fifteen patients with large rectoceles were selected for repair using a 10 × 5-cm graft, and were followed for 1 to 4 years. All patients were symptomatically improved, and only 1 of 15 had anatomic failure.

Glazener and colleagues[23] performed a large multicenter, randomized trial (PROSPECT) that included a total of 1352 women, 735 of whom were included in comparing biological graft material versus native tissue repair. The material used included use of either porcine acellular collagen matrix, porcine small intestinal submucosa, or bovine dermal grafts. These grafts were inserted below the fascial layer and secured with peripheral sutures. Of the 735 patients, 367 were assigned to native tissue repair, and 368 were assigned to graft augmentation. The study found that the mean pelvic organ prolapse symptom scores and quality of life did not differ substantially between the comparison groups at 1 year. Objective assessment of treatment failure, which was defined as the leading edge greater than 0 cm beyond the hymen, was found to be higher in the biological graft treatment group (18%) compared with native tissue repair (16%); however, this was not statistically significant. The study, however, included women

Table 1
Absorbable mesh and biologic graft versus native tissue repair

Article	Type of Augment	No. of Patients Assigned	Prolapse Location	Anatomic Success Rate[a]
Sand et al,[21] 2001	Absorbable mesh No augment	161	Posterior only	119/132 (90%) overall. 13/132 recurrence: 7 without augment, 6 with absorbable mesh
Oster and Astrup,[22] 1981	Biological (dermal autograft)	15	Posterior only	14/15 (93%)
Glazener et al,[23] 2017	Biological (porcine acellular collagen)	368	Anterior and posterior combined	244/298 (82%)
	No augment	367		256/303 (84%)
Paraiso et al,[24] 2006	Biological (porcine small intestinal submucosa)	37	Posterior only	20/37 (54%)
	No augment	69		44/69 (64%)
Sung et al,[25] 2012	Biological (porcine subintestinal submucosa)	80	Posterior only	59/67 (88%)
	No augment	80		64/70 (91%)

[a] The definition of anatomic success varied between articles, ranging from the leading edge 0 to −2 on Pelvic Organ Prolapse Quantification System assessment.

with both anterior and posterior compartment prolapse, so the results cannot be attributed solely to posterior compartment repair.

Paraiso and colleagues[24] performed a study using 3 different surgical techniques in the repair of rectoceles, including posterior colporrhaphy, site-specific rectocele repair, and site-specific repair augmented with a porcine small intestinal submucosa graft. The graft was a 4 × 8-cm piece that was secured superiorly to the posterior vaginal fibromuscularis and epithelium, laterally to the levator ani fascia, and inferiorly to the perineal body. A total of 106 patients were randomly assigned to the 3 groups, with 37 having undergone graft augmented repair. Failure was defined as having a postoperative Pelvic Organ Prolapse Quantification System (POPQ) point Bp ≥ -2 at 1 year. The subjects who received graft augmentation had a significantly greater anatomic failure rate (46%) compared with site-specific (22%) or posterior colporrhaphy (14%). The study concluded that although all 3 methods of posterior compartment repair improved symptoms, quality of life, and sexual function overall, the addition of biological graft did not improve anatomic outcomes compared with posterior colporrhaphy or site-specific rectocele repair alone.

Sung and colleagues[25] performed a randomized controlled trial comparing the effects of porcine subintestinal submucosal graft augmentation for rectocele repairs. The patients had at least a stage 2 rectocele, and were followed up at 2 weeks, 6 weeks, 6 months, and 12 months. The graft was a 4 × 7-cm piece secured over the native tissue repair, trimmed to appropriate size, sutured superiorly to the rectovaginal connective tissue, laterally to the levator ani fascia, and inferiorly to the perineal body. Anatomic failure was defined as having a postoperative POPQ point Ap or Bp ≥ -1 cm. A total of 160 women were randomized, of which 67 received the biologic graft. The study showed 8 (12%) of 67 experienced anatomic failure, compared with 6 (8.6%) of 70 failure in the native tissue repair group, showing no significant difference in graft augmented repair. Symptomatically, there was no difference in subjective measurements including vaginal bulge or defecatory symptoms.

Overall, these studies (see **Table 1**) comparing biologic graft with native tissue repair showed no difference between native tissue and augmented repair for symptomatic outcomes. The latest Cochran review[26] assessed the surgical management of posterior vaginal wall prolapse with biological graft. Evidence was insufficient in showing any difference between the 2 groups in rates of prolapse recurrence, repeat surgery, dyspareunia, symptomatic defecation, or awareness of prolapse.

SYNTHETIC VERSUS NATIVE TISSUE

Although there are numerous studies regarding synthetic mesh placement in the posterior compartment, not many have separated the results of anterior and posterior compartment repair. Even fewer studies have directly compared augmented repair with native tissue repair (**Table 2**), making it difficult to make any conclusions regarding the efficacy of synthetic mesh.

The PROSPECT study[23] compared synthetic mesh with native tissue repair in a total of 865 women with pelvic organ prolapse, among whom 435 women were included in the synthetic mesh augmented group. As with the previously discussed study of biological graft augment, this study included both anterior and posterior compartment repairs, and as such the results could not be attributed solely to the posterior compartment. A higher proportion of women had objective failure in the synthetic mesh arm (16%) compared with native tissue repair (14%), but did not reach statistical significance.

Lim and colleagues[18] performed a retrospective review on 90 patients assessing the safety and efficacy of posterior colporrhaphy using composite Vicryl-Prolene without primary repair, and reported a success rate of 84% at a 6-month follow-up. They initially concluded that posterior colporrhaphy with synthetic mesh is effective in treating posterior compartment prolapse in the short term; however, on longer follow-up[27] revealed that the complication rate was unacceptably high, discussed later in this article.

Khandwala[20] performed a review of 48 patients with posterior compartment prolapse of at least POPQ stage 2 were repaired with a composite Monocryl-Prolene mesh. The mean follow-up was 13 months, and 93% of patients had anatomic success defined as POPQ stage 1 or less.

Song and colleagues[28] assessed 163 patients, 53 of whom had combined anterior and posterior Prolift mesh placed. Satisfactory anatomic outcomes, defined as POPQ stage 1 or better, occurred in 83.3% of cases for the posterior compartment after a mean follow-up of 40.4 months. Meyer and colleagues[29] assessed 70 patients, of whom 37 had received only the posterior Prolift (23/70) or combined anterior and posterior (14/70). On 5-year follow-up, 100% of the patients (26/26) had anatomic POPQ stage 2 or less, although the percentage dropped to 42% (11/26) if the criteria were changed to POPQ stage 1 or less. de Tayrac and colleagues[30] also performed an assessment of rectocele repairs on 26 women using a combined bilateral sacrospinous suspension and polypropylene mesh at a median follow-up of 9.2 months; 92.3% of women were deemed cured, with 1 patient having asymptomatic stage 2 rectocele.

Overall, the anatomic cure rates with synthetic mesh were comparable with those for traditional

Table 2
Synthetic mesh versus native tissue repair

Article	Type of Augment	No. of Patients Assigned	Prolapse Location	Anatomic Success Rate[a]
Glazener et al,[23] 2017	Synthetic mesh (polypropylene)	435	Anterior and posterior combined	282/336 (84%)
	No augment	430		291/338 (86%)
Lim et al,[18] 2005	Synthetic mesh (composite Vicryl-Prolene)	90	Posterior only	26/31 (84%)
Song et al,[28] 2016	Synthetic mesh (polypropylene)	163	Anterior and posterior combined	100/120 (83%)
de Tayrac et al,[30] 2006	Synthetic mesh (polypropylene)	26	Posterior only	24/26 (92%)
Meyer et al,[29] 2016	Synthetic mesh (polypropylene)	37	Anterior and posterior combined	26/26 (100%)
Khandwala,[20] 2013	Synthetic mesh (composite Monocryl-Prolene)	48	Posterior only	40/43 (93%)

[a] The definition of anatomic success varied between papers, ranging from stage 0 to 2 on Pelvic Organ Prolapse Quantification System assessment.

nonmesh repairs,[31] reported to be between 76% and 90%.[32–34] The use of synthetic mesh, however, resulted in significant complications, such as erosion, decrease in sexual activity, chronic pain, and dyspareunia resulting in the US Food and Drug Administration (FDA) issuing a safety concern.[35]

COMPLICATIONS

The use of vaginal mesh has come under public scrutiny due to debilitating complications such as erosion, chronic pain, and dyspareunia. Vaginal mesh erosion was reported in 12.0% to 36.0% of patients, de novo dyspareunia in 3.4% to 27.0%, worsened dyspareunia in up to 63.0%, and rectocele recurrence in 22.0%.[27,31,36,37] The FDA issued a safety concern in 2008, and again in 2011, regarding the complications associated with transvaginal mesh, stating that serious complications associated with surgical mesh for transvaginal repair are not rare.[35] In 2016, the FDA reclassified transvaginal mesh systems from a moderate-risk device to a high-risk device. Approximately 10% of women undergoing pelvic organ prolapse surgery experienced mesh erosion within 12 months of surgery.[38] More than half of women with erosion from a nonabsorbable synthetic mesh required surgical excision in the operating room, with some requiring multiple surgeries.[38] Even after surgery for these complications, the symptoms may not have completely resolved.[39]

An Interventional Procedures review of 503 women drew attention to a high incidence of serious adverse effects in women who were having mesh inserted with blind introducer devices included in mesh kits. They concluded that until benefits and risks have been properly evaluated, mesh kits using nonabsorbable synthetic mesh should be reserved for more complex cases of prolapse.

CURRENT RECOMMENDATIONS

The Society of Gynecologic Surgeons Systematic Review group[40,41] previously published a systematic review noting the relative lack of data regarding the use of graft and mesh for pelvic organ prolapse. Since then, the number of studies regarding the use of transvaginal augment material has increased. Schimpf and colleagues[42] performed a review of outcomes of augmented posterior compartment prolapse, stating that there is no difference in anatomic and quality-of-life outcomes using any of the different augments, including synthetic absorbable, synthetic nonabsorbable, or biologic graft compared with native tissue repair. It did not show any significant improvement on urinary and sexual function. The FDA has stated that mesh in transvaginal prolapse repair introduces additional risks not present in other types of repair. Regarding posterior repair, they stated that there is no evidence that mesh augment provides any added benefit compared with traditional surgery without mesh,[35] and encouraged recognition by physicians that most pelvic organ prolapse can be treated successfully without mesh.

SUMMARY

With the given results and recommendations, native tissue repair may be preferable to the use of mesh or graft for posterior compartment prolapse, as the use of augment material has not shown to have superior outcomes.

REFERENCES

1. Winters JC. Vaginal and abdominal reconstructive surgery for pelvic organ prolapse. 11th edition. Campbell-Walsh Urology; 2016. p. 1939–86.
2. Kudish BI. Posterior wall prolapse and repair. Clin Obstet Gynecol 2010;53(1):59–71.
3. Wu JM, Kawasaki A, Hundley AF, et al. Predicting the number of women who will undergo incontinence and prolapse surgery, 2010 to 2050. Am J Obstet Gynecol 2011;205:230.e1-e5.
4. Shah AD, Kohli N, Rajan SS, et al. The age distribution, rates, and types of surgery for pelvic organ prolapse in the USA. Int Urogynecol J Pelvic Floor Dysfunct 2008;19:421–8.
5. Lisi G, Campanelli M, Grande S, et al. Transperineal rectocele repair with biomesh: updating of a tertiary refer center prospective study. Int J Colorectal Dis 2018. https://doi.org/10.1007/s00384-018-3054-2.
6. Cundiff GW, Weidner AC, Visco AG, et al. An anatomic and functional assessment of the discrete defect rectocele repair. Am J Obstet Gynecol 1998; 179:1451–6.
7. Oversand SH, Staff AC, Spydslaug AE, et al. Long-term follow-up after native tissue repair for pelvic organ prolapse. Int Urogynecol J 2014;25:81–9.
8. Miedel A, Tegerstedt G, Mörlin B, et al. A 5-year prospective follow-up study of vaginal surgery for pelvic organ prolapse. Int Urogynecol J Pelvic Floor Dysfunct 2008;19(12):1593–601.
9. Løwenstein E, Møller LA, Laigaard J, et al. Reoperation for pelvic organ prolapse: a Danish cohort study with 15-20 years' follow-up. Int Urogynecol J 2018; 29(1):119–24.
10. Cundiff GW, Fenner D. Evaluation and treatment of women with rectocele: focus on associated

defecatory and sexual dysfunction. Obstet Gynecol 2004;104(6):1403–21.
11. Kleeman D. Posterior pelvic floor prolapse and a review or the anatomy, preoperative testing, and surgical management. Minerva Ginecol 2008;60: 165–82.
12. Richardson AC. The anatomic defects in rectocele and enterocele. J Pelvic Surg 1995;4:214–21.
13. DeLancey JO. Anatomic aspects of vaginal eversion after hysterectomy. Am J Obstet Gynecol 1992;166: 1717–24 [discussion: 1724–8].
14. DeLancey JO. Structural anatomy of the posterior pelvic compartment as it relates to rectocele. Am J Obstet Gynecol 1999;180:815–23.
15. Richardson AC. The rectovaginal septum revisited: its relationship to rectocele and its importance in rectocele repair. Clin Obstet Gynecol 1993;36: 976–83.
16. Rovner ES. Pelvic organ prolapse, a review. Ostomy Wound Manage 2000;46(12):24–37.
17. Allahdin S, Glazener C, Bain C. A randomised controlled trial evaluating the use of polyglactin mesh, polydioxanone and polyglactin sutures for pelvic organ prolapse surgery. J Obstet Gynaecol 2008;28(4):427–31.
18. Lim YN, Rane A, Muller R. An ambispective observational study in the safety and efficacy of posterior colporrhaphy with composite Vicryl-Prolene mesh. Int Urogynecol J Pelvic Floor Dysfunct 2005;16: 126–31.
19. El Haddad R, Martan A, Masata J, et al. Long-term review on posterior colporrhaphy with levator ani muscles plication and incorporating a Vypro II mesh. Ceska Gynekol 2009;74(4):282–5.
20. Khandwala S. Transvaginal mesh surgery for pelvic organ prolapse: one-year outcome analysis. Female Pelvic Med Reconstr Surg 2013;19(2): 84–9.
21. Sand PK, Koduri S, Lobel RW, et al. Prospective randomized trial of polyglactin 910 mesh to prevent recurrence of cystoceles and rectoceles. Am J Obstet Gynecol 2001;184(7):1357–62 [discussion: 1362–4].
22. Oster S, Astrup A. A new vaginal operation for recurrent and large rectocele using dermis transplant. Acta Obstet Gynecol Scand 1981;60: 493–5.
23. Glazener CM, Breeman S, Elders A, et al. Mesh, graft, or standard repair for women having primary transvaginal anterior or posterior compartment prolapse surgery: two parallel-group, multicentre, randomised, controlled trials (PROSPECT). Lancet 2017; 389(10067):381–92.
24. Paraiso MF, Barber MD, Muir TW, et al. Rectocele repair: a randomized trial of three surgical techniques including graft augmentation. Am J Obstet Gynecol 2006;195(6):1762–71.
25. Sung VW, Rardin CR, Raker CA, et al. Porcine subintestinal submucosal graft augmentation for rectocele repair: a randomized controlled trial. Obstet Gynecol 2012;119(1):125–33.
26. Mowat A, Maher D, Baessler K, et al. Surgery for women with posterior compartment prolapse. Cochrane Database Syst Rev 2018;(3): CD012975.
27. Lim YN, Muller R, Corstiaans A, et al. A long-term review of posterior colporrhaphy with Vypro 2 mesh. Int Urogynecol J Pelvic Floor Dysfunct 2007;18(9): 1053–7.
28. Song W, Kim TH, Chung JW, et al. Anatomical and functional outcomes of prolift transvaginal mesh for treatment of pelvic organ prolapse. Low Urin Tract Symptoms 2016;8(3):159–64.
29. Meyer I, McGwin G, Swain TA, et al. Synthetic graft augmentation in vaginal prolapse surgery: long-term objective and subjective outcomes. J Minim Invasive Gynecol 2016;23(4): 614–21.
30. de Tayrac R, Picone O, Chauveaud-Lambling A, et al. A 2-year anatomical and functional assessment of transvaginal rectocele repair using a polypropylene mesh. Int Urogynecol J Pelvic Floor Dysfunct 2006;17:100–5.
31. Richardson ML, Elliot CS, Sokol ER. Posterior compartment prolapse: a urogynecology perspective. Urol Clin North Am 2012;39(3):361–9.
32. Kahn MA, Stanton SL. Posterior colporrhaphy: its effects on bowel and sexual function. Br J Obstet Gynaecol 1997;104(1):82–6.
33. Arnold MW, Stewart WR, Aguilar PS. Rectocele repair: four years' experience. Dis Colon Rectum 1990;33(8):684–7.
34. Janssen L, van Dijke C. Selection criteria for anterior rectal wall repair in symptomatic rectocele and anterior rectal wall prolapse. Dis Colon Rectum 1994; 37(11):1100–7.
35. U.S. Food and Drug Administration. Urogynecologic surgical mesh: update on the safety and effectiveness of transvaginal placement for pelvic organ prolapse. Available at: https://www.fda.gov/downloads/MedicalDevices/Safety/AlertsandNotices/UCM262760.pdf.
36. Milani R, Salvatore S, Soligo M, et al. Functional and anatomical outcome of anterior and posterior vaginal prolapse repair with Prolene mesh. BJOG 2005;112:107–11.
37. Dunn GE, Hansen BL, Egger MJ, et al. Changed women: the long-term impact of vaginal mesh complications. Female Pelvic Med Reconstr Surg 2014; 20:131–6.
38. Abed H, Rahn DD, Lowenstein L, et al. Incidence and management of graft erosion, wound granulation, and dyspareunia following vaginal prolapse repair with graft materials: a systematic review. Int Urogynecol J 2011;22(7):789–98.

39. Crosby EC, Abernethy M, Berger MB, et al. Symptom resolution after operative management of complications from transvaginal mesh. Obstet Gynecol 2014;123:134–9.
40. Sung VW, Rogers RG, Schaffer JI, et al. Graft use in transvaginal pelvic organ prolapse repair: a systematic review. Obstet Gynecol 2008;112:1131–42.
41. Murphy M. Clinical practice guidelines on vaginal graft use from the Society of Gynecologic Surgeons. Obstet Gynecol 2008;112:1123–30.
42. Schimpf MO, Abed H, Sanses T, et al. Society of Gynecologic Surgeons systematic review group: graft and mesh use in transvaginal prolapse repair: a systematic review. Obstet Gynecol 2016;128(1):81–91.

Surgery for Apical Vaginal Prolapse

Transvaginal Suture-Based Repair

Ekene A. Enemchukwu, MD, MPH[a,b,*]

KEYWORDS

• Apical prolapse • Transvaginal repair • Native tissue repair • Posthysterectomy

KEY POINTS

- An estimated 300,000 women undergo pelvic organ prolapse (POP) surgery in the United States every year at a cost of more than 1 billion dollars per year.
- Apical support is required to achieve successful prolapse repair.
- Transvaginal native tissue repairs have the advantage of providing minimally invasive surgical repairs without the added risk of abdominal, laparoscopic, or robotic surgery while avoiding the risk of mesh augmentation.

INTRODUCTION

An estimated 300,000 women undergo pelvic organ prolapse (POP) surgery in the United States every year at an annual cost of more than 1 billion dollars.[1–3] The prevalence of POP is approximately 2.9% to 8% and increases with age.[4–6] POP is often associated with urinary, anorectal, and/or sexual dysfunction, all of which can negatively affect a woman's quality of life. As the population ages and women live longer and more active lives, the search for safe, durable surgical repairs continues. The estimated lifetime risk of undergoing POP surgery is as high as 20% with reoperation rates up to 30%.[7–9]

Risk factors for POP are well-defined, including advanced age, parity, obesity, and postmenopausal status.[7,10] POP occurs as a result of pelvic floor support defects. Defects in the level 1 support (uterosacral and cardinal ligament) can cause uterine prolapse or, in the posthysterectomy woman, descent of the vaginal cuff with herniation of the small or large bowel, also known as an enterocele.

Apical support is required to achieve successful prolapse repair.[11–13] Chen and colleagues,[12] confirmed the importance of good apical support for successful POP repair surgery in a study involving dynamic MRI.[12] The investigators radiographically demonstrated the significance of apical support disruption on the magnitude of anterior wall prolapse.[14]

Surgical management options are divided into obliterative or restorative techniques. Obliterative repairs have high success rates; however, they are reserved for women who no longer wish to be sexually active. Restorative repairs aim to restore vaginal length, axis, and function. These repairs can be approached vaginally or abdominally, and performed with or without biological or synthetic mesh augmentation. The surgical approach should be individualized based on patient factors, including suitability for surgical approach, desire for future sexual function, and past surgical history. The goal is to relieve bothersome symptoms. Historically, success was defined based on anatomic outcomes. However, among the most important recent developments

Disclosure Statement: None.

[a] Department of Urology, Stanford University, 300 Pasteur Drive, Grant Building, 2nd Floor, S287, Stanford, CA 94304, USA; [b] Department of Obstetrics & Gynecology, 300 Pasteur Drive- HG332 Stanford, CA 94305, USA
* 300 Pasteur Drive, Grant Building, 2nd Floor, S287, Stanford, CA 94304.
E-mail address: enemche@stanford.edu

Urol Clin N Am 46 (2019) 97–102
https://doi.org/10.1016/j.ucl.2018.08.004
0094-0143/19/© 2018 Elsevier Inc. All rights reserved.

in POP outcomes research is the realization that patient-reported outcomes are perhaps more important than anatomic outcomes.[15]

The open abdominal sacrocolpopexy is considered the gold standard approach for apical POP repair due to its superior anatomic outcomes, long-term durability, and lower rates of dyspareunia.[16] However, the open approach has largely been replaced by minimally invasive techniques using laparoscopic and robotic techniques. Diwadkar and colleagues[17] performed a systematic review and found that abdominal sacrocolpopexy and mesh-augmented repairs have superior outcomes. However, they also reported higher reoperation rates in mesh-augmented repairs than in native tissue transvaginal repairs. Transvaginal native tissue repairs have the advantage of providing minimally invasive surgical repairs without the added risk of abdominal, laparoscopic, or robotic surgery while avoiding the risk of mesh augmentation.[2] This article reviews transvaginal native tissue repairs for posthysterectomy vault prolapse.

TRANSVAGINAL NATIVE TISSUE TECHNIQUES

Historically, native tissue transvaginal techniques have involved suspension of the vaginal cuff to the sacrotuberous, sacrospinous, or uterosacral ligaments. Currently, the most commonly performed transvaginal vaginal vault repairs are the sacrospinous ligament fixation (SSLF) and the uterosacral ligament suspension (ULS). The iliococcygeus suspension is a modification of the SSLF that was originally developed to address the high rates of postoperative cystocele repair.[14] However, the procedure is typically performed bilaterally in the woman with a foreshortened vagina that fails to reach the sacrospinous ligament or with significant scarring that precludes safe exposure of the sacrospinous ligament.

Sacrospinous Ligament Fixation

The sacrospinous ligament extends from the ischial spine to the lateral sacrum, dividing the sciatic notch into the greater and lesser sciatic foramen. Numerous vessels and nerves lie posterior and lateral to the sacrospinous ligament, including the inferior gluteal vessels, the hypogastric venous plexus, the sciatic nerve, and the pudendal nerve and vessels. The sciatic nerve courses superior and lateral to sacrospinous ligament, whereas the pudendal nerve and vessels lie directly posterior to the ischial spine.

The SSLF procedure was first described in 1958 by Sederl.[18] Indications include total procidentia, posthysterectomy vaginal vault prolapse,[19] and hysteropexy. Traditionally, the SSLF is approached posteriorly. The extraperitoneal approach provides the added advantage of avoiding the peritoneal cavity, particularly in women with prior abdominal surgery and risk of pelvic adhesions. In the post-hysterectomy setting, an enterocele sac is often encountered and should be dissected off the vaginal wall. The enterocele sac can be entered and the abdominal contents reduced. The peritoneum is then closed in a purse-string fashion, incorporating the uterosacral ligaments and the anterior or posterior peritoneum. When the sacrospinous ligament is identified, 2 narrow retractors (eg, Breisky-Navratil) can be placed to protect the rectum and expose the ligament. The surgical technique then involves fixation of the vaginal vault using a combination of 2 to 4 nonabsorbable or delayed absorbable sutures and a Miya hook, Deschamps ligature carrier, Capio automatic suture capturing device (Boston Scientific, Marlborough, MA, USA), or (alternatively) suture passage under direct visualization. The sutures are placed 2 cm medial to the ischial spine and 0.5 cm below the superior edge of the sacrospinous ligament. Avoidance of an intervening suture bridge is important to allow adequate fibrosis and scarring. Therefore, vaginal length and the position of the vaginal apex should be assessed before attempting this approach to ensure the vaginal cuff is able to make direct contact with the sacrospinous ligament. If indicated, anterior colporrhaphy is performed and the SSLF sutures are subsequently passed through the posterior surface of the vaginal apex. The procedure can be performed either unilaterally or bilaterally. Bilateral placement has been reported in patients with recurrent vault prolapse or desire to maintain symmetry and a wide vaginal vault.[20] Jones and colleagues[21] performed a retrospective review of 103 women undergoing SSLF. Sixty-two women (60%) underwent bilateral suspension, whereas the remaining 41 (40%) underwent unilateral suspension. Although the follow-up was short (mean 4.6–8.6 months), the investigators observed no difference in anatomic cure rates in the unilateral and bilateral groups (90.2% and 85.5%, respectively) and did not observe increased morbidity or anterior prolapse recurrence in the bilateral group.

Alternatively, the sacrospinous ligament can be approached anteriorly using a paravaginal dissection. The Michigan 4-wall technique describes an apical approach that differs from the original technique by attaching both the anterior and posterior walls to the sacrospinous ligament. The investigators report that this allows proper selection of suspension points and reduces the risk of anterior vaginal wall recurrence.[22]

When the vaginal cuff does not reach the sacrospinous ligament, an iliococcygeus suspension can be performed. The dissection is performed in a similar fashion to the SSLF, with the dissection extending toward the ischial spine. Rather than exposing the SSLF, the tissue overlying the iliococcygeus muscle and fascia are mobilized bilaterally and a delayed absorbable suture is placed in the muscle and fascia.

Several retrospective cohort studies examine and report single-center SSLF safety and outcomes. Overall, success rates are high, except for an outlier that reports 8% success rate.[23] Sze and Karram[24] published a review in which surgical success varied widely depending on the definition used. They found success rates up to 94% (mean 75%) in more than 1000 subjects. Paraiso and colleagues[25] followed 243 women for a mean time of 73 months and observed apical recurrences in 8.2% of women and prolapse-free survival rates of 88.3%, 79.7%, and 51.9% at 1, 5, and 10 years, respectively. Maher and colleagues[26] compared the outcomes of SSLF and iliococcygeus suspension in a matched case controlled study and found no difference in recurrence or complication rates. For the SSLF group, the investigators reported a 94% success rate at a mean follow-up time of 19 months, with recurrence rates of 3%, 25%, and 6% for the apical, anterior, and posterior compartments, respectively. They observed similar rates of buttock pain, intraoperative hemorrhage, and subsequent cystocele in both groups.[26]

Randomized controlled trials comparing SSLF to mesh techniques are lacking. Maher and colleagues[27] randomized 95 women to SSLF or abdominal sacral colpopexy (ASC). After 2 years, they found no statistically significant difference in subjective (94% ASC and 91% SSLF) or objective success rates (76% ASC and 69% SSLF). They reported higher cost, slower return to activity, and longer operating room time with ASC. The group did not report reoperation rates. In a multicenter randomized controlled trial, Halaska and colleagues[28] randomized 168 women with posthysterectomy vaginal vault prolapse to SSLF or vaginal mesh (VM) repair. At 1-year follow-up, prolapse recurrence was 16.9% in the VM group and 39.4% in the SSLF group (P = .003). They observed no difference in quality of life improvements but observed a 20.8% mesh exposure rate in the VM group. In a single-center randomized controlled trial, Svabik and colleagues [29] randomized 142 women with posthysterectomy vaginal vault prolapse and levator ani avulsion injury to VM or SSLF. At 1 year, they observed objective success rates of 97% in the VM group and 35% in the SSLF group on clinical examination and ultrasound (P<.001). However, they did not detect any difference in subjective outcomes, which they attributed to being under- powered. The mesh erosion rate was 8.3% in the VM group.

Marguiles and colleagues[30] performed a systematic review of vaginal SSLF and reported anatomic cure rates of 98.3% apically, and 81.2% and 87.4% in the anterior and posterior vaginal compartments, respectively. POP symptoms resolved in 82% to 100% of subjects in 5 of the 11 studies reviewed.

Complications

Serious intraoperative and postoperative complications, such as hemorrhage, nerve injury, and rectal injury, are uncommon. The most common complication reported is buttock pain (0.4%–9.3%), which can be caused by injury or entrapment of a small nerve that runs through the SSLF-iliococcygeus muscle complex.[31] Buttock pain should be self-limited with complete resolution within 6 weeks. The pain is often managed expectantly with reassurance, antiinflammatory medications, and donut pillows to relieve discomfort while sitting. Pain that radiates down the leg is more likely caused by sciatic nerve or root entrapment. This occurs as a result of suture placement cephalad to the SSLF and warrants immediate reoperation for suture removal. Vulvovaginal pain and/or numbness can occur as a result of pudendal nerve injury or entrapment. Immediate reoperation for suture removal should be performed. Persistent buttock pain and paresthesia suggest nerve injuries and warrant reoperation to remove the sutures.

Other complications are relatively rare. Risk of intraoperative hemorrhage requiring blood transfusions is low (~2%). Intraoperative hemorrhage can occur as a result of inferior gluteal vessel, hypogastric venous plexus, pudendal vessel injuries, and perirectal veins. These injuries can often be managed with tight vaginal packing and hemostatic agents. Given the location of the SSLF, bleeding in this area is difficult to manage abdominally or with selective embolization.[24,31] Due to the proximity of the sacrospinous ligament to the rectum, a rectal injury can occur during dissection of the perirectal space or dissection of the SSLF. Rectal examination should always be performed. Intraoperative recognition and repair using standard technique is imperative to avoid complications. Pelvic infections, urinary retention, and urinary tract infections are uncommon and short-lived, as long the issue is identified and treated in a timely fashion. Finally, sexual dysfunction and dyspareunia due to vaginal shortening or narrowing have been reported in case series.[32,33] Avoidance of excessive vaginal wall trimming and prescribing postoperative estrogen cream can minimize this risk. Finally, although ureteral obstruction or injury is a rare complication of the SSLF procedure, intraoperative cystoscopy should always be performed if there is any concern for ureteral injury.

Uterosacral Ligament Suspension

The uterosacral ligament and cardinal ligaments are fascial condensations that suspend the vaginal apex. In 1927, Miller[34] first described plication and suspension of vaginal vault using these ligaments. In 2000, Shull and colleagues[35] described a modification of the technique. Although the original technique described an intraperitoneal approach, an extraperitoneal approach can be taken. However, an intraperitoneal allows proper palpation and, in some cases, visualization of important structures and landmarks. If performed concomitantly with hysterectomy, the ligaments should be tagged for subsequent identification. In the posthysterectomy setting, an enterocele sac may be encountered. The sac should be dissected off the vaginal cuff, the peritoneum carefully entered, and the bowels reduced. The ischial spines are important landmarks. The uterosacral ligament is located posterior and medial to the ischial spines, whereas the ureter is located ventral and lateral to the ischial spines. Occasionally, the ureters can be palpated. Intraoperative ureteral catheters can also aid in identification of the ureters, if needed. 2 to 3 delayed absorbable sutures are placed through each ligament bilaterally, with or without the assistance of an Allis clamp. The sutures can then be passed through the layers of anterior and posterior vaginal walls. Nonabsorbable suture can be placed using a pulley-type stitch to avoid the presence of permanent suture in the vaginal lumen. The pulley stitch technique is performed by including the muscular layer of the vaginal wall while excluding the epithelial layer. Finally, cystoscopy should always be performed to ensure patency of bilateral ureters before and after tying the sutures.

Similar to the SSLF technique, numerous outcomes studies exist in the medical literature. Silva and colleagues[34] observed a recurrence rate of 15% in a single-center cohort study in which failure was defined as symptomatic prolapse of stage 2 or greater. Shull and colleagues[35] performed a retrospective review of 298 women undergoing ULS and reported a recurrence rate of 13% in 1 or more compartment.

In a cohort of 983 subjects, Unger and colleagues[36] observed that 14.4% of cases had POP recurrences, 11% had recurrences beyond the hymen, 10.6% were symptomatic with bulge symptoms, and 3.4% required reoperation.

Complications

Serious complications are infrequent. Ureteral obstruction was the most commonly reported complication (4.8%) in 1 large cohort.[36] A metaanalysis by Marguiles and collegues [30] reported a rate of 1.8%. In most cases, removal of the offending suture relieved the obstruction. In rare cases, ureteral reimplantation was required (0%–0.6%). Cystotomy (1%), small bowel obstruction (0.8%) and ileus (0.1%) were also reported.[36]

SACROSPINOUS LIGAMENT FIXATION VERSUS UTEROSACRAL LIGAMENT SUSPENSION

One randomized controlled trial comparing the efficacy and safety of the ULS and SSLF has been reported in the literature. In the randomized multicenter Operations and Pelvic Muscle Training in the Management of Apical Support Loss (OPTIMAL) trial, Barber and colleagues[37] randomized 374 women with stage 2 to 4 POP to ULS or SSLF. Success was defined as (1) no apical descent greater than one-third in the vaginal vault, (2) no bothersome vaginal bulge symptoms, and (3) no retreatment for POP. At 24 months, no significant differences were observed in anatomic outcomes, length of hospitalization, blood loss, and surgical time. Anatomic success rates were 59.2% and 60.5% for ULS and SSLF, respectively. Recently, the same group published a follow-up in which 285 (86%) women completed the 5-year extension of the OPTIMAL trial.[38] Overall, 5.1% required reoperation at 2 years. Combined, 18% developed bulge symptoms, and 17.5% developed anterior or posterior POP beyond the hymen.

Adverse events were unique to each repair. For SSLF, neurologic pain occurred more frequently, at a rate of 12.4% compared with 6.9% in the ULS group. Ureteral obstruction was more common in the ULS group, with a rate of 3.2%. Five cases (2.7%) resolved with suture removal, 1 (0.5%) required stent placement, and 1 (0.5%) was not recognized intraoperatively.

SUMMARY

Transvaginal apical native tissue POP repairs are safe and effective. Although studies suggest transvaginal mesh-augmented repairs are more durable, the risk of mesh-related complications is not insignificant. The risk and benefits of each technique should be discussed with the patient and weighed against individual patient factors.

REFERENCES

1. Wu JM, Kawasaki A, Hundley AF, et al. Predicting the number of women who will undergo incontinence and prolapse surgery, 2010 to 2050. Am J Obstet Gynecol 2011;205(3):230.e1–5.
2. Boyles SH, Weber AM, Meyn L. Procedures for pelvic organ prolapse in the United States, 1979–1997. Am J Obstet Gynecol 2003;188:108–15.
3. Subak LL, Waetjen LE, van den Eden S, et al. Cost of pelvic organ prolapse surgery in the United States. Obstet Gynecol 2002;98:646–51.
4. Nygaard I, Barber MD, Burgio KL, et al. Prevalence of symptomatic pelvic floor disorders in US women. JAMA 2008;300:1311–6.
5. Rortveit G, Brown JS, Thom DH, et al. Symptomatic pelvic organ prolapse: prevalence and risk factors in a population-based, racially diverse cohort. Obstet Gynecol 2007;109:1396–403.
6. Tegerstedt G, Maehle-Schmidt M, Nyrén O, et al. Prevalence of symptomatic pelvic organ prolapse in a Swedish population. Int Urogynecol J Pelvic Floor Dysfunct 2005;16:497–503.
7. Olsen AL, Smith VJ, Bergstrom JO, et al. Epidemiology of surgically managed pelvic organ prolapse and urinary incontinence. Obstet Gynecol 1997;89:501–6.
8. Wu JM, Matthews CA, Conover MM, et al. Lifetime risk of stress urinary incontinence or pelvic organ prolapse surgery. Obstet Gynecol 2014;123(6):1201–6.
9. Committee on Practice Bulletins-Gynecology, American Urogynecologic Society. Practice bulletin No. 185: pelvic organ prolapse. Obstet Gynecol 2017;130(5):e234–50.
10. Jelovsek JE, Maher C, Barber MD. Pelvic organ prolapse. Lancet 2007;369:1027.
11. Marchionni M, Bracco GL, Checcucci V, et al. True incidence of vaginal vault prolapse. Thirteen years of experience. J Reprod Med 1999;44(8):679–84.
12. Chen L, Ashton-Miller JA, Hsu Y, et al. Interaction between apical supports and levator ani in anterior vaginal support: theoretical analysis. Obstet Gynecol 2006;108(2):324–32.
13. Summers A, Winkel LA, Hussain HK, et al. The relationship between anterior and apical compartment support. Am J Obstet Gynecol 2006;194(5):1438–43.
14. Shull BL. Pelvic organ prolapse. Am J Obstet Gynecol 1999;181(1):6–11.
15. Barber MD, Brubaker L, Nygaard I, et al. Defining success after surgery for pelvic organ prolapse. Obstet Gynecol 2009;114:600–9.
16. Maher C, Feiner B, Baessler K, et al. Surgery for women with apical vaginal prolapse. Cochrane Database Syst Rev 2016;(10):CD012376.
17. Diwadkar GB, Barber MD, Feiner B, et al. Complication and reoperation rates after apical vaginal prolapse surgical repair: a systematic review. Obstet Gynecol 2009;113(2 Pt 1):367–73.
18. Sederl J. Zur operation des prolapses der blind endigenden sheiden. Geburtshilfe Frauenheilkd 1958;18:824–8.
19. Morley GW, DeLancey JOL. Sacrospinous ligament fixation for eversion of the vagina. Am J Obstet Gynecol 1988;158:872.
20. Pohl JF, Frattarelli JL. Bilateral transvaginal sacrospinous colpopexy: preliminary experience. Am J Obstet Gynecol 1997;177:1356.
21. Jones CM, Hatch K, Harrigill K. Unilateral and Bilateral Sacrospinous Ligament Fixation for Pelvic Prolapse: A Nonconcurrent Cohort Comparison. Female Pelvic Med Reconstr Surg 2001;7(1):27–33.
22. Kearney R, DeLancey JO. Selecting suspension points and excising the vagina during Michigan four-wall sacrospinous suspension. Obstet Gynecol 2003;101:325–30.
23. Holley RJ, Varner RE, Gleason BP, et al. Recurrent pelvic support defects after sacrospinous ligament fixation for vaginal vault prolapse. J Am Coll Surg 1995;180:444–8.
24. Sze EH, Karram MM. Transvaginal repair of vault prolapse: a review. Obstet Gynecol 1997;89:466e75.
25. Paraiso MFR, Ballard LA, Walters MD, et al. Pelvic support defects and visceral and sexual function in women treated with sacrospinous ligament suspension and pelvic reconstruction. Am J Obstet Gynecol 1996;175:1423e30 [discussion: 1430e1].
26. Maher CF, Murray CJ, Carey MP, et al. Iliococcygeus or sacrospinous fixation for vaginal vault prolapse. Obstet Gynecol 2001;98:40e4.
27. Maher CF, Qatawneh AM, Dwyer PL, et al. Abdominal sacral colpopexy or vaginal sacrospinous colpopexy for vaginal vault prolapse: a prospective randomized study. Am J Obstet Gynecol 2004;190(1):20–6.
28. Halaska M, Maxova K, Sottner O, et al. A multicenter, randomized, prospective, controlled study comparing sacrospinous fixation and transvaginal mesh in the treatment of posthysterectomy vaginal vault prolapse. Am J Obstet Gynecol 2012;207(4):301.e1-7.
29. Svabik K, Martan A, Masata J, et al. Comparison of vaginal mesh repair with sacrospinous vaginal colpopexy in the management of vaginal vault prolapse after hysterectomy in patients with levator ani avulsion: a randomized controlled trial. Ultrasound Obstet Gynecol 2014;43(4):365–71.
30. Marguiles RU, Rogers MA, Morgan DM. Outcomes of transvaginal uterosacral ligament suspension: systematic review and metaanalysis. Am J Obstet Gynecol 2010;202:124.
31. Karram MM, Ridway BM, Walters MD. Surgical treatment of vaginal apex prolapse. In: Walters MD, Karram MM, editors. Urogynecology and female

pelvic reconstructive surgery. 4th edition. Philadelphia: Elsevier Saunders; 2015. p. 372–4.
32. Given FT Jr, Muhlendorf IK, Browning GM. Vaginal length and sexual function after colpopexy for complete uterovaginal eversion. Am J Obstet Gynecol 1993;169:284e7.
33. Holley RL, Varner RE, Gleason BP, et al. Sexual function after sacrospinous ligament fixation for vaginal vault prolapse. J Reprod Med 1996;41(5):355–8.
34. Silva WA, Pauls RN, Segal JL, et al. Uterosacral ligament vault suspension: five-year outcomes. Obstet Gynecol 2006;108:255–63.
35. Shull BL, Bachofen C, Coates KW, et al. A transvaginal approach to repair of apical and other associated sites of pelvic organ prolapse with uterosacral ligaments. Am J Obstet Gynecol 2000;183(6):1365–73.
36. Unger CA, Walters MD, Ridgeway B, et al. Incidence of adverse events after uterosacral colpopexy for uterovaginal and posthysterectomy vault prolapse. Am J Obstet Gynecol 2015;212(5):603.e1–7.
37. Barber MD, Brubaker L, Burgio KL, et al. Comparison of 2 transvaginal surgical approaches and perioperative behavioral therapy for apical vaginal prolapse: the OPTIMAL randomized trial. JAMA 2014;311(10):1023–34.
38. Jelovsek JE, Barber MD, Brubaker L, et al. Effect of uterosacral ligament suspension vs sacrospinous ligament fixation with or without perioperative behavioral therapy for pelvic organ vaginal prolapse on surgical outcomes and prolapse symptoms at 5 years in the OPTIMAL randomized clinical trial. JAMA 2018;319(15):1554–65.

Surgery for Apical Vaginal Prolapse after Hysterectomy

Transvaginal Mesh-Based Repair

Shannon L. Wallace, MD[a,*], Raveen Syan, MD[b], Eric R. Sokol, MD[c,d]

KEYWORDS

• Transvaginal mesh • Apical prolapse • Outcomes • Vaginal vault prolapse • Prolapse repair

KEY POINTS

- Numerous mesh products have been made available for transvaginal apical prolapse repair.
- Although data are limited, studies indicate that transvaginal mesh placement does not result in superior anatomic or subjective outcomes compared with native tissue for apical prolapse.
- Given unique complications specific to mesh use, it is reasonable to reserve mesh use for high-risk cases.
- Current trials are underway comparing native tissue with ultralightweight mesh for transvaginal apical prolapse repair.
- American Urogynecologic Society (AUGS) and the Society of Urodynamics, Female Pelvic Medicine and Urogenital Reconstruction have recommended that surgeons thoroughly counsel their patients, and those performing these procedures should have additional specialized expertise.

INTRODUCTION

There has been a rapid development of surgical innovations to improve outcomes and reduce prolapse recurrence rates in female pelvic reconstructive surgery.[1] The success of mesh-augmented repairs in abdominal hernia surgeries led vaginal prolapse surgeons to hypothesize that synthetic mesh would improve the durability of apical repair,[2] especially given consistent and robust evidence that mesh use in the sacrocolpopexy approach provides superior anatomic outcomes for apical vaginal prolapse compared with native tissue vaginal prolapse repair. Given the requirement for abdominal entry and a longer operating time with sacrocolpopexy, surgeons adapted this mesh-based technology to a transvaginal approach.[3] In 2001, the Food and Drug Administration (FDA) approved the use of commercial mesh kits for transvaginal prolapse repair. Vaginal mesh and associated kits were first introduced in the United States in 2005 for augmentation of

Disclosure Statement: No disclosures (S.L. Wallace, R. Syan). Board of Directors, American Urogynecologic Society. Grant support: National Institutes of Health, ACell, Coloplast, Cook MyoSite, and Foundation for Female Health Awareness. Equity - Pelvalon (E.R. Sokol).

[a] Department of Obstetrics and Gynecology, Division of Urogynecology and Pelvic Reconstructive Surgery, Stanford University School of Medicine, 300 Pasteur Drive, Grant S287, Stanford, CA 94305, USA; [b] Department of Urology, Stanford University School of Medicine, 300 Pasteur Drive, Grant S287, Stanford, CA 94305, USA; [c] Department of Obstetrics and Gynecology (by Courtesy), Division of Urogynecology and Pelvic Reconstructive Surgery, Stanford University School of Medicine, 300 Pasteur Drive, Room G304a, Stanford, CA 94305, USA; [d] Department of Urology (by Courtesy), Stanford University School of Medicine, 300 Pasteur Drive, Room G304a, Stanford, CA 94305, USA

* Corresponding author.

E-mail address: shanwall@stanford.edu

Urol Clin N Am 46 (2019) 103–111
https://doi.org/10.1016/j.ucl.2018.08.005
0094-0143/19/© 2018 Elsevier Inc. All rights reserved.

suture-based native tissue repair of anterior, posterior, and apical vaginal prolapse.

Initial observational studies of synthetic implants suggested comparable apical anatomic results, lower failure rates, shorter operative time, and lower morbidity. However, short-term safety data and long-term outcome data were insufficient when these products were brought to market. Increasing reports of mesh-related complications including vaginal erosions, infections, granulomas, dyspareunia, vesicovaginal fistulas, and chronic pain, and a lack of superior functional outcomes, led to public warnings from the FDA about their safety.[4]

The future of transvaginal mesh in female pelvic reconstructive surgery is uncertain and placement has become controversial in the face of complications and litigation. Here we review the history of the introduction of transvaginal mesh, mesh classifications, outcome data, the FDA investigations and warnings, and finally statements from the American Congress of Obstetricians and Gynecologists, the American Urogynecologic Society (AUGS), the Society of Gynecologic Surgeons, and the Society of Urodynamics, Female Pelvic Medicine and Urogenital Reconstruction.

TYPES OF MESH PRODUCTS

Synthetic and biologic grafts have been used for the treatment of pelvic organ prolapse. Although mesh is usually used to refer to synthetic mesh, "transvaginal mesh" is used to describe synthetic mesh, xenografts, allografts, and autografts.

SYNTHETIC MESH

Synthetic meshes were initially categorized into four types based on pore size (macroporous or microporous), filament type (monofilament or multifilament), surface properties (coated or non-coated), and architecture (knit or woven). Pore size determines which cells can enter the mesh and affects infection risk, mesh density, and flexibility. Transvaginal mesh is usually classified by pore size, where pore size greater than 75 μm is considered macroporous, and less than 10 μm is considered microporous. Type 1 mesh is macroporous, type 2 mesh is microporous, type 3 has macroporous and microporous components, and type 4 has very small pores. Most mesh used in pelvic floor reconstruction is type 1 monofilament, macroporous, polypropylene mesh. The large pore size and monofilaments in this mesh encourage tissue ingrowth and integration, and also allow macrophages to permeate through the mesh and prevent bacterial adherence. Synthetic meshes have minimal risk of donor-to-host immune reactions but have increased risk of foreign body bacterial colonization leading to infections and erosions.[5–9]

Initially, only anterior and posterior compartment repairs were augmented with mesh. Mesh was placed between the vaginal epithelium and underlying endopelvic connective tissue. Mesh was then developed to augment apical suspensions with attachment to pelvic supportive connective tissue structures, including the sacrospinous-coccygeus ligament complex, arcus tendineus fascia pelvis (ATFP), iliococcygeus fascia, and obturator membrane.[10]

Mesh Patches

Small mesh patches were first used in transvaginal prolapse repair of a single compartment. In apical repair, these small patches were fixed to the iliococcygeus fascia, the ATFP, or the sacrospinous ligament. Mesh patches were then developed into tension-free vaginal kits.

Early Mesh Kits

Early transvaginal mesh kits used metal trocars to guide placement of mesh arms through the obturator membrane. These kits used a standardized piece of mesh and a consistent approach reducing the likelihood of excessive tension on the mesh arms. In some cases, once the mesh was placed, the endopelvic fascia was sutured, creating a double-layer closure to reinforce the apical mesh suspension. The vagina was then closed without trimming the vaginal wall to minimize the occurrence of vaginal mesh exposure. The first kits that targeted apical vaginal compartment repair included the Gynecare Prolift (Ethicon, Inc, Somerville, NJ), the Perigee and the Apogee (American Medical Systems, Minnetonka, MN), and the Avaulta (BARD, Covington, GA). Currently, all early mesh kits have been discontinued and withdrawn from the market.

- The Prolift system was available as a four-armed anterior implant, a two-armed posterior implant, or a six-armed combined implant. This system used a metal trocar with a flexible mesh retrieval device that was passed through the obturator foramen and through the sacrospinous ligament bilaterally to correct apical vaginal wall defects.
- The Perigee system was designed to treat anterior and apical vaginal compartment defects. This system used four transobturator side-specific trocars that were passed through the ATFP just proximal to the level of the ischial spine and to the level of the bladder neck.

- The Apogee system was designed to treat posterior and apical vaginal compartment defects. This system used two side-specific trocars passed through the ATFP to the level of the ischial spines via the ischiorectal fossa.
- The Avaulta anterior system was designed to treat anterior and apical vaginal compartment defects. This system had compartment-specific trocars with a flexible InSnare retrieval device that was passed anteriorly through the obturator foramen to place the proximal mesh arms near the ischial spine and the distal arms at the level of the bladder neck. There were two additional distal posterior arms that attached bilaterally to the junction of the bulbocavernosus and transverse perineal muscles. The mesh was available with or without an acellular collagen barrier.

Second-Generation Mesh Kits

The subsequent second-generation mesh kits use either a pulley stitch or self-fixating tips to attach mesh to the sacrospinous ligament and ATFP. These newer kits include the Pinnacle (Boston Scientific, Marlborough, MA), the Elevate (American Medical Systems, Minnetonka, MN), the Uphold system (Boston Scientific, Marlborough, MA) and Coloplast Restorelle Direct Fix (Coloplast, Minneapolis, MN). The Prosima (Ethicon, Inc, Somerville, NJ) system was a single-incision, fixation-less system that was held into place by a pessary-like vaginal support device for 3 weeks postoperatively.

- The Pinnacle system was designed to treat anterior and apical prolapse. The Capio needle driver device secured four mesh arms through the sacrospinous ligament and the ATFP bilaterally. This system has been withdrawn from the market.
- The Elevate system was designed to treat apical and either anterior or posterior prolapse. The mesh was placed with self-fixating tips through the sacrospinous ligaments (and the obturator foramen for the anterior system) bilaterally. This system has been withdrawn from the market.
- The anterior Prosima was the first fixation-less vaginal mesh system. The mesh was laid in place with an inserter such that the arms extended just anterior and superior to the ischial spines and lay across the ATFP. A pessary-like vaginal support device was sewn into place at the time of surgery and stayed in place for 3 to 4 weeks to allow tissue ingrowth into the graft. This system has been withdrawn from the market.
- The Uphold system is designed to treat apical prolapse with or without the uterus in situ. The Capio needle driver secures two mesh arms through the sacrospinous ligament and the mesh is secured to the vaginal vault or cervix and under the bladder. This system is currently on the market and is the subject of an FDA 522 postmarket surveillance study.
- The Coloplast Restorelle Direct Fix is designed to treat apical and either anterior or posterior prolapse. This ultralightweight mesh is secured by two mesh arms to the sacrospinous ligament with the Digitex suture delivery device. Additional mesh arms are secured to the obturator internus fixation point for distal anterior fixation or to the ATFP for distal posterior fixation. This system is currently on the market and is the subject of an FDA 522 postmarket surveillance study.

BIOLOGIC MESH GRAFTS

Several biologic grafts have been marketed to augment vaginal prolapse repair. Surgeons may choose to use biologic mesh in patients who have a high recurrence risk, such as those with poor tissue quality, increased intra-abdominal pressure from obesity, chronic constipation, chronic coughing or heavy lifting, or those who have failed previous native tissue repairs. The complications and success rates of biologic mesh grafts are varied because these meshes differ in origin (autograft, allograft, xenograft) and source (dermis, fascia, pericardium, small intestinal submucosa) with different degradation rates and tissue rebuilding processes.[11] However, there is currently no evidence that biologic grafts improve prolapse outcomes or reduce risks compared with native-tissue prolapse repair.

XENOGRAFT MESH

Xenograft meshes consist of acellular extracts of collagen harvested from nonhuman (bovine, porcine) sources. They pose a foreign body infection risk and some patients may refuse the implantation of animal-derived material because of cultural or religious beliefs.

ACell MatriStem

MatriStem Pelvic Floor Matrix (ACell, Columbia, MD) is composed of a porcine-derived extracellular matrix and is intended for implantation during anterior, posterior, and apical defect repair to reinforce soft tissue. The device is supplied in a multilayer sheet configuration in sizes up to 10 cm × 15 cm. ACell MatriStem is currently being compared with native tissue prolapse repair as part of an FDA 522 postmarket surveillance study, but the company recently announced that it was putting pursuit of the pelvic organ prolapse market on hold.

ALLOGRAFTS

Allograft mesh is composed of tissue transplanted between genetically nonidentical individuals of the same species and is most often derived from cadaveric fascia of human donors. Allograft mesh is biocompatible, but still may trigger a host immunologic response, even after decellularization removes nonhost antigens. By using allograft mesh, the morbidity of autologous fascia harvest is avoided but multiple prospective studies have shown that outcomes are less beneficial when compared with autologous fascia and synthetic meshes.

AUTOGRAFTS

Autograft meshes are donor tissues that are harvested from a different site on the same individual's body. The most commonly used autografts are fascia lata and rectus fascia. Autograft mesh does not trigger a host-immune response but clear disadvantages are that a surgical procedure is necessary to harvest an unpredictable quantity and quality of tissue.[12]

INDICATIONS AND CONTRAINDICATIONS OF TRANSVAGINAL MESH FOR APICAL PROLAPSE

Transvaginal mesh for apical vaginal repair still remains a durable option for high-risk patients with severe or recurrent prolapse. There are no evidence-based guidelines regarding absolute contraindications for the use of vaginal mesh, so surgeons performing apical repair with transvaginal mesh should use good judgment when selecting patients. Increasing body mass index has been associated with increased risk of mesh exposure and wound infections.[13] Diabetes and smoking are associated with decreased vascularity, poor tissue healing, and increased mesh exposure, so placement of a foreign body may not be recommended in these patients. Additionally, patients with severe vaginal atrophy or chronic pelvic pain may not be candidates for mesh because placement may exacerbate these symptoms.[13] Patients undergoing transvaginal mesh prolapse surgery should be thoroughly counseled and informed about the risks and benefits of mesh use.[14,15]

OUTCOMES ASSOCIATED WITH TRANSVAGINAL APICAL MESH REPAIR

The benefit of transvaginal mesh placement has been assessed with respect to the separate compartments of repair. A large meta-analysis performed by the Society of Gynecologic Surgeons' Systematic Review Group[16] found that, when directly comparing the benefit of transvaginal apical mesh-based repair with suture-based repair, outcomes were similar. The benefit of mesh-based repair was only obvious in the anterior compartment, but the group notes that high-quality studies directly comparing apical suspension alone are limited. Overall, 3% to 10% of patients who undergo apical surgical repair have recurrent vaginal vault prolapse.[17,18] It is difficult to directly compare studies because of differences in type of mesh, type of repair, and surgical technique, although overall trends can be elucidated.[19]

ANATOMIC AND SUBJECTIVE OUTCOMES

Type of Apical Repair

There have been limited studies comparing the role of transvaginal mesh placement for treatment of apical prolapse with different types of apical suspension. A study by de Tayrac and colleagues[20] compared fixation of a polypropylene intravaginal sling with an infracoccygeal sacropexy versus a sacrospinous suspension for uterine or vaginal vault suspension. With 24 patients randomized to infracoccygeal sacropexy and 25 patients randomized to sacrospinous suspension, they found that prolapse cure rates and symptom scores were equivalent between the groups. They did note that infracoccygeal sacropexy was associated with a reduced rate of postoperative pain and cystocele recurrence.

Comparison with Native Tissue Repair

Only one study compared the role of mesh with native repair for the treatment of the apical compartment alone. Cosma and colleagues[21] performed a retrospective case control study of outcomes in patients with stage III-IV pelvic organ prolapse who underwent uterosacral ligament suspension without mesh with those who received posterior intravaginal slingplasty (included multifilament and monofilament polypropylene mesh types). At a mean follow-up of more than 4 years, they found recurrent vault prolapse rates were higher in patients who had uterosacral ligament suspension without mesh in stage IV prolapse; however, reoperation rates and subjective cure rates were equivalent. They concluded that the first-line intervention should be a non-mesh-based vault repair, with mesh reserved for select severe cases.

Vaginal Kits

Several vaginal kits that involved apical suspension have been created. Of these, a couple are still on the market and are proceeding with FDA-mandated postmarket surveillance studies. However, we provide a brief summary of the findings of these kits before their removal, because they help to understand the role of vaginal mesh in apical repairs.

Prolift

Many studies have been performed that examine the benefit of the Prolift vaginal kit. Iglesia and colleagues[22] randomized patients with stage 2 to 4 prolapse to vaginal colpopexy with or without synthetic monofilament polypropylene mesh. Sixty-five patients were recruited before the study was halted, as vaginal mesh erosion rates reached 15.6% (the predetermined stopping criteria was 15%). They showed at 3 months that objective and subjective cure rates were similar between the groups. Equivalency was confirmed in this study population at 12-month follow-up[23]; however, repeat operations at 1 year were performed only in the mesh group because of mesh erosion. Given this finding, the authors concluded that risks associated with the Prolift system may outweigh the benefits of its use. A subsequent 3-year outcomes study by this group confirmed that long-term cure rates remained similar between groups.[24]

Withagen and colleagues[19] compared native tissue repair (sacrospinous or uterosacral ligament suspension) with Prolift and similarly showed that 6- and 12-month outcomes for treatment of the apical compartment and failure rates (defined as stage II prolapse or greater or repeat surgery in the apical compartment) were similar between groups. Improvements in symptoms and quality of life were the same between the groups.

Halaska and colleagues[25] showed that patients randomized to Prolift had lower prolapse recurrence rates than patients who underwent a sacrospinous ligament fixation (SSLF) at 12 months, where the most common compartment of recurrence was anterior. Svabik and colleagues[26] compared patients with known levator ani avulsion injury who were randomized to Prolift or SSLF native tissue repair, and also found higher recurrence rates with SSLF at 12 months follow-up. They do note, however, that subjective cure rates were equivalent. Dos Reis Brandão da Silveira and colleagues[27] also showed higher recurrence rate in the anterior compartment at 12 months when comparing patients randomized to Prolift versus native tissue repair. Similar to other studies, subjective improvement was similar between groups, although they did note that improvements in the Prolapse Quality-of-Life Questionnaire were higher in the mesh group compared with the native tissue group.

Elevate

The Elevate anterior and posterior mesh kit was compared with native tissue repair for stage 2 or higher prolapse.[28] Anatomic success rates in the anterior compartment were significantly higher in the Elevate group, as seen in Prolift studies. This was not maintained for the apical compartment.

Perigee

A retrospective review was performed comparing patients who underwent Perigee anterior repair with synthetic mesh plus SSLF versus patients with native tissue anterior repair and SSLF.[29] At 3 years follow-up, they showed that cumulative cure rates were higher in the anterior compartment and the apical compartment in the mesh group. They also found higher subjective success rates in the mesh group.

Uphold

The Uphold system is still available on the market and is part of an FDA-mandated multicenter post-market surveillance study. This product has been assessed in multiple prospective studies but has not been compared with native tissue alone. A 5-year follow-up of patients treated with Uphold apical repair, with or without anterior repair, reported good anatomic outcomes (Pelvic Organ Prolapse Quantification (POPQ) stage <2 in 83%) and improvements in quality of life.[30] However, they note that three patients (1.5% of the study group) had severe pain that persisted despite treatment. This same group showed that Uphold without anterior colporrhaphy had significantly higher risk of prolapse-related bother compared with those who received concomitant anterior colporrhaphy.[31]

Comparison of Vaginal Kits

Despite the previously mentioned retrospective review showing subjective and objective improvements in the Perigee group compared with native tissue,[29] which was not seen in most Prolift studies, a prospective study by Long and colleagues[32] showed that success rates were similar between patients receiving Perigee or Prolift systems, as were mesh-related complications. A prospective study comparing Prolift and Gynecare mesh found that despite similar anatomic outcomes, patients reported higher improvements on the Pelvic Floor Disability Index-20 questionnaire in the Prolift group.[33] Mesh complications were similar. The authors conclude that Gynecare mesh should be considered more than Prolift given the lower cost of this product.

Studies comparing different mesh kits are limited, but they seem to have similar anatomic outcomes and cure rates. There is not sufficient evidence to consider one superior to the other.

Biologic Grafts

Studies examining outcomes with biologic grafts are limited. Ramanah and colleagues[34] performed a retrospective review comparing the use of InteXen (American Medical Systems) porcine dermis graft with native tissue repair and noted equivalent objective and subjective recurrence rates. No mesh erosion was seen in the graft group. A retrospective review of cystocele repair using porcine dermis interposition grafts noted no apical recurrences in the 71% of patients who had received concomitant vaginal vault prolapse repair.[35]

Sexual Outcomes

There have been mixed findings regarding sexual outcomes with use of transvaginal mesh placement. When comparing polypropylene mesh placement with an infracoccygeal sacropexy versus sacrospinous suspension, there was no difference in dyspareunia rates.[20] When comparing patients who had posterior intravaginal slingplasty versus native tissue, Cosma and colleagues[21] showed that there was no overall difference in questionnaire data looking at urinary, sexual health, and quality of life measures between the groups. However, they noted that in the five patients who had mesh erosion, this resulted in worsening quality of life measures and sexual function.

Several studies examining the use of the Prolift system showed no difference in sexual questionnaires or dyspareunia rates.[19,22,23] By comparison, Milani and colleagues[36] specifically focused on sexual function outcomes when patients were randomized to native tissue versus mesh-based repair (Prolift). All patients were sexually active at time of enrollment. They found that despite equivalency in total scores from the Pelvic Organ Prolapse/Urinary Incontinence Sexual Function Questionnaire (PSIQ-12), sexual function actually improved in the native tissue repair group, which did not occur in the mesh group. They also noted that mesh exposure seemed to be independently associated with lower PSIQ-12 scores, which was similar to what was described by Cosma and colleagues.[21] This study suggests that complications related to mesh use may worsen sexual outcomes.

With regards to the Uphold system, the Nordic TVM Group found that in patients who completed preoperative sexual function questionnaires (PISQ-12), 66% had a worsening of sexual function.[31] This was mainly related to a decline in scores in the partner-related domain. They found that performing a concomitant anterior repair did not predict worse sexual function.

With regards to biologic mesh, Ramanah and colleagues[34] showed no vaginal erosion or retraction with biologic graft (InteXen porcine dermis graft).

COMPLICATIONS

Numerous complications have been described that are specific to use of mesh, which include vaginal erosion, urinary tract erosions, immobility of the vagina, pain, and vaginal shortening.[17]

Erosion rates in the VAMP Study using Prolift were 15.6% at 3 months, and some patients required intraoperative intervention.[22] At 12 months, the only patients who required reoperation were in the mesh group, for mesh erosion.[23] Withagen's group reported similar rates of erosion of 16.9%.[19]

With regards to pain, Withagen and colleagues[19] reported similar rates of de novo pain between native tissue repair and the Prolift repair system. The Nordic TVM Group showed that 1.5% of their study population who received Uphold had persistent severe pain despite treatment, although they did not have a comparison group to determine pain attributable to the Uphold system.[30] Bowel injury was seen in one patient in the Prolift study performed by Dos Reis Brandão da Silveira and colleagues.[27] They also reported a single case of rectal extrusion at 6 months postoperatively that, although asymptomatic, did require vaginal and transrectal surgical removal, with reported uneventful recovery. Su and colleagues[28] showed that the Elevate system had longer hospital stay and higher estimated intraoperative blood loss. Type of vaginal kit was not associated with worse mesh-related complications.[16,17]

Outcomes following a 1-year prospective study of use of Uphold for treatment of apical prolapse with or without concomitant anterior repair reported rates of serious complications to be 4.7%, and minor complications 9.7%.[31] They comment that these rates are comparable with complication rates seen in other transvaginal mesh kits.

Overall, several studies comparing mesh use with native tissue repair report similar overall complication rates; however, mesh-specific complications, such as erosion/extrusion, pain, and rectal extrusion, have been reported, and must be considered when using transvaginal mesh.

FOOD AND DRUG ADMINISTRATION HISTORY

When transvaginal mesh was presented to the FDA, it was approved as a class II medical device. A class II device (low- to moderate-risk) poses slightly higher risks than a class I device (low-risk) and has special controls concerning labeling and postmarket surveillance. However, class II devices do not need premarket long-term safety and efficacy trials as would have been needed for a class III device (high-risk device). In 2001, the FDA found vaginal mesh to be similar to mesh used for abdominal hernia repair and approved its use without premarket clinical data or scientific review.

Between 2005 and 2008, the FDA received more than 1000 reports of complications from nine surgical mesh manufacturers. In October 2008, the FDA issued a Public Health Notification warning that "although rare, these complications can have serious consequences, including erosion, infection, and perforation of bowel and vessels associated with the kits designed for transvaginal placement." The FDA issued recommendations on how to properly counsel patients about complications and how to report nonserious adverse events, such as mesh erosion and dyspareunia.

After reviewing data from its Manufacturer and User Device Experience database, the FDA released an update in July 2011 stating that "serious complications associated with surgical mesh for transvaginal repair of pelvic organ prolapse are not rare and it is not clear that transvaginal prolapse repair with mesh is more effective than traditional nonmesh repair."[37] In the 2011 update, the FDA listed recommendations for patients that included specific questions to ask their surgeon regarding mesh, alternative options, how complications are handled, and surgical follow-up. After the FDA notification, estimates of transvaginal mesh procedures significantly declined. In 2014, the FDA reclassified surgical mesh for transvaginal prolapse repair from class II to class III.[38] This new reclassification required manufacturers of transvaginal mesh for pelvic organ prolapse to obtain premarket approval and undergo rigorous testing of their devices to increase assurance of safety and efficacy. Of note, this reclassification excluded mesh used for either stress urinary incontinence or transabdominal pelvic organ prolapse repair, such as sacrocolpopexy.

SOCIETY OPINIONS

In December 2011, The American Congress of Obstetricians and Gynecologists and the AUGS released a committee opinion offering recommendations for safe and effective use of vaginal mesh for pelvic organ prolapse repair. They recommended restricting transvaginal mesh to high-risk patients with recurrent prolapse or medical conditions. They also agreed with the FDA assessment that long-term clinical trials and follow-up were needed to compare the benefits and safety of transvaginal mesh repair with native tissue repair.[39]

Since the initial FDA statements, public awareness of mesh complications has been raised and numerous litigious claims have been filed against surgeons and device manufacturers. Many hospitals and surgeons have moved away from transvaginal mesh use because of fears of litigation. In response to the FDA warnings and the decrease in transvaginal mesh procedures, AUGS and the Society for Urodynamics, Female Pelvic Medicine and Urogenital Reconstruction published a joint position statement on vaginal mesh.[40] In their position statement they emphasized that these devices should not be removed from the market or restricted because they may be a good option in the right patient. They encouraged surgeons to thoroughly counsel their patients and recommended that surgeons performing these procedures should have additional specialized expertise. Finally, they specified that the FDA warnings exclude mesh placed transvaginally for midurethral slings or abdominally for sacrocolpopexy.

The transvaginal mesh litigation and controversy also shrouds the international pelvic surgery community. In 2017, Australia removed transvaginal mesh and single-incision mesh slings from the market and New Zealand has banned all manufacturers of mesh, including midurethral slings. Many countries are considering waiting for evidence of safety and efficacy before allowing the marketing of these products.

SUMMARY

Many transvaginal mesh products have been created to address vaginal vault suspension. These synthetic-based mesh products have not been shown to reliably improve outcomes with respect to apical compartment repair. Although data are limited, recurrence rates and subjective measures of improvement are equivalent compared with native tissue repair, and the different types of vaginal kits have not proven superior to one another. Given the known unique complications specific to mesh with equivalent outcomes with respect to the apical compartment, it is reasonable to reserve mesh use for specific cases, such as recurrence after native-tissue repair or for patient-specific risk factors, where mesh may have a more defined benefit.

REFERENCES

1. Jelovsek JE, Maher C, Barber MD. Pelvic organ prolapse. Lancet 2007;369:1027–38.
2. Sung VW, Rogers RG, Schaffer JI, et al. Graft use in transvaginal pelvic organ prolapse repair: a systematic review. Obstet Gynecol 2008;112:1131–42.
3. Barber MD, Maher C. Apical prolapse. Int Urogynecol J 2013;24:1815–33.
4. Maher C, Feiner B, Baessler K, et al. Transvaginal mesh or grafts compared with native tissue repair for vaginal prolapse. Cochrane Database Syst Rev 2016;(2):CD012079.
5. Amid P. Classification of biomaterials and their related complications in abdominal wall hernia surgery. Hernia 1997;1:15–21.
6. Greca FH, Souza-Filho ZA, Giovanini A, et al. The influence of porosity on the integration histology of two polypropylene meshes for the treatment of abdominal wall defects in dogs. Hernia 2008;12:45–9.
7. Klinge UKB. Modified classification of surgical meshes for hernia repair based on the analysis of 1000 explanted meshes. Hernia 2011;16:251–8.
8. Weyhe D, Schmitz I, Belyaev O, et al. Experimental comparison of monofile light and heavy polypropylene meshes: less weight does not mean less biological response. World J Surg 2006;30:1586–91.
9. Dietz HP, Vancaillie P, Svehla M, et al. Mechanical properties of urogynecologic implant materials. Int Urogynecol J Pelvic Floor Dysfunct 2003;14:239–43.
10. Larouche M, Merovitz L, Correa JA, et al. Outcomes of trocar-guided Gynemesh PS™ versus single-incision trocarless Polyform™ transvaginal mesh procedures. Int Urogynecol J 2015;26:71–7.
11. Schimpf MO, Abed H, Sanses T, et al. Graft and mesh use in transvaginal prolapse repair: a systematic review. Obstet Gynecol 2016;28:81–91.
12. Patel H, Ostergard D, Sternschuss G. Polypropylene mesh and the host response. Int Urogynecol J Pelvic Floor Dysfunct 2012;23:669–79.
13. Bako A, Dhar R. Review of synthetic mesh-related complication in pelvic floor reconstructive surgery. Int Urogynecol J Pelvic Floor Dysfunct 2008;20: 103–11.
14. Deffieux X, Letouzey V, Savary D, et al. Prevention of complications related to the use of prosthetic meshes in prolapse surgery: guidelines for clinical practice. Eur J Obstet Gynecol Reprod Biol 2012; 165:170–80.
15. Miller D, Milani AL, Sutherland SE, et al. Informed surgical consent for a mesh/graft-augmented vaginal repair of pelvic organ prolapse. Consensus of the 2nd IUGA Grafts Roundtable: optimizing safety and appropriateness of graft use in transvaginal pelvic reconstructive surgery. Int Urogynecol J 2012;23:S33–42.
16. Schimpf MO, Abed H, Sanses T, et al. Society of gynecologic surgeons systematic review group. graft and mesh use in transvaginal prolapse repair: a systematic review. Obstet Gynecol 2016;128:81–91.
17. Klauschie JL, Cornella JL. Surgical treatment of vaginal vault prolapse: a historic summary and review of outcomes. Female Pelvic Med Reconstr Surg 2012;18:10–7.
18. Prodigalidad LT, Peled Y, Stanton SL, et al. Longterm results of prolapse recurrence and functional outcome after vaginal hysterectomy. Int J Gynaecol Obstet 2013;120(1):57–60.
19. Withagen MI, Milani AL, den Boon J, et al. Trocar-guided mesh compared with conventional vaginal repair in recurrent prolapse: a randomized controlled trial. Obstet Gynecol 2011;117:242–50.
20. de Tayrac R, Mathe ML, Bader G, et al. Infracoccygeal sacropexy or sacrospinous suspension for uterine or vaginal vault prolapse. Int J Gynaecol Obstet 2008;100:154–9.
21. Cosma S, Menato G, Preti M, et al. Advanced uterovaginal prolapse and vaginal vault suspension: synthetic mesh vs native tissue repair. Arch Gynecol Obstet 2014;289:1053–60.
22. Iglesia CB, Sokol AI, Sokol ER, et al. Vaginal mesh for prolapse: a randomized controlled trial. Obstet Gynecol 2010;116:93–303.
23. Sokol AI, Iglesia CB, Kudish BI, et al. One-year objective and functional outcomes of a randomized clinical trial of vaginal mesh for prolapse. Am J Obstet Gynecol 2012;206:86.e1-9.
24. Gutman RE, Nosti PA, Sokol AI, et al. Three-year outcomes of vaginal mesh for prolapse: a randomized controlled trial. Obstet Gynecol 2013;122:770–7.
25. Halaska M, Maxova K, Sottner O, et al. A multicenter, randomized, prospective, controlled study comparing sacrospinous fixation and transvaginal mesh in the treatment of posthysterectomy vaginal vault prolapse. Am J Obstet Gynecol 2012;207: 301.e1-7.
26. Svabik K, Martan A, Masata J, et al. Comparison of vaginal mesh repair with sacrospinous vaginal colpopexy in the management of vaginal vault prolapse after hysterectomy in patients with levator ani avulsion: a randomized controlled trial. Ultrasound Obstet Gynecol 2014;43:365–71.
27. Dos Reis Brandão da Silveira S, Haddad J, de Jármy-Di Bella ZI NF, et al. Multicenter, randomized

trial comparing native vaginal tissue repair and synthetic mesh repair for genital prolapse surgical treatment. Int Urogynecol J 2015;26:335–42.

28. Su TH, Lau HH, Huang WC, et al. Single-incision mesh repair versus traditional native tissue repair for pelvic organ prolapse: results of a cohort study. Int Urogynecol J 2014;25:901–8.
29. Lo TS, Pue LB, Tan YL, et al. Long-term outcomes of synthetic transobturator nonabsorbable anterior mesh versus anterior colporrhaphy in symptomatic, advanced pelvic organ prolapse surgery. Int Urogynecol J 2014;25:257–64.
30. Rahkola-Soisalo P, Mikkola TS, Altman D, et al. Pelvic organ prolapse repair using the uphold vaginal support system: 5-year follow-up. Female Pelvic Med Reconstr Surg 2017. [Epub ahead of print].
31. Rahkola-Soisalo P, Altman D, Falconer C, et al. Quality of life after Uphold™ Vaginal Support System surgery for apical pelvic organ prolapse-A prospective multicenter study. Eur J Obstet Gynecol Reprod Biol 2017;208:86–90.
32. Long CY, Hsu CS, Jang MY, et al. Comparison of clinical outcome and urodynamic findings using "Perigee and/or Apogee" versus "Prolift anterior and/or posterior" system devices for the treatment of pelvic organ prolapse. Int Urogynecol J 2011; 22:233–9.
33. Chen YS, Cao Q, Ding JX, et al. Midterm prospective comparison of vaginal repair with mesh vs Prolift system devices for prolapse. Eur J Obstet Gynecol Reprod Biol 2012;164:221–6.
34. Ramanah R, Mairot J, Clement MC, et al. Evaluating the porcine dermis graft InteXen in three-compartment transvaginal pelvic organ prolapse repair. Int Urogynecol J 2010;21:1151–6.
35. Gomelsky A, Rudy DC, Dmochowski RR. Porcine dermis interposition graft for repair of high grade anterior compartment defects with or without concomitant pelvic organ prolapse procedures. J Urol 2004;171:1581–4.
36. Milani AL, Withagen MI, The HS, et al. Sexual function following trocar-guided mesh or vaginal native tissue repair in recurrent prolapse: a randomized controlled trial. J Sex Med 2011;8:2944–53.
37. FDA update on serious complications associated with transvaginal placement of surgical mesh for pelvic organ prolapse: FDA safety communication. Silver Spring (MD): United States Food and Drug Administration; 2011.
38. FDA reclassification of surgical mesh for transvaginal pelvic organ prolapse repair and surgical instrumentation for urogynecologic surgical mesh procedures; designation of special controls for urogynecological surgical mesh instrumentation. Silver Spring (MD): United States Food and Drug Administration; 2014.
39. ACOG Committee Opinion No.513. Vaginal placement of synthetic mesh for pelvic organ prolapse. Obstet Gynecol 2011;118(6):1459–64.
40. AUGS (American Urogynecological Society). Position statement on restriction of surgical options for pelvic floor disorders. Female Pelvic Med Reconstr Surg 2013;19(4):199–201.

Surgery for Apical Vaginal Prolapse After Hysterectomy

Abdominal Sacrocolpopexy

Wai Lee, MD[a,*], Justina Tam, MD[b], Kathleen Kobashi, MD[a]

KEYWORDS

• Apical vaginal prolapse • Abdominal sacrocolpopexy • Female urology • Urogynecology
• Review paper

KEY POINTS

- Although patient selection for abdominal sacrocolpopexy has evolved, the appropriate surgical approach for apical pelvic organ prolapse should align with patient goals.
- Minimally invasive approaches for abdominal sacrocolpopexy provide clear benefits to patient recovery, albeit at a higher cost.
- Other advances in surgical technique for abdominal sacrocolpopexy have been described, but further studies are needed before making recommendations.
- Controversies still exist with the use of both vaginal and abdominal mesh, rendering it imperative that the surgeon stay well-informed of these issues.

INTRODUCTION

Pelvic organ prolapse (POP) affects nearly one-half of the female population.[1] Approximately 11% to 19% of women with POP will undergo surgery for their prolapse.[2,3] In 1997, there were 225,964 women who underwent surgery for POP at an estimated cost of $1 trillion to the United States economy.[4] This number is expected to increase with the aging population, giving attention to quality of life issues, and an increased awareness of pelvic floor disorders. One estimate has the annual number of surgeries for POP increasing by 48% from 210,700 in 2010 to 310,050 in 2050.[5]

In cases of symptomatic apical prolapse, there are obliterative and restorative approaches to corrective surgery. Restorative approaches can be performed either transvaginally or abdominally (**Fig. 1**). The principle abdominal approach to address apical prolapse is the abdominal sacrocolpopexy (SCP), which remains the gold standard for healthy patients desiring a restorative procedure.[6–8] This finding may be attributed to findings that the SCP was more durable than vaginal approaches or had less postoperative dyspareunia.[9] Moreover, the advent of minimally invasive approaches has resulted in decreased morbidity to the procedure with similar anatomic outcomes compared with the open SCP, albeit at a higher cost.[7] Among urologists, there has been an exponential rise in SCPs performed (8 cases in 2003 to 398 cases in 2012) and this has been noted particularly with minimally invasive approaches (282 cases in 2012).[10] The advantages and limitations

Disclosure Statement: J. Tam has a research grant with Medtronic for a study on overactive bladder. W. Lee's spouse has a research grant with Medtronic. K. Kobashi serves on the advisory board and speakers' bureau and/or is an investigator for Medtronic, Allergan, Axonics, and Avadel.

[a] Virginia Mason Medical Center, 1100 Ninth Avenue, Seattle, WA 98111, USA; [b] Department of Urology, Stony Brook Medicine, 101 Nicolls Road, HSC Level 9-040, Stony Brook, NY 11794, USA
* Corresponding author.
E-mail address: WaiLee@gmail.com

Urol Clin N Am 46 (2019) 113–121
https://doi.org/10.1016/j.ucl.2018.08.006
0094-0143/19/© 2018 Elsevier Inc. All rights reserved.

Abbreviations	
CARE	Colpopexy and Urinary Reduction Efforts
LSCP	Laparoscopic sacrocolpopexy
POP	Pelvic organ prolapse
RSCP	Robotic sacrocolpopexy
SCP	Sacrocolpopexy
SUI	Stress urinary incontinence

of the SCP are discussed in this article along with recent advances in surgical technique, preoperative evaluation, and patient selection.

PATIENT EVALUATION

Abdominal SCP is an ideal surgical approach for women with symptomatic apical POP desiring a restorative repair. Patients who have high-grade anterior and/or posterior compartment prolapse are also excellent candidates for SCP given the high probability that the apical compartment is involved.[11] Those who have failed prior vaginal repairs or require concomitant abdominal surgery are also particularly well-suited for SCP.[12] Surgical candidates should undergo a thorough history and physical examination, including pelvic examination to evaluate for anterior, apical, and posterior compartment prolapse. This may be graded using the POP quantification system POP-Q, an objective and reproducible grading system.[13] For those who have not undergone a hysterectomy, further evaluation should be considered. This process may entail a gynecologic examination including a Pap smear and/or transvaginal ultrasound examination in postmenopausal women or in patients with abnormal uterine bleeding.[12]

A patient with POP may describe symptoms of vaginal pressure, heaviness, and/or the presence of a vaginal bulge, with or without concomitant urinary, bowel, and/or sexual functional disorders. Regarding urinary symptoms, stress and urgency urinary incontinence are common, and lower urinary tract symptoms such as urgency, frequency, sensation of incomplete bladder emptying, urinary intermittency, and hesitancy may also be present. Bowel dysfunction, including the need to perform manual reduction of prolapse to facilitate complete evacuation of the bowels, and sexual dysfunction, such as dyspareunia or fear of being active in the face of prolapse, may also be problematic. Quality of life questionnaires may be helpful to quantify bothersome symptoms, and a voiding diary may provide valuable objective information. A postvoid residual assessment should also be performed. Hydronephrosis owing to ureteral kinking from prolapse occurs in an estimated 7.1% to 22.4% of patients with severe POP. Accordingly, abdominal ultrasound examination should also be considered in women with high-grade POP. Treatment of advanced POP has been shown to result in improvement or resolution of the hydronephrosis.[14–16]

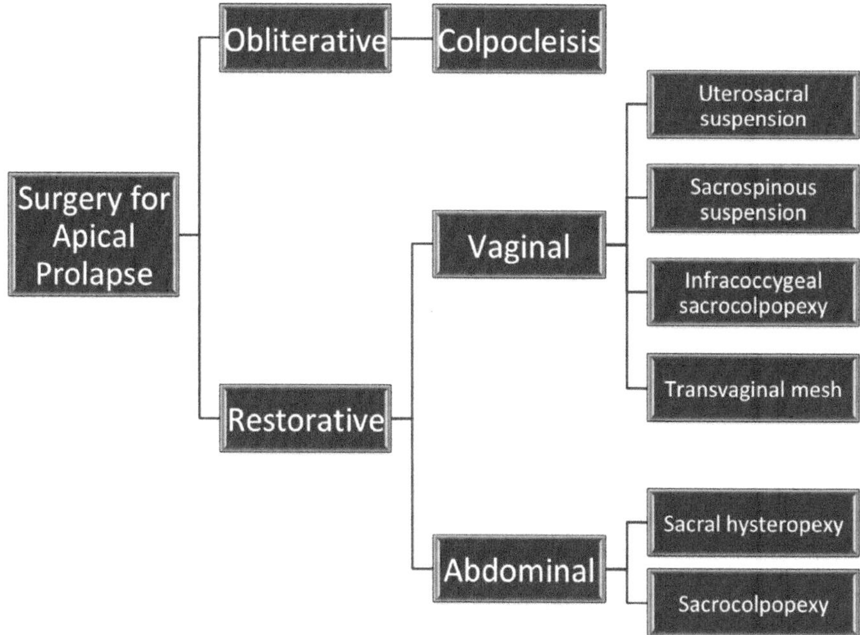

Fig. 1. Surgical approach to apical pelvic organ prolapse.

Urodynamic evaluation may be considered in women with lower urinary tract symptoms, especially in those with high-grade prolapse and incomplete bladder emptying, which may be due to the prolapse or an underlying element of detrusor underactivity.[12] In addition, as stress urinary incontinence (SUI) may develop in approximately 25% of patients after prolapse repair,[17] evaluation for occult SUI with the prolapse reduced should also be performed.[18–20] Women who exhibited urodynamic SUI during prolapse reduction were more likely to report postoperative SUI after prolapse repair. This information is important in the counseling of patients considering SCP because a concomitant antiincontinence procedure may be warranted to minimize the risk of de novo SUI.[20,21] The long-term outcome of the Colpopexy and Urinary Reduction Efforts (CARE) trial reported that urethropexy during open SCP prevented SUI for a longer time (median, 3.11 years) when compared with no urethropexy (median, 0.94 years).[22] A large retrospective study including 7000 patients found that concomitant antiincontinence procedures in patients undergoing minimally invasive SCP did not increase the risk of clinically important surgical complications other than urinary tract infection.[23]

A patient's prior surgical history should also be reviewed, with particular attention to prior antiincontinence procedures, pelvic floor reconstruction or mesh, which may impact surgical decision making.[19] It should also be considered that patients might be unable to accurately recall their surgical history. Prior studies have demonstrated that patient recall of mesh placement after midurethral sling decreased right after informed consent was performed (98% could recall mesh was being placed) to just 6 weeks postoperatively (84% could recall mesh was placed; $P = .01$). This well-designed study demonstrated that patients are prone to forgetting critical components of their surgery, despite high health literacy or a regimented consent protocol.[24] This finding necessitates obtaining a patient's prior surgical records before undertaking POP surgery when possible.

Physicians are often less inclined to offer SCP to older women, instead opting for more conservative approaches such as a pessary or vaginal procedures. For minimally invasive ASC, the cardiopulmonary strain from insufflation and Trendelenburg positioning must be considered during surgical planning.[19] However, appropriately selected elderly patients may be suitable candidates for surgical treatment after obtaining proper medical clearance.[6,14,19,25] Moreover, Robinson and colleagues[25] (2013) found that women 65 years or older with apical POP had low rates of perioperative morbidity regardless if they underwent robotic or transvaginal repairs of their prolapse. They also found that risk classification systems such as the American Society of Anesthesiologists physical classification system or the Charlson Comorbidity Index were inadequate predictors of perioperative complications.

There may also be a reluctance to offer surgery to obese patients who may pose a greater technical challenge in the operating room or who may be at increased risk for perioperative complications and/or prolapse recurrence.[26,27] There are conflicting data on whether obese patients undergoing SCP have increased operative time.[28,29] A large, retrospective study including nearly 5000 women found that obese and overweight patients had significantly longer operative times in both laparoscopic and open SCPs.[28] In contrast, a retrospective study of patients undergoing robotic-assisted SCP (RSCP) found that there were no significant differences in operative time, intraoperative complications, blood loss, or hospital stay in obese patients compared with those with a normal body mass index. The authors suggest that these findings may be due to the advantages that robotic surgery offers that may allow surgeons to overcome issues encountered in open and laparoscopic procedures such as impaired visualization, limited space, and compromised dexterity.[30]

In addition to a thorough patient history and physical examination, a critical component in the patient evaluation is an understanding of their goals of treatment. A prospective study revealed that resolution of urinary symptoms, ability to perform daily activities, and sexual function are at least as important as the resolution of prolapse symptoms regardless of the severity of the patient's prolapse, suggesting that understanding the patient's goals is essential. Indeed, this may be at least as important as anatomic cure in providing good care and achieving patient satisfaction.[31] Once the patient's goals are identified, appropriate counseling to allow patients to make an informed decision regarding their treatment plan is necessary.[32]

DEFINITION OF SUCCESS

As with many surgeries performed with the goal of alleviating a patient's symptoms and improving quality of life, there exists a dichotomy in the definition of success after surgery for POP. Objective measures for success may be based upon anatomy (correction of prolapse on physical examination) or the need for eventual reoperation or pessary device (recurrence of prolapse).

Subjective assessment may include patient self-reported degree of bother, presence or absence of a bulge, level of activity, dyspareunia, quality of life and/or overall satisfaction. There is however, no standardized definition of success following surgery for POP, leading to widely variable outcomes in the literature.[33]

During long-term follow-up of the CARE trial, outcomes were stratified into subjective, anatomic or composite (either subjective or anatomic) failure. Anatomic failure after SCP was defined as postoperative POP requiring reoperation or pessary or recurrent prolapse on POP-Q, defined as the vaginal apex descending to below the upper third of the vagina (C <- $^{2}/_{3}$ TVL) or anterior or posterior vaginal wall prolapse beyond the hymen (Ba >0 or Bp >0 cm). Interestingly, half of the anatomic failures at 7 years follow-up denied symptoms and did not require further treatment.[22] Moreover, up to 17% of symptomatic patients had no significant POP (Stage 0 or 1) on examination.[33]

The discordance between anatomic and symptomatic success in POP surgery remains a source of challenge when evaluating the literature.[34] A standardized definition of success after SCP that emphasizes subjective improvement or cure while accounting for bothersome prolapse or reoperation is needed.

ABDOMINAL SACROCOLPOPEXY VERSUS VAGINAL APPROACHES

A Cochrane meta-analysis by Maher and colleagues[9] (2013) demonstrated that open SCP had superior anatomic durability when compared with transvaginal approaches. However, only 3 randomized studies were included for vaginal sacrospinous ligament fixation, and these studies reported no significant difference in subjective improvement. Open SCP was also found to have superior reduction in apical prolapse when compared with high vaginal uterosacral suspension (100% vs 82.5%, P = .033) at 12 months follow-up.[35] In another meta-analysis, Siddiqui and colleagues[36] (2015) found no difference in postoperative dyspareunia between open SCP and transvaginal approaches. Open SCP was also associated with higher rates of ileus and small bowel obstruction (OR 9.45, 95% CI 3.39–26.4) as well as mesh and suture complications (OR 3.26, 95% CI 1.62–6.56, P<.001).

The abdominal approach was also demonstrated to have superior objective outcomes when compared with vaginal mesh. In a randomized control trial, Maher and colleagues (2011) found laparoscopic SCP (LSCP) had a 77% objective success rate (POP-Q sites Aa Ba C Ap and Bp <−1 cm individually or in total) whereas the anatomic success rate of total vaginal mesh (Prolift) using the same definition was only 43% (P<.001). Patients in the LSCP group also had higher satisfaction rates, shorter hospital stays, and lower reoperation rates at 2-year follow-up. The vaginal mesh group did however, have significantly shorter operative times when compared with the LSCP group (50 vs 97 minutes, P<.001).[37]

MINIMALLY INVASIVE VERSUS OPEN APPROACHES

Although abdominal SCP is considered the gold standard procedure in the treatment of apical POP with success rates ranging from 58% to 100%,[6] it is associated with high rates of morbidity,[38] and new techniques such as LSCP and robotic SCP (RSCP) have gained in popularity. Retrospective studies have found that, compared with minimally invasive SCP, open SCP was associated with higher rates of complications (7.6% vs 5.1%),[39] longer duration of hospitalization, shorter operative time, higher rate of perioperative blood transfusion and blood loss, higher rate of 30-day hospital readmission, and higher rates of 30-day reoperation.[38,39] Recurrence rates have been found to be similar between minimally invasive SCP and open SCP groups.[38] A randomized study by Costantini and colleagues[40] (2016) showed that both open SCP and LSCP were efficacious; however, more apical recurrences occurred following LSCP, albeit without the need for reoperation, at an average follow-up of 41.7 months. Based on these findings and the results of an equivalence trial performed by Freeman and colleagues[41] (2013), LSCP and open SCP can be performed with similar outcomes.[40]

Robotic technology has improved the ability to perform laparoscopic pelvic surgery by improving dexterity and precision of instrumentation, as well as allowing 3-dimensional visualization. A video of robotic-assisted laparoscopic SCP by Jennifer Anger, Ja-Hong Kim, and Peter Schulam is available at: https://www.youtube.com/watch?v=v3uzF2J1Rh8. Not surprisingly, RSCP has gained popularity. There have been conflicting results when comparing LSCP and RSCP. A retrospective study by Nosti and colleagues[38] (2014) suggested that, compared with RSCP, LSCP was associated with greater overall complication rates and greater likelihood of conversion to an open approach (4.0% vs 0.4%; P<.01). In contrast, a retrospective study by Unger and colleagues[42] suggested that RSCP was associated with a higher rate of bladder injury, greater blood loss, and a higher reoperation rate for recurrent POP. However, there was no statistically significant difference in anatomic failure rates between RSCP and LSCP.[38] Randomized studies have demonstrated that RSCP is associated with longer operative time and increased pain and cost when compared with LSCP; however, both groups result in improvement in pelvic floor symptoms and quality of life measures.[43–45]

In conclusion, minimally invasive techniques have been demonstrated to have equivalent efficacy when compared with the traditional open abdominal SCP. Accordingly, with comparable efficacy regardless of approach, both RSCP and LSCP have become increasingly popular.

ADVANCES IN ROBOTIC SACROCOLPOPEXY

Technological advancements have led to the use of robotic techniques, and these techniques continue to evolve. There is no consensus on the amount of vaginal dissection that should be performed, or the number, type, or location of sutures that should be placed to secure the suspending mesh.[46] Traditionally permanent suture was used to prevent detachment of the mesh from the vagina. However, a retrospective study demonstrated that the use of delayed absorbable monofilament suture resulted in a reduced rate of mesh exposure when compared with permanent braided suture (0% vs 3.7%, respectively; $P = .002$) as well as no significant difference in POP recurrence. This method has resulted in a shift by some surgeons to use absorbable suture options.[47]

The use of barbed sutures has also been reported in the literature. In a randomized study by Tan-Kim and colleagues[48] (2015), women undergoing LSCP or RSCP were randomized to have their mesh secured using either running barbed suture or nonbarbed interrupted sutures. The barbed suture was found to take significantly less time to place (29 minutes vs 42 minutes; $P<.001$), and at the 12-month follow-up there was no significant difference in anatomic failure between the 2 groups. Other studies have found the use of barbed sutures for SCP mesh fixation to the vaginal wall to be safe with reduced operative times.[49] Despite these results, surgeons reported better ease of suture placement and greater intraoperative satisfaction with mesh appearance when using nonbarbed sutures.[48] A video of RSCP using V-Loc may be viewed at: https://www.youtube.com/watch?v=TC5Ke2fZY9w.

Retroperitonealization of mesh during SCP has been recommended to prevent formation of adhesions. There have been studies, however, that seem to contradict the need for this step. A retrospective study performed by Kulhan and colleagues[50] (2018) suggested that patients who underwent retroperitonealization of the mesh had worse pain and higher rates of postoperative de novo dyspareunia and urinary urgency than those who did not undergo retroperitonealization of the mesh. There was no difference in postoperative complications between the 2 groups. Elneil and colleagues[51] (2005) performed a prospective case series of 128 patients who underwent LSCP, hysteropexy, or cervicopexy with mesh. The peritoneum was not closed over the mesh and, at a median follow-up of 19 months, there were no bowel-related complications as a result of leaving the mesh uncovered. The authors suggest that the dissection required to retroperitonealize the mesh may result in inadvertent injuries such that can cause retroperitoneal hematoma, bowel injury, ureteral injury, or ureteral kinking during reapproximation of the peritoneum. Conversely, although these results suggest that retroperitonealization of the mesh is not necessary, there have been reports of bowel ischemia as a result of exposed mesh causing small bowel adhesions and resultant strangulation.[52] Indeed, on follow-up laparoscopy, women who had undergone prior laparoscopic hysteropexy with uncovered mesh were noted to have adhesions of bowel to the mesh.[53] At our institution, we routinely retroperitonealize the mesh during RSCP with running barbed sutures to prevent any potential adhesions or bowel-related complications.

A completely retroperitoneal approach has also been described. Onol and Onol (2012)[54] reported on the use of a retroperitoneal approach, in which a Pfannenstiel or midline incision is made, and the peritoneum over the bladder is retracted to allow vesicovaginal dissection. The sacral promontory is exposed by mobilizing the right parietal peritoneum and the mesh is secured to the anterior vaginal wall at the vaginal cuff or cervix and to the anterior longitudinal ligament. The authors reported objective and subjective cure rates of 91.3% and 86.9%, respectively. This technique is intended to avoid the risks of transperitoneal access and the need for the Trendelenburg positioning that is required in traditional approaches to SCP. This surgical approach was also performed by Anding and colleagues[55] (2018) on 15 patients using polyvinylidenfluoride mesh loaded with iron particles to visualize the mesh on subsequent MRI. All patients had complete anatomic and functional cure after surgery without any complications. Radiographic correction of prolapse on MRI was also demonstrated. Further long-term studies on the extraperitoneal SCP are still necessary at this point.

Matanes and colleagues[56] (2017) reported on a single-port RSCP in which the procedure is performed through a single entry point, usually at the umbilicus, that allows for improved cosmesis. The authors reported improvement in the learning curve over time by the single surgeon in regard to operative time (median of 226 minutes for first 15 cases vs a median of 156 minutes for the next 10 cases). There were no adverse intraoperative events, although 1 of the 25 patients required reoperation for small bowel obstruction. Of note, this patient did not have her mesh retroperitonealized and this event altered the surgeon's approach toward subsequent patients, who had their meshes retroperitonealized. Further long-term data are required to evaluate the usefulness of this modality.

One advantage of minimally invasive techniques is decreased length of hospital stay over open approaches, although patients are generally kept in the hospital for observation overnight after an RSCP. A retrospective study explored the safety of same day discharge after RSCP suggesting that this practice is safe and does not result in increased health care utilization such as phone calls or clinic, urgent care, or emergency department visits, or 30-day readmission rates.[57] Such cost-saving measures may be needed as the trend toward more minimally invasive techniques continues. Further research on the various techniques and new technologies is needed, because the technique of SCP will continue to evolve and improve.

MULTICOMPARTMENT PROLAPSE

Although abdominal SCP is considered the gold standard for apical prolapse, apical prolapse often occurs concomitantly with anterior and posterior vaginal wall prolapse. In most instances, apical repair also restores anterior and posterior support. In cadaveric studies, LSCP provided excellent apical suspension and anterior vaginal wall support.[58] There was also resolution of posterior POP with SCP alone in the extended CARE trial. Ninety-six percent of women (23/24) with apical and posterior (Ap $\geq$0) prolapse at baseline had resolution of their posterior prolapse with SCP alone at 5-year follow-up. No patients required further surgery for their posterior compartment.[59]

Another study by Kaser and colleagues[60] (2012) found similar anatomic and functional outcomes between women who underwent SCP alone versus those who underwent SCP with posterior colporrhaphy. It should be noted, however, that in this retrospective study the women in the SCP with posterior colporrhaphy group had significantly worse posterior prolapse at baseline compared with the group that only underwent SCP. Although these studies are prone to selection bias because the criteria for concurrent posterior repair is left up to the surgeon, there seems to be adequate evidence that SCP alone provides enough posterior vaginal compartment support and alleviation of functional outcomes, such as defecatory dysfunction.[7]

REGARDING MESH

In 2011, the United States Food and Drug Administration released a statement acknowledging lower rates of mesh complications in abdominally placed mesh for POP repair when compared with vaginal mesh.[61] However, mesh-related complications remain a consideration after SCP. In the CARE trial, the 7-year estimated risk for vaginal mesh exposure after abdominal SCP was 10%, with 65% of these patients requiring surgical excision.[22] Some investigators have suggested that this rate may be inflated secondary to increased detection from close follow-up of patients[62] or because many patients in this trial received non–type I polypropylene mesh.[7]

Strategies to minimize mesh complications include smoking cessation, avoiding perioperative infections, and avoiding the use of postoperative vaginal estrogen when no contraindications exist. Some authors have also advocated for the use of delayed absorbable suture material for mesh attachment to the vagina and sacral promontory.[7] Another strategy has been the avoidance of mesh altogether. Culligan and colleagues[63] (2005) randomized patients to receive either cadaveric fascia lata or polypropylene mesh during open SCP. Objective cure rates were significantly higher in the mesh group (91%) when compared with the fascial group (68%; P = .007) at the 1-year follow-up. The mesh group had higher (26%) rates of graft-related events, such as erosions, wound breakdown, postoperative fever, or ileus, when compared with the cadaveric fascia group (15%), but this difference was not significant (P = .19).

The use of autologous fascia for SCP has also been described in the literature. Latini and colleagues[64] (2004) performed open SCP using autologous fascia lata on 10 women with no morbidity associated with the harvest site. Patients also had sustained improvement of POP (stage II or lower) at a mean follow-up of 30.5 months. Maloney and colleagues[65] (1990) reported a 90% cure rate of vaginal vault prolapse using rectus fascia as graft material in open SCP. However, this small case series only reported on 10 women and long-term follow-up is unknown. The use of autologous rectus fascia has also been described during open SCP when there is a high risk for infection[66] or in the salvage setting in patients after complete excision of SCP mesh.[67] A video of transabdominal SCP with autologous rectus fascia graft by Adrienne Quirouet, Nitya Abraham, and Howard B. Goldman may be downloaded from: https://link.springer.com/article/10.1007%2Fs00192-016-2987-7. Autologous fascia has also been used in RSCP in the primary setting. Twiss and colleagues[68] (2018) harvested autologous fascia lata in 5 patients via lateral upper thigh incisions that were shaped into a Y-mesh for RSCP. Only short-term follow-up of 5 weeks was reported, but the technique seemed to be a safe and feasible alternative. A video of total autologous fascia lata RSCP: A new technique (video abstract V10–05) by Christian Twiss, Frank Lin, and Joel Funk may be accessed with subscription through the 2018 American Urologic Association meeting surgical video library: https://auau.auanet.org/. It will be very interesting to see the long-term follow-up for this cohort.

The litigious atmosphere surrounding the use of mesh in POP has influenced patient attitudes toward surgical mesh.[69] A survey of 170 female urology patients found that as many as 88% had seen a mesh-related attorney advertisement in the past 6 months and more than one-half of the respondents are exposed to such ads more than once a week.[70] Physician awareness of the heightened anxiety regarding mesh may help to answer patient questions during preoperative counseling. It is important to guide patient concerns and to educate them about distinctions between the risks of transvaginal mesh and the safety and efficacy of abdominal mesh or midurethral sling.[71]

SUMMARY

With the number of ASCs performed by urologists increasing, it is important for the surgeon to stay well-informed of advances and controversies surrounding this surgical technique.[10] For patients who opt for definitive repair of their apical prolapse, the surgical approach should align with the patient goals. Based on the strong objective and subjective outcomes, ASC for apical POP remains the gold standard for women desiring a restorative repair. Although minimally invasive approaches have a higher cost than open surgery, they have excellent patient outcomes and should be considered. Variations in minimally invasive techniques are described, but the overarching principles of SCP have remained unchanged over the years. During this evolving era in pelvic floor medicine, it is imperative that surgeons partner with their patients to find the optimal solution for their POP and pelvic floor dysfunction.

REFERENCES

1. Beck R. Pelvic relaxational prolapse. Principles and practice of clinical gynecology. New York: John Wiley & Sons; 1983. p. 677–85.
2. Wu JM, Matthews CA, Conover MM, et al. Lifetime risk of stress urinary incontinence or pelvic organ prolapse surgery. Obstet Gynecol 2014;123(6):1201–6.
3. Smith FJ, Holman CD, Moorin RE, et al. Lifetime risk of undergoing surgery for pelvic organ prolapse. Obstet Gynecol 2010;116(5):1096–100.
4. Subak LL, Waetjen LE, van den Eeden S, et al. Cost of pelvic organ prolapse surgery in the United States. Obstet Gynecol 2001;98(4):646–51.
5. Wu JM, Kawasaki A, Hundley AF, et al. Predicting the number of women who will undergo incontinence and prolapse surgery, 2010 to 2050. Am J Obstet Gynecol 2011;205(3):230.e1-5.
6. Nygaard IE, McCreery R, Brubaker L, et al. Abdominal sacrocolpopexy: a comprehensive review. Obstet Gynecol 2004;104(4):805–23.
7. Oliver JL, Kim JH. Robotic sacrocolpopexy-is it the treatment of choice for advanced apical pelvic organ prolapse? Curr Urol Rep 2017;18(9):66.
8. Serati M, Bogani G, Sorice P, et al. Robot-assisted sacrocolpopexy for pelvic organ prolapse: a systematic review and meta-analysis of comparative studies. Eur Urol 2014;66(2):303–18.
9. Maher C, Feiner B, Baessler K, et al. Surgical management of pelvic organ prolapse in women. Cochrane Database Syst Rev 2013;(4):CD004014.
10. Elterman DS, Chughtai BI, Vertosick E, et al. Changes in pelvic organ prolapse surgery in the last decade among United States urologists. J Urol 2014;191(4):1022–7.
11. Lowder JL, Park AJ, Ellison R, et al. The role of apical vaginal support in the appearance of anterior and posterior vaginal prolapse. Obstet Gynecol 2008;111(1):152–7.
12. White WM, Pickens RB, Elder RF, et al. Robotic-assisted sacrocolpopexy for pelvic organ prolapse. Urol Clin North Am 2014;41(4):549–57.

13. Bump RC, Mattiasson A, Bo K, et al. The standardization of terminology of female pelvic organ prolapse and pelvic floor dysfunction. Am J Obstet Gynecol 1996;175(1):10–7.
14. Farthmann J, Watermann D, Zamperoni H, et al. Pelvic organ prolapse surgery in elderly patients. Arch Gynecol Obstet 2017;295(6):1421–5.
15. Wee WW, Wong HF, Lee LC, et al. Incidence of hydronephrosis in severe uterovaginal or vault prolapse. Singapore Med J 2013;54(3):160–2.
16. Leanza V, Ciotta L, Vecchio R, et al. Hydronephrosis and utero-vaginal prolapse in postmenopausal women: management and treatment. G Chir 2015; 36(6):251–6.
17. Brubaker L, Cundiff GW, Fine P, et al. Abdominal sacrocolpopexy with Burch colposuspension to reduce urinary stress incontinence. N Engl J Med 2006;354(15):1557–66.
18. Collins CW, Winters JC. AUA/SUFU adult urodynamics guideline: a clinical review. Urol Clin north Am 2014;41(3):353–62.
19. Glass D, Brucker B, Nitti V. Treatment of pelvic organ prolapse in the frail elderly patient. AUA Update Ser 2017;36(3).
20. Visco AG, Brubaker L, Nygaard I, et al. The role of preoperative urodynamic testing in stress-continent women undergoing sacrocolpopexy: the Colpopexy and Urinary Reduction Efforts (CARE) randomized surgical trial. Int Urogynecol J Pelvic Floor Dysfunct 2008;19(5):607–14.
21. Brubaker L, Cundiff G, Fine P, et al. A randomized trial of Colpopexy and Urinary Reduction Efforts (CARE): design and methods. Control Clin Trials 2003;24(5):629–42.
22. Nygaard I, Brubaker L, Zyczynski HM, et al. Long-term outcomes following abdominal sacrocolpopexy for pelvic organ prolapse. JAMA 2013;309(19): 2016–24.
23. Clancy AA, Mallick R, Breau RH, et al. Complications after minimally invasive sacrocolpopexy with and without concomitant incontinence surgery: a National Surgical Quality Improvement Program (NSQIP) database study. Neurourol Urodyn 2018. [Epub ahead of print].
24. McFadden BL, Constantine ML, Hammil SL, et al. Patient recall 6 weeks after surgical consent for mid-urethral sling using mesh. Int Urogynecol J 2013; 24(12):2099–104.
25. Robinson BL, Parnell BA, Sandbulte JT, et al. Robotic versus vaginal urogynecologic surgery: a retrospective cohort study of perioperative complications in elderly women. Female Pelvic Med Reconstr Surg 2013;19(4):230–7.
26. Kawasaki A, Corey EG, Laskey RA, et al. Obesity as a risk for the recurrence of anterior vaginal wall prolapse after anterior colporrhaphy. J Reprod Med 2013;58(5–6):195–9.
27. Rappa C, Saccone G. Recurrence of vaginal prolapse after total vaginal hysterectomy with concurrent vaginal uterosacral ligament suspension: comparison between normal-weight and overweight women. Am J Obstet Gynecol 2016;215(5):601. e1–4.
28. Halder GE, Salemi JL, Hart S, et al. Association between obesity and perioperative morbidity in open versus laparoscopic sacrocolpopexy. Female Pelvic Med Reconstr Surg 2017;23(2):146–50.
29. Thubert T, Naveau A, Letohic A, et al. Outcomes and feasibility of laparoscopic sacrocolpopexy among obese versus non-obese women. Int J Gynaecol Obstet 2013;120(1):49–52.
30. Kissane LM, Calixte R, Grigorescu B, et al. Impact of obesity on robotic-assisted sacrocolpopexy. J Minim Invasive Gynecol 2017;24(1):36–40.
31. Adams SR, Dramitinos P, Shapiro A, et al. Do patient goals vary with stage of prolapse? Am J Obstet Gynecol 2011;205(5):502.e1-6.
32. Chu CM, Agrawal A, Mazloomdoost D, et al. Patients' knowledge of and attitude toward robotic surgery for pelvic organ prolapse. Female Pelvic Med Reconstr Surg 2018. [Epub ahead of print].
33. Barber MD, Brubaker L, Nygaard I, et al. Defining success after surgery for pelvic organ prolapse. Obstet Gynecol 2009;114(3):600–9.
34. Lee U, Raz S. Emerging concepts for pelvic organ prolapse surgery: what is cure? Curr Urol Rep 2011;12(1):62–7.
35. Rondini C, Braun H, Alvarez J, et al. High uterosacral vault suspension vs Sacrocolpopexy for treating apical defects: a randomized controlled trial with twelve months follow-up. Int Urogynecol J 2015; 26(8):1131–8.
36. Siddiqui NY, Grimes CL, Casiano ER, et al. Mesh sacrocolpopexy compared with native tissue vaginal repair: a systematic review and meta-analysis. Obstet Gynecol 2015;125(1):44–55.
37. Maher CF, Feiner B, DeCuyper EM, et al. Laparoscopic sacral colpopexy versus total vaginal mesh for vaginal vault prolapse: a randomized trial. Am J Obstet Gynecol 2011;204(4):360.e1-7.
38. Nosti PA, Umoh Andy U, Kane S, et al. Outcomes of abdominal and minimally invasive sacrocolpopexy: a retrospective cohort study. Female Pelvic Med Reconstr Surg 2014;20(1):33–7.
39. Linder BJ, Occhino JA, Habermann EB, et al. A national contemporary analysis of perioperative outcomes for open versus minimally-invasive sacrocolpopexy. J Urol 2018 [pii:S0022-5347(18)42906-0].
40. Costantini E, Mearini L, Lazzeri M, et al. Laparoscopic versus abdominal sacrocolpopexy: a randomized, controlled trial. J Urol 2016;196(1):159–65.
41. Freeman RM, Pantazis K, Thomson A, et al. A randomised controlled trial of abdominal versus

laparoscopic sacrocolpopexy for the treatment of post-hysterectomy vaginal vault prolapse: LAS study. Int Urogynecol J 2013;24(3):377–84.

42. Unger CA, Paraiso MF, Jelovsek JE, et al. Perioperative adverse events after minimally invasive abdominal sacrocolpopexy. Am J Obstet Gynecol 2014;211(5):547.e1-8.
43. Anger JT, Mueller ER, Tarnay C, et al. Robotic compared with laparoscopic sacrocolpopexy: a randomized controlled trial. Obstet Gynecol 2014; 123(1):5–12.
44. Kenton K, Mueller ER, Tarney C, et al. One-year outcomes after minimally invasive sacrocolpopexy. Female Pelvic Med Reconstr Surg 2016;22(5):382–4.
45. Paraiso MF, Jelovsek JE, Frick A, et al. Laparoscopic compared with robotic sacrocolpopexy for vaginal prolapse: a randomized controlled trial. Obstet Gynecol 2011;118(5):1005–13.
46. Matthews CA. Minimally invasive sacrocolpopexy: how to avoid short- and long-term complications. Curr Urol Rep 2016;17(11):81.
47. Shepherd JP, Higdon HL 3rd, Stanford EJ, et al. Effect of suture selection on the rate of suture or mesh erosion and surgery failure in abdominal sacrocolpopexy. Female Pelvic Med Reconstr Surg 2010;16(4):229–33.
48. Tan-Kim J, Nager CW, Grimes CL, et al. A randomized trial of vaginal mesh attachment techniques for minimally invasive sacrocolpopexy. Int Urogynecol J 2015;26(5):649–56.
49. Kallidonis P, Al-Aown A, Vasilas M, et al. Laparoscopic sacrocolpopexy using barbed sutures for mesh fixation and peritoneal closure: a safe option to reduce operational times. Urol Ann 2017;9(2):159–65.
50. Kulhan M, Kulhan NG, Ata N, et al. Should the visceral peritoneum be closed over mesh in abdominal sacrocolpopexy? Eur J Obstet Gynecol Reprod Biol 2018;222:142–5.
51. Elneil S, Cutner AS, Remy M, et al. Abdominal sacrocolpopexy for vault prolapse without burial of mesh: a case series. BJOG 2005;112(4):486–9.
52. Vulliamy P, Berner AM, Farooq MS, et al. Near-fatal small bowel ischaemia secondary to sacrocolpopexy mesh. BMJ Case Rep 2013;2013 [pii: bcr2012008179].
53. Rahmanou P, White B, Price N, et al. Laparoscopic hysteropexy: 1- to 4-year follow-up of women postoperatively. Int Urogynecol J 2014;25(1):131–8.
54. Onol FF, Onol SY. Review of extraperitoneal sacrocolpopexy as a technique for advanced uterine and vault prolapse. Curr Opin Obstet Gynecol 2012;24(4):253–8.
55. Anding R, Latz S, Mueller S, et al. MP33-10 complete extraperitoneal sacrocolpopexy with PVDF visible mesh implant. J Urol 2018;199(4):e432.
56. Matanes E, Lauterbach R, Mustafa-Mikhail S, et al. Single port robotic assisted sacrocolpopexy: our experience with the first 25 cases. Female Pelvic Med Reconstr Surg 2017;23(3):e14–8.
57. Kisby CK, Polin MR, Visco AG, et al. Same-day discharge after robotic-assisted sacrocolpopexy. Female Pelvic Med Reconstr Surg 2018. [Epub ahead of print].
58. Ercoli A, Campagna G, Delmas V, et al. Anatomical insights into sacrocolpopexy for multicompartment pelvic organ prolapse. Neurourol Urodyn 2016; 35(7):813–8.
59. Grimes CL, Lukacz ES, Gantz MG, et al. What happens to the posterior compartment and bowel symptoms after sacrocolpopexy? Evaluation of 5-year outcomes from E-CARE. Female Pelvic Med Reconstr Surg 2014;20(5):261–6.
60. Kaser DJ, Kinsler EL, Mackenzie TA, et al. Anatomic and functional outcomes of sacrocolpopexy with or without posterior colporrhaphy. Int Urogynecol J 2012;23(9):1215–20.
61. Food U, Administration D. Urogynecologic surgical mesh: update on the safety and effectiveness of transvaginal placement for pelvic organ prolapse. July 2011. 2012.
62. Brubaker L, Nygaard I, Richter HE, et al. Two-year outcomes after sacrocolpopexy with and without burch to prevent stress urinary incontinence. Obstet Gynecol 2008;112(1):49.
63. Culligan PJ, Blackwell L, Goldsmith LJ, et al. A randomized controlled trial comparing fascia lata and synthetic mesh for sacral colpopexy. Obstet Gynecol 2005;106(1):29–37.
64. Latini JM, Brown JA, Kreder KJ. Abdominal sacral colpopexy using autologous fascia lata. J Urol 2004;171(3):1176–9.
65. Maloney JC, Dunton CJ, Smith K. Repair of vaginal vault prolapse with abdominal sacropexy. J Reprod Med 1990;35(1):6–10.
66. Abraham N, Quirouet A, Goldman HB. Transabdominal sacrocolpopexy with autologous rectus fascia graft. Int Urogynecol J 2016;27(8):1273–5.
67. Oliver JL, Chaudhry ZQ, Medendorp AR, et al. Complete excision of sacrocolpopexy mesh with autologous fascia sacrocolpopexy. Urology 2017; 106:65–9.
68. Twiss C, Lin F, Funk J. V10-05 total autologous fascia lata robotic sacrocolpopexy: a new technique. J Urol 2018;199(4):e1073–4.
69. Koski ME, Chamberlain J, Rosoff J, et al. Patient perception of transvaginal mesh and the media. Urology 2014;84(3):575–82.
70. Tippett E, King J, Lucent V, et al. Does attorney advertising influence patient perceptions of pelvic mesh? Urology 2018;111:65–71.
71. Winters J, Smith A, Krlin R. 11th edition. Vaginal and abdominal reconstructive surgery for pelvic organ prolapse. Campbell-Walsh urology, 3. Philadelphia: Elsevier Saunders; 2016. p. 1939–86.

Surgery for Vesicovaginal Fistula

Vaginal Approach to Vesicovaginal Fistula

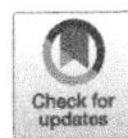

Dominic Lee, FRACS (Urology)[a], Philippe Zimmern, MD, FPMRS[b,*]

KEYWORDS

• Vesicovaginal fistula • Transvaginal approach • Tissue interposition • Outcomes
• Minimally invasive • Surgical technique

KEY POINTS

- Vesicovaginal fistula (VVF) is a socially devastating condition in both developed and developing countries, although etiology differs.
- Proper evaluation, with imaging for confirmation of VVF and postoperative repair, may be required for medico-legal purposes.
- There is no consensus on the route of approach or surgical technique for optimal outcomes, rather there are decisions based on surgeon experience and mitigating circumstances, such as concurrent ureteric injury.
- Strict adherence to the principles of repair is required to ensure a successful outcome.
- There is growing interest in minimally invasive techniques to repair VVF.

 **Video content accompanies this article at http://www.urologic.theclinics.com.**

INTRODUCTION

Vesicovaginal fistula (VVF) is a pathologic connection between the bladder and the vagina. It is a socially devastating condition that can affect women across a vast age range. The incidence in the developed world is estimated between 0.3% and 2.0%.[1,2] Most cases arise as a consequence of trauma to the genitourinary tract from pelvic surgeries usually unrecognized during the time of hysterectomy, endometrioma excision, or prolapse surgery. Less common causes include radiation injury and advanced pelvic cancer. In the developing world, the commonest cause relates to childbirth (>90%), where early marriage coupled with poor socioeconomic conditions are a large contributor, especially in Africa.[3] This article aims to discuss the preoperative workup and diagnosis of VVF with the illustration of a clinical case. We also discuss the relevant controversies in VVF management and focus on the surgical technique for repair via a transvaginal approach and its surgical outcomes.

CLASSIFICATION

Depending on the etiology, various classifications exist to characterize VVF. Classification of VVF in general can be divided into simple or complex. Simple VVFs are ≤2 cm and often solitary and not induced by radiation. Complex VVFs are when the VVF exceeds 2 cm, involves the ureter, is related to a recurrence after previous failed repairs, or is due to radiation damage.[4] In obstetric fistulae, the 2 commonly used classification systems include the Goh and Waaldijk systems. In

Disclosure Statement: None.

[a] Department of Urology, St George Hospital, 28A Gray Street, Kogarah, New South Wales 2217, Australia; [b] Department of Urology, UT Southwestern Medical Center at Dallas, 5323 Harry Hines Boulevard, JA5- 130 C, Dallas, TX 75390-9110, USA
* Corresponding author.
E-mail address: Philippe.Zimmern@utsouthwestern.edu

Urol Clin N Am 46 (2019) 123–133
https://doi.org/10.1016/j.ucl.2018.08.010
0094-0143/19/© 2018 Elsevier Inc. All rights reserved.

a recent comparative analysis, the Goh classification system demonstrated a significantly better prediction of fistula closure than the Waaldijk system, $P = .0421$.[5] Cross application of the Goh classification to nonobstetric VVF has been examined by Beardmore-Gray and colleagues[6] in a retrospective series of 63 cases in a single surgeon series. Although the Goh classification of types 1 to 4 VVF was not predictive of successful closure outcomes, the continence outcomes deteriorated with increasing Goh classification type. The most significant predictor of outcome success in this series was the age and size of the fistula.[6]

CLINICAL SCENARIO

A 51-year-old woman referred from an outside institution with mid-vaginal VVF following transvaginal mesh placement and transobturator mid-urethral sling for cystocele and recurrent stress urinary incontinence (SUI), respectively. Intraoperative bladder injury with trocar at the time of prolapse repair was managed conservatively. The patient had a complicated surgical history with concurrent laparoscopic-assisted vaginal hysterectomy and tension-free vaginal tape mid-urethral sling for SUI 5 years ago. Obstructive voiding confirmed on urodynamics with revision sling surgery 1 month before prolapse repair with a sling incision was followed by recurrent SUI.

Vaginal examination revealed a narrow but well-healed anterior colporrhaphy scar with mesh extrusion evident (**Fig. 1**). There was no secondary prolapse. Sub-urethral sling was palpable with no extrusion.

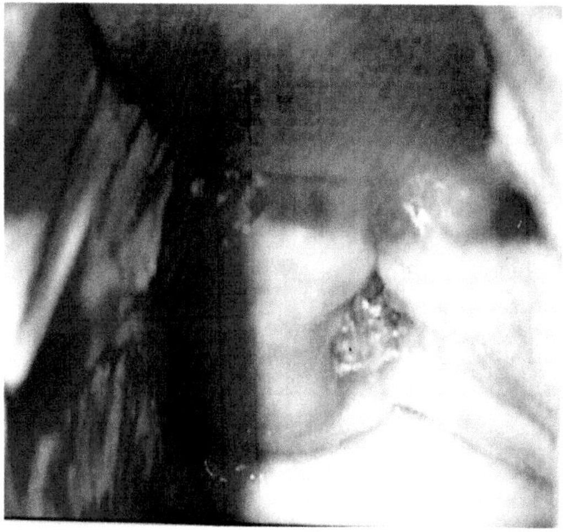

Fig. 1. Vaginal examination revealed a narrow but well-healed anterior colporrhaphy scar with mesh extrusion evident.

At cystoscopy, the urethra was found to be narrowed distally consistent with mid-urethral sling placement. A large fistula tract was noted with exposed mesh just above the inter-ureteric ridge away from the ureteric orifices. Both retrograde pyelograms were normal to exclude concurrent ureteric injury/ureterovaginal fistula. A voiding cysto-urethrogram (VCUG) showed the presence of the VVF (**Fig. 2**A). The patient underwent a transvaginal VVF repair with broad mesh excision, multilayer fistula closure, Martius flap interposition, and maximum bladder drainage with urethral catheter and suprapubic (SP) tube placement. She made a full recovery. At 4 weeks, VCUG confirmed no fistula, reflux, or prolapse.

CLINICAL EVALUATION

A distinction should be made between nonirradiated and irradiated/malignant VVF, as the complexities of surgery, route of repair, and types of tissue interposition used are often different depending on the expertise of the surgeon. In most cases, a post-hysterectomy VVF is less surgically challenging than irradiated VVF, in which the potential for reconstruction maybe compromised by poor tissue quality and subsequent urinary diversion with an ileal or transverse colonic diversion being possibly the only viable option.

The clinical history is often with continuous vaginal leakage of urine. Most VVFs present early following gynecologic or obstetric surgery. For a small VVF, a small amount of watery discharge associated with normal urinary voids maybe the only symptom. Surgical operation reports should be thoroughly evaluated at the time of original surgery to exclude a bladder injury. Any history of 1 or more cesarean deliveries should be noted, as this is a risk factor for VVF at the time of hysterectomy. Furthermore, this can inform that surgical repair may be difficult with potential loss of tissue vascularity and obvious surgical planes. Previous treatments with cobalt radiation for cervical cancer should be noted. Delayed presentation from radiation-induced VVF may occur many years after the inciting event.

A detailed pelvic examination is of utmost importance to ascertain the location, quantity, and size of fistula. In addition, the quality of the surrounding vaginal tissues should be assessed for infection, necrosis, presence or absence of foreign body (vaginal mesh), radiation change, or any significant loss of suppleness, scarring, or tethering to surrounding structures, as it is paramount for surgical planning.

In cases in which the diagnosis of fistula is uncertain, testing for VVF can be achieved after

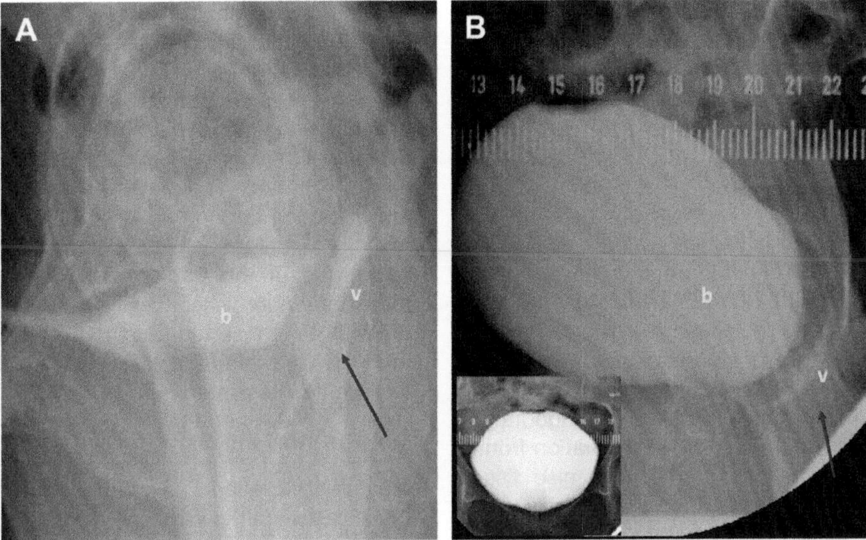

Fig. 2. Investigations are performed to confirm the presence of the VVF. (*A*) Voiding cystourethrogram (VCUG) - lateral voiding views confirming high VVF indicated by arrow with contrast evident in vagina. (*B*) Distended bladder with fistula identified on filling phase of voiding VCUG. b, bladder; v, vagina (showing contrast from bladder to vagina); fistula (*arrow*).

instillation of a diluted methylene blue dye to observe for vaginal leak and/or a tampon test with insertion of a vaginal tampon and bladder filling with ambulation to observe for tampon wetness with the blue dye.

Computed tomography (CT) urogram or retrograde pyelogram to exclude ureteric injury/ureterovaginal fistula is mandatory (**Fig. 3**); however, a negative CT urogram does not exclude a ureterovaginal fistula, as the ureter may drain well and display no evidence of hydronephrosis. Ten percent of VVFs have associated ureteral fistulas.[7] If a ureterovaginal fistula is suspected, a retrograde pyelogram is best for confirmation and localization at the time of cystoscopy. A cystoscopic examination is required to confirm the diagnosis and also to evaluate the position of the fistula with regard to the ureteric orifice. Any suspicion of malignancy in the bladder or vagina will require biopsy for histologic confirmation.

Other investigations, including voiding cystourethrogram (VCUG) with lateral voiding views (not anteroposterior view), to confirm preoperative confirmation of VVF and postoperative closure are important, especially when medico-legal documentation is necessary (**Fig. 2**B). Less frequently used

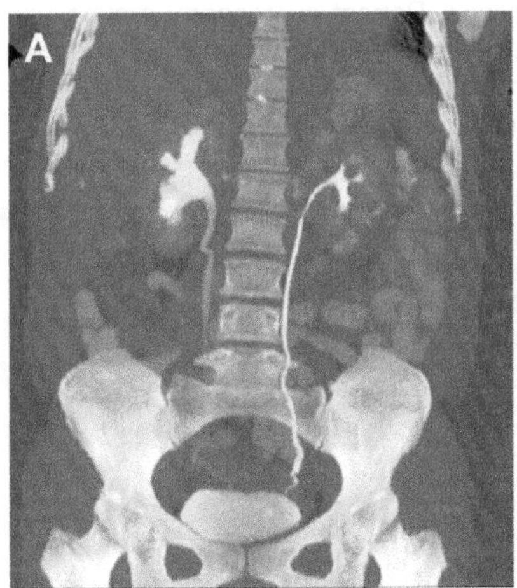

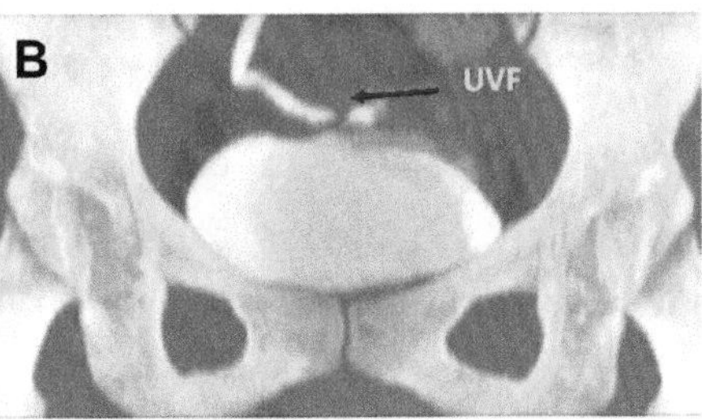

Fig. 3. CT urogram or retrograde pyelogram to exclude ureteric injury/ureterovaginal fistula is mandatory. (*A*) CT pyelogram demonstrating ureterovesical fistula (UVF). (*B*) Opacification of the distal ureter showing ureterovaginal fistula on close up with CT pyelogram (delayed phase). UVF, uretero-vaginal fistula.

imaging modalities, such as magnetic resonance fistulography[8] or transvaginal ultrasound evaluation,[9] although operator dependent, may be used depending on the availability and expertise of the radiology service.

PREOPERATIVE WORKUP

Ensure the patient is stable, as most repairs are undertaken electively. If there is urosepsis or if a urinoma is present, allow 6 weeks to pass after drainage before considering operative repair. Also consider that postpartum uterus may take several weeks to involute and repair should be delayed in this instance. Catheter management is important, as further bladder inflammation from a Foley catheter balloon can compromise tissue quality for repair. It is advised that a catheter be removed at least 4 weeks before repair.

TREATMENT

Conservative Options

Nonsurgical management techniques have been reported mainly in the management of uncomplicated and small (<1 cm) VVFs. Various techniques including injection of fibrin sealant/cyanoacrylic glue and/or electrocautery with laser or coagulation diathermy have been used, with reported success ranging from 67% to 100%. Most of these series have small patient numbers and no significant long-term follow-up.[10–13] Selection of suitable patients is based on the premise of a small uncomplicated VVF with early detection and no fistula resolution despite continuous urinary drainage and anticholinergic medications over a 4-week to 12-week period. Importantly, patients should be counseled that surgical intervention maybe required should any of these conservative measures fail. The injection of sealant serves to plug and stabilize the fistula until tissue ingrowth occurs for permanent closure. This must be balanced with judicious use of electrocoagulation to avoid further devitalization of adjacent tissue and risk failure.

The McKay transurethral procedure is a rarely performed technique that can be considered in patients with small VVFs (**Fig. 4**). In a small case series of 5 patients, 80% of the cases were successful. The technique involves the placement of a cystoscope through an established suprapubic tract for visualization. A 32-Fr Amplatz sheath is passed per urethra and a rubber cap placed over the open-ended sheath. A laparoscopic needle driver is then inserted, and transurethral closure of the fistula performed with a few absorbable sutures in an interrupted fashion.[14]

Surgical Options

Treatment of patients with VVF is often dictated by the expertise of the individual treating surgeon, as a standardized treatment algorithm is lacking. Optimization of preoperative patient factors, including nutrition, urinary drainage, and skin care should be taken into consideration when a delayed approach to surgery is intended.

CONTROVERSIES

Timing of Surgery

There is no consensus on the timing of repair for successful outcome; however, the timing of surgery should be balanced between attainment of optimal tissue conditions and liberation of urinary leak for the patient. For optimization of repair, any infections should be fully treated, inflammation should be given sufficient time to resolve, and all devitalized tissues debrided along with clearance of any foreign body (**Box 1**). The classic strategy is repair within 1 week of injury or a delay of 3 to 6 months to allow for healing of the traumatized tissue. Repeat cystoscopy maybe undertaken to assess for healing within the bladder and scar formation before VVF repair, as regular pelvic examinations maybe less reliable.

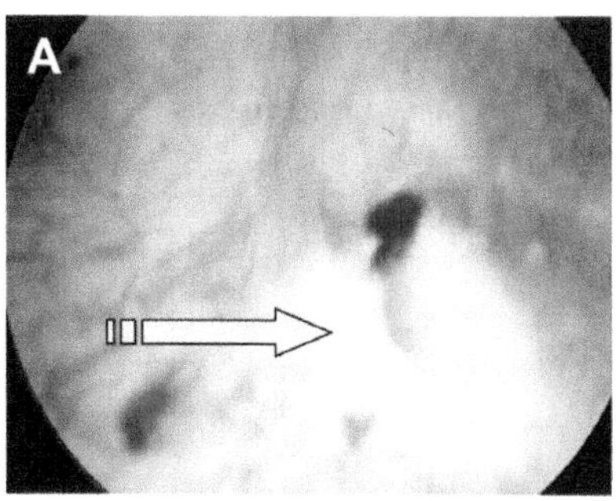

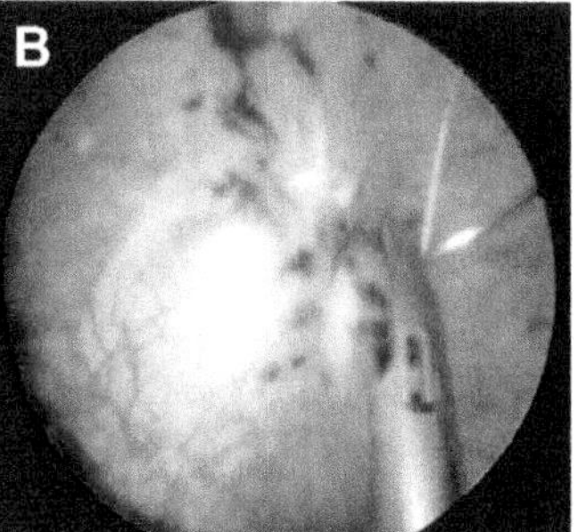

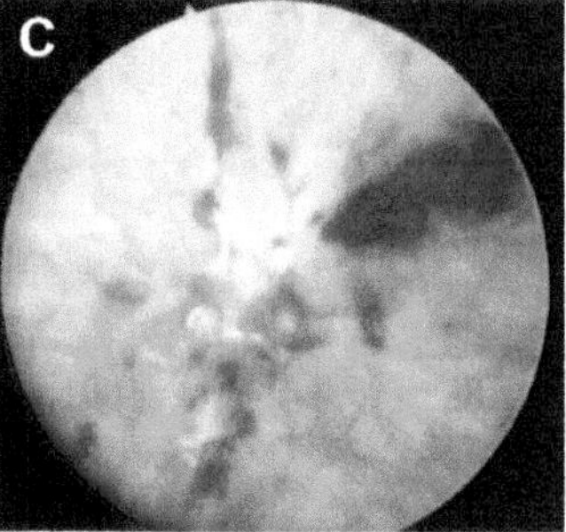

Fig. 4. The McKay transurethral procedure is a rarely performed technique that can be considered in patients with small VVF (*A*) Fistula on view indicated by arrow (*B*) Closure with laparoscopic instrument with the transurethral technique (*C*) Closure of the VVF following repair.

Box 1
Principles of vesicovaginal fistula repair

- Treat infection/anemia/malnutrition
- Ensure no foreign nondissolving material or malignancy
- Nonoverlapping suture lines
- Tension-free
- Watertight
- Consider well-vascularized interposed flap
- Uninterrupted bladder drainage

Excision of Fistulous Tract

Should the fistulous tract be excised? Although this was standard practice at the turn of the twentieth century, it is a controversial subject. Current thinking argues against fistulous tract excision to (1) minimize fistula size, (2) minimize bleeding, (3) avoid ureteric injury, and (4) retain fibrous ring to allow for tension-free closure. Cruikshank[15] and Raz[16] reported a 100% success rate in their respective series of 11 and 65 patients without tract excision. More recently, we also reported similar outcomes from our series, as we routinely leave the fistulous tract intact at the time of transvaginal VVF repair.[17]

Routes of Repair

It is debatable as to whether the abdominal or vaginal route is the most appropriate for fistula repair. The most commonly used approach reported in a recent meta-analysis was transvaginal (n = 534/1379; 39%), followed by transabdominal/transvesical approach (n = 493/1379; 36%) and laparoscopic/robotic approach (n = 207/1379; 15%), respectively.[18] The abdominal approach is indicated after a failed VVF vaginal repair, for ureteric involvement, and when vaginal access is limited. Furthermore, this approach allows for omental and peritoneal flap interposition. The transvaginal approach is favored due to its minimally invasive nature, shorter hospital stay, limited blood loss and postoperative pain, and various tissue interposition options, such as peritoneal flap, Martius fat pad, or gracilis muscle flap.[19]

The chosen technique usually depends on the competency and expertise of the treating physician. Competency aside, the selection of patients for transvaginal repair depends on patient and fistula factors. The transvaginal technique is preferable due to its minimally invasive nature. See **Table 1** for comparison between transvaginal and transabdominal routes of repair. The disadvantage of a transvaginal repair includes potential vaginal shortening and generation of a dead space with a Latzko technique.[20] Contraindications to vaginal approach include concurrent ureteral reimplantation, involvement of other pelvic structures, vaginal stenosis, or inability to obtain proper exposure.[21,22]

Table 1
Abdominal versus transvaginal repair

Variables	Transvaginal	Transabdominal
Indication	Simple	Complex
Vaginal access/ exposure	Limited	No
Blood loss	Limited	More
Invasiveness	Minimal	Maximal
Postoperative pain	Mild	Moderate-severe
Vaginal shortening	Possible	No
Associated pelvic pathology	No	Yes
Ureteric involvement	No	Yes

TRANSVAGINAL ROUTE

Latzko Technique

The Latzko procedure has long been championed for small noncomplicated fistulas and remains relevant in the current age, although its popularity has waned somewhat over the years. It is in effect a partial colpocleisis. An elliptical portion of vaginal mucosa is mobilized and denuded around the fistula tract, at least 2 cm in all directions. The pubovesical fascia and vaginal mucosa are closed in layers, using interrupted sagittally oriented sutures imbricating one over the other. The vesical edges of the fistula are not disturbed with no tension across the suture lines. The major disadvantage is vaginal shortening with potential interference with sexual activity and risk of failure. The success rate ranges from 89% to 100%.[23–25]

Flap-Splitting Technique

A catheter placed through the fistula tract aides in pulling down the fistula and in dissecting it all around. This catheter is usually a council tip catheter with a guidewire in its center to avoid losing the direction of the fistula tract during the dissection and subsequent closure (**Fig. 5**A). The flap-splitting technique involves raising a wide anterior vaginal wall flap whose apex reaches and circumscribes the fistula opening. Then a wide circular mobilization of the vaginal mucosa from the edge

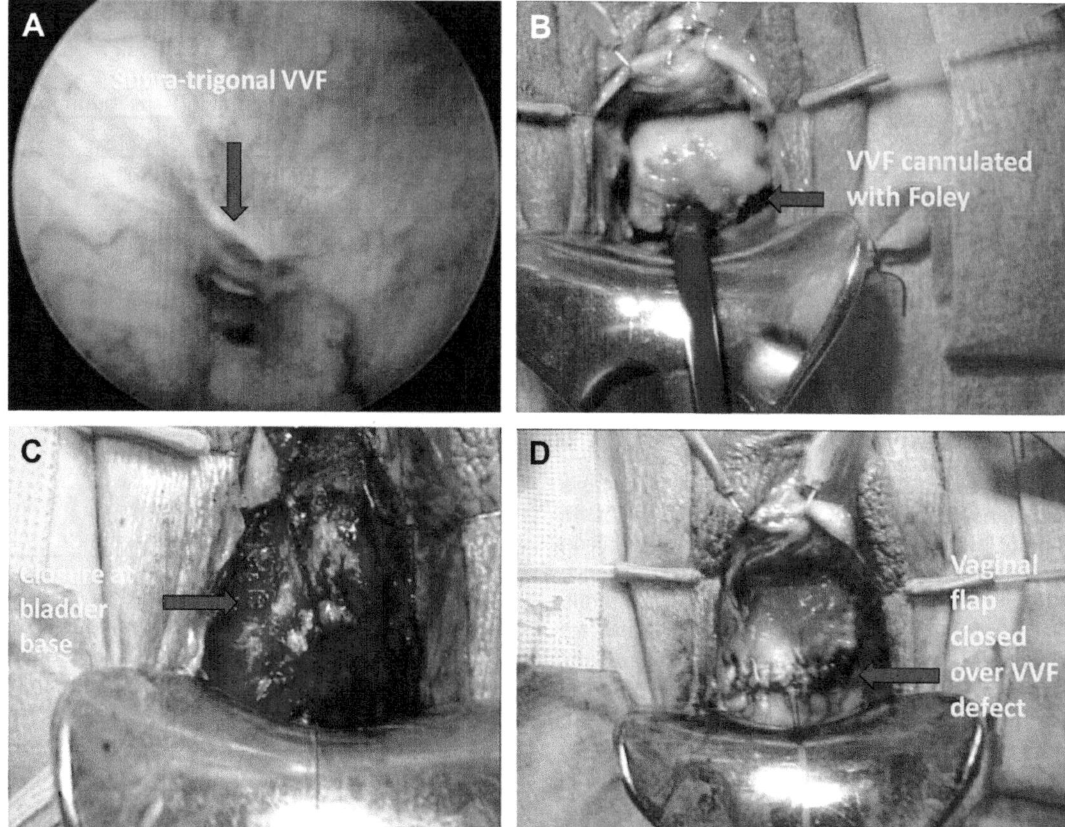

Fig. 5. A catheter placed through the fistula tract aides in pulling down the fistula and in dissecting it all around. (*A*) High VVF seen on cystoscopy. (*B*) Fistula cannulated with Foley catheter via vagina for transvaginal repair. (*C*) Closure of bladder detrusor layer of VVF. (*D*) Completion of VVF with vaginal advancement flap as part of multilayer closure. VVF, vesico-vaginal fistula.

of the fistula is undertaken, anteriorly, laterally, and then posteriorly. The bladder is closed in 2 layers. The first is submucosal with running sutures in a nontensioned fashion. Typically, the closure is started at each corner of the fistula with a U-shaped stitch to avoid the risk of breakdown that could lead to a recurrence (**Fig. 5**B). The 2 half-running sutures are tied up at the midpoint of the defect and the guidewire, which has been left in place, is withdrawn as the fistula nears complete closure. The watertightness of this repair is tested by filling the bladder under gravity via the suprapubic tube catheter. A second layer is used to close the muscularis and reduce tension on the first suture line. This second line of closure entails preplacing several interrupted sutures at a right angle with the preceding suture line, and then tying them from back to front to completely cover and support the underlying closure line. Then a decision should be made as to whether or not an interposition graft is needed before closure of the vaginal incision (**Fig. 5**C, D). Likewise, a trigonal area VVF should be repaired in a transverse direction to avoid kinking or obstructing the ureters from medialization.

INTERPOSITION

Tissue interposition over the VVF repair site may serve as an adjunct to improve outcomes. Such an interposition delivers a vascularized pedicle flap that enhances healing. Not all patients require tissue interposition after the completion of the VVF repair. Decision for tissue graft interposition depends largely on the characteristics of the fistula. Large VVF and/or high location of the vaginal fistula in addition to the quality of the surrounding tissue dictates what type of graft is used. Of note, if the repair is not watertight, tissue graft interposition will not be sufficient to prevent a fistula recurrence.

For the transvaginal technique, tissue grafts that have been used include the following:

- Martius flap
- Peritoneal flap
- Omental flap

In the current era in which most fistulae are post-hysterectomy and located high in the vaginal vault (see **Fig. 2**A), peritoneal and omental flaps are the most commonly performed ones.

MARTIUS GRAFT

First described in 1928, the Martius labial graft is probably the most common graft used for reconstruction in the female lower urinary tract. Its versatility has been used for urethra, vaginal, and rectal reconstruction.[26] The fibro-adipose tissue has dual vascular supply to the graft: inferiorly from the internal pudendal artery and superiorly from the external pudendal artery. Care must be exercised in the preservation of at least one of these vascular branches on harvest. The original technique included the incorporation of the underlying bulbo-cavernosus muscle as part of the repair. This was associated with significant morbidity and has been subsequently modified. The current approach uses the labial fibro-adipose fat pad harvested from the labia majora alone. We have previously published our technique and outcomes and a brief summary of the surgical technique is provided as follows.[27]

MARTIUS GRAFT TECHNIQUE

An 8-cm to 10-cm-long vertical incision over the labia majora from the level of the mons pubis down toward the level of the fourchette is performed (Video 1). This is a typical incision for a high-vault VVF to allow sufficient length of the fat pad to reach the vaginal apex. When the procedure is indicated for a urethral or bladder neck pathology, the incision can be shorter and start midway over the labia majora, still extending down to the level of the posterior fourchette.

The labia majora incision is deepened to the level of the labial fat pad, which is gently grasped with an Allis clamp and mobilized on an inferior pedicle providing a postero-inferior blood supply to the graft based on branches from the internal pudendal artery. To avoid medial labial skin distortion or retraction, the fat medially beneath the labial skin is spared and the fat pad dissection is carried slightly obliquely and away from the inner labial folds. Once a sufficient length has been obtained with medial and lateral dissection, the flap is gradually divided superiorly. Large veins can supply the apex of the flap coming from the mons pubis and they may require careful ligature to avoid retraction and a secondary labial hematoma. Final mobilization continues by detaching the fat pad posteriorly off the underlying ischiocavernosus and bulbocavernosus muscles, ensuring a broad base inferiorly to protect the blood supply. The Martius fat pad is tunneled beneath and along the lateral vaginal wall to finally reach and overlay the 2-layer bladder closure, to which it is secured. The tunnel should be widened to accept at least 2 fingers to prevent compression of the blood supply of the fat pad, which could compromise its survival. A drain (small Penrose or #7 Jackson-Pratt drain) is placed. The incision is closed in 2 layers, a running subcutaneous deep absorbable suture over the drain, and then interrupted absorbable sutures on the skin. In case of vaginal wall defect precluding primary vaginal wall closure, a skin island can be included with the fibro-adipose graft to form a full-thickness fascio-cutaneous flap to close any deficiencies within the vagina in a tension-free manner.

PERITONEAL/OMENTUM FLAP

This technique was first described by Raz and colleagues[28] in 1993, and is suitable for a high vaginal or trigonal VVF. With a flap-splitting technique, the anterior and posterior vaginal wall flaps are dissected to widely expose the fistula tract. During the posterior dissection of the fistula tract, it is important to recognize the location of the rectum, which can be aided by Betadine-soaked gauze inserted rectally at the start of the procedure to mold it over and facilitate its recognition. Behind the bladder base, the peritoneum at the bottom of the pouch of Douglas can be easily entered. This peritoneal window can give access to a tongue of omentum (**Fig. 6**) left by the prior surgeon, epiploic fronds from the sigmoid, or a free flap of peritoneum with its adjacent fat. The peritoneal flap is mobilized carefully and advanced to reach beyond the fistula site to cover over the fistula repair suture line, where it is tacked in place with several absorbable sutures. The vaginal incision is then closed over by advancing the anterior vaginal flap to meet the posterior vaginal flap, thus avoiding overlapping of suture lines.

GRACILIS FLAP

The gracilis muscle flap is seldom used except in total vaginal reconstruction following pelvic exenteration or in case of radiation damage. Its major blood supply is a branch of the profunda femoris entering the upper one-third of the muscle. This long muscular flap reaches to cover the medial portion of the groin, the vulva, the perineum, and the lower abdomen. Consultation with Plastic surgery is recommended in these infrequent situations.

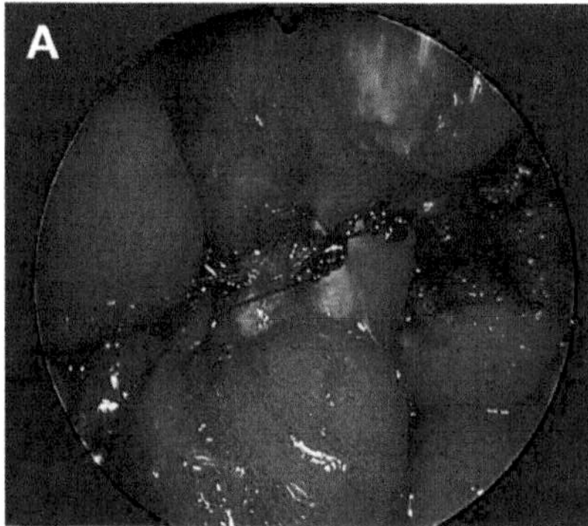

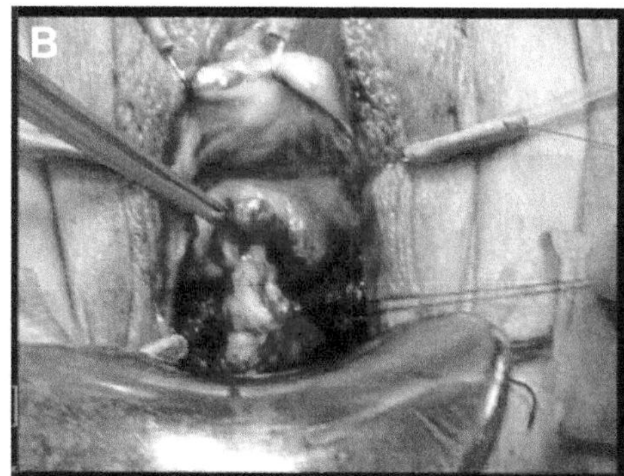

Fig. 6. Peritoneal/omental flap technique by Raz is suitable for a high vaginal or trigonal VVF. (*A*) Peritoneal flap as described by Raz used for interposition in VVF repair. (*B*) Omentum harvested for interposition for VVF repair.

TRANSVAGINAL REPAIR TECHNIQUE

We outline our preferred modified transvaginal approach in Video 2. The surgeon will need a good set of headlights and long instruments for high vaginal vault fistulae cases. The patient is placed in high lithotomy position, although some centers prefer a prone position for fistula access. Choice of supporting stirrups is a matter of physician preference. A thorough examination under anesthesia is performed. Occasionally the VVF can be seen on vaginoscopy that is too small to see on cystoscopy (**Fig. 7**A). For a high fistula, it is prudent to pack the rectum with Betadine-soaked vaginal gauze. Cystoscopy at this stage confirms the location and proper efflux from each ureteric orifice. If a ureter is in very close proximity to the fistula, a ureteric catheter can be placed or the decision for vaginal repair aborted to proceed transabdominally with possible ureteral reimplantation in the same setting. A large-bore suprapubic catheter (SPC) is placed at this point. An episiotomy or Schuchardt incision may be helpful for a small introitus to gain better access to the vaginal vault. The patient is placed in Trendelenburg position and a Lone star retractor is set up for exposure. Weighted posterior vaginal retractors maybe used for optimal vaginal visualization and access. A 5-Fr open-ended catheter is used to place a guidewire through the fistula (vaginally or cystoscopically), and the wire is retained until the very end of the fistula closure (**Fig. 7**B). The insertion and inflation of a Foley balloon catheter passed over the guidewire (council tip catheter) or Fogarty catheter for tiny fistula tract helps to identify the fistula's edges and will bring the tract down to ease the surgeon's dissection of this tract.

A U-shape incision incorporating the opening of the fistula is used, and a plane between the vaginal mucosa and the perivesical fascia is carefully developed. The rest of the repair was described earlier in this article in the "Flap-splitting Technique" section. After complete mobilization of the fistula tract to ensure a tension-free closure, the tract is closed, the watertightness of the repair is checked, and a second layer is performed at right angle with the first one. A cystoscopy is repeated to check for ureteric efflux. If there are concerns, methylene blue or fluorescein can be injected intraoperatively. When indicated, a peritoneal or omental flap for high-vault vaginal VVF or a Martius flap for a lower-tract VVF is secured over the repair

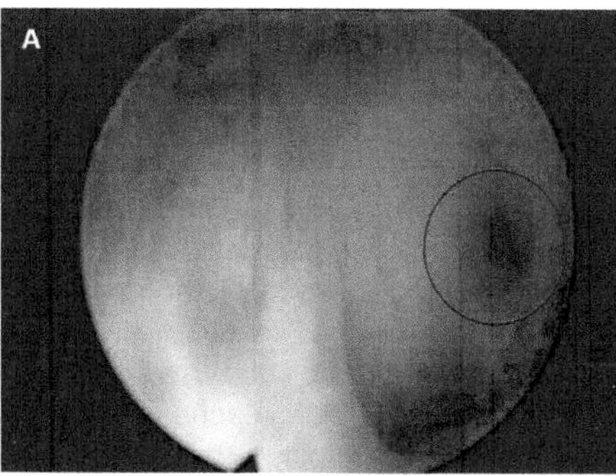

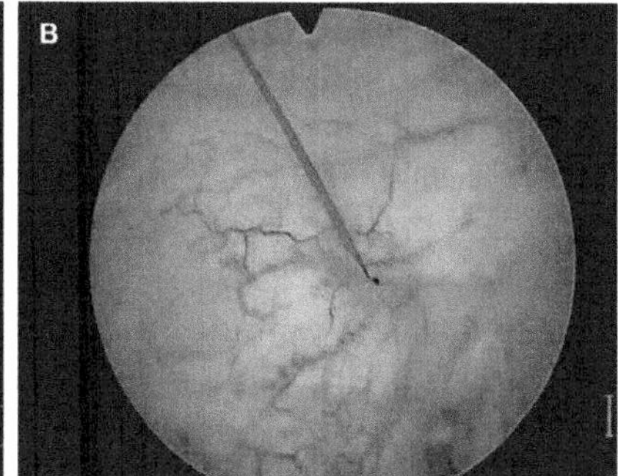

Fig. 7. Occasionally the VVF (*Circle*) can be seen on vaginoscopy that is too small to see on cystoscopy. (*A*) Vaginoscopy identifying small VVF. Image taken by inserting cystoscope transvaginally. (*B*) Small VVF cannulated with guide wire showing the small defect on cystoscopy.

site with absorbable sutures. The anterior vaginal flap is advanced over the repair and/or tissue interposition and the incision is closed. A urethral Foley catheter is left indwelling. A vaginal pack is then inserted. Perioperative antibiotics are continued.

POSTOPERATIVE CARE

Uninterrupted bladder drainage is recommended with a urethral Foley and a suprapubic tube catheter. To prevent secondary bladder spasms, anticholinergic medications, as well as belladonna and opium (BNO) suppositories can be used. Low-dose prophylactic antibiotics can be used to decrease the rate of catheter-induced infection. A voiding cystourethrogram with lateral views is obtained at 4 weeks after repair. If the fistula is healed, then a voiding trial can be performed with the suprapubic tube used for post-void residual monitoring. This suprapubic catheter can be removed as soon as adequate bladder emptying has returned. Sexual activity is avoided until complete vaginal healing (2–3 months).

RESULTS

Despite evolving and modification of existing surgical techniques, retrospective data analysis has not supported which technique is superior for VVF repair (**Table 2**). To date, there are no randomized controlled trials comparing route of repair (transvaginal vs transabdominal) or tissue interposition versus no interposition. Therefore, the nominated approach is dependent on the characteristics, size, and location of the fistula and the expertise of the surgeon in adhering to the principles of VVF repair outlined in **Table 1**. A transvaginal approach should be in the arsenal of a pelvic reconstructive surgeon.

Most of the outcomes of transvaginal VVF are based on retrospective series. The heterogeneity of the fistula (size, location) and the occasional use of an interposition graft makes standardization of outcomes difficult; however, the estimated success of repair ranges from 83% to 100%.[17,29–34] **Box 2** highlights outcomes from some of the major contemporary series documenting transvaginal technique.

Box 2
Complications related to vesicovaginal fistula repairs

Acute

- Urinary tract infection
- Ureteral injury/obstruction: may require reimplantation
- Urine leak: stress or urge urinary incontinence
- Vaginal bleeding
- Bladder spasms: anticholinergics are generally administered

Chronic

- Fistula recurrence: requires waiting for complete healing, then re-repair with a vascularized flap, usually an abdominal approach is preferred
- Change in vaginal caliber where vaginal stenosis maybe an issue
- Incontinence: ensure it is not a recurrent fistula; imaging is useful

NEOBLADDER-VAGINA FISTULA

An infrequently seen but rare complication following radical cystectomy and ileal orthotopic neobladder, the estimated incidence of neobladder-vaginal fistula has been reported at approximately 5%.[35] An intraoperative injury to the anterior vaginal wall remains an important predisposing factor.[36] An abdominal approach is particularly daunting, given the posterior position of the fistula and risk of potential devascularization of the mesenteric blood flow from an aggressive dissection for fistula access. A transvaginal

Table 2
Outcomes of vesicovaginal fistula repair via transvaginal route

Study	N	Tissue Graft	Outcome, %	Follow-up, y
Eilber et al,[29] 2003	207	Peritoneal/Martius/Labia	97	10
Kochakarn et al,[30] 2007	19	N/A	83	8
Hilton,[31] 2012	201	Martius	96.1	N/A
Pshak et al,[32] 2013	49	None	100	1
Lee et al,[17] 2014	50	Martius	97	4.5
Gedik et al,[33] 2015	25	None	100	1
Malde et al,[34] 2017	43	Martius	95	3.2

Abrreviation: N/A, not available.

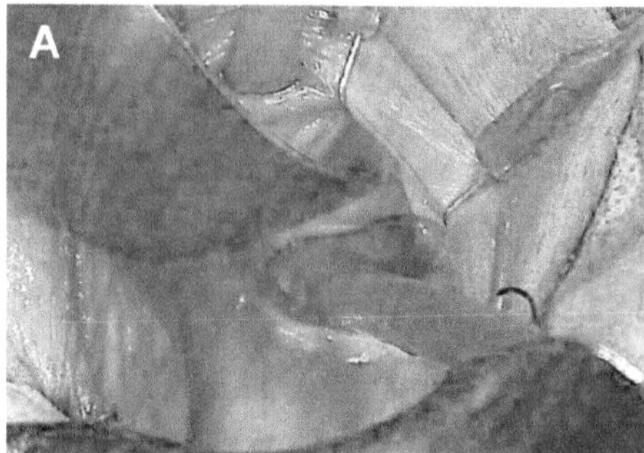

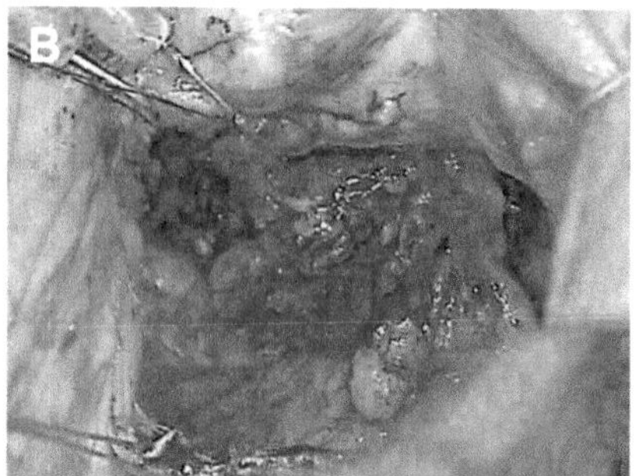

Fig. 8. A transvaginal approach has been documented in a few retrospective series. (*A*) Large VVF identified with Foley catheter passing through defect to aid in transvaginal repair. (*B*) Repair of VVF completed in multiple layers.

approach has been documented in a few retrospective series (**Fig. 8**A, B).[37] A Martius interposition flap is often used in these series. The technique was reported by Carmel and colleagues[38] in their small series of 8 patients using either a Martius or Omental flap with a success rate of 100% with a mean follow-up of 33 months.

ROBOTIC/LAPAROSCOPIC APPROACH

Finally, minimally invasive surgery has seen a surge in popularity over the years. Traditional laparoscopic techniques introduced in the 1990s required advanced skills. The arrival of the robotic platform has revolutionized the approach, making intracorporeal suturing better and more efficient and hence a higher uptake in utilization of the technology, which translates to less pain and blood loss with quicker recovery and shorter hospital length of stay. There are 2 approaches described. The first is a transvesical technique in keeping with principles of the open technique described initially by O'Conor and Collegues[39] the second is an extravesical technique. A recent meta-analysis by Miklos and colleagues[40] reviewed both laparoscopic and robotic techniques in a pooled series of 44 articles accounting for 256 patients. Extravesical and transvesical approaches were comparable. Follow-up varied between 1 and 74 months. The overall success of laparoscopic/robotic VVF repairs was 80% to 100%, with a slightly higher success in the extravesical group, although this did not reach statistical significance. Surprisingly, those who had tissue interposition did worse than those without tissue interposed (80%–100% versus 97%–100%, respectively).

SUMMARY

Management of VVF requires a detailed knowledge of vaginal anatomy and surgical skills, with the ability to operate vaginally or abdominally to achieve optimal outcomes. Although no one technique is superior, and the evidence is lacking with regard to which approach is best for the patient, the onus is on the surgeon to choose a technique of repair that he or she is most facile with while keeping the tenets of VVF repair principles.

SUPPLEMENTARY DATA

Supplementary data related to this article can be found online at https://doi.org/10.1016/j.ucl.2018.08.010.

REFERENCES

1. Thompson JD. Vesicovaginal and urethrovaginal fistula. In: rock JA, Thompson JD, editors. Te Linde's operative gynecology. 8th edition. Philadelphia: JB Lippincott; 1997. p. 1175–205 [chapter: 41].
2. Härkki-Sirén P, Sjöberg J, Tiitinen A. Urinary tract injuries after hysterectomy. Obstet Gynecol 1998; 92(1):113–8.
3. Wall LL. Obstetric vesicovaginal fistula as an international public-health problem. Lancet 2006;368: 1201–9.
4. Stamatakos M, Sargedi C, Stasinou T, et al. Vesicovaginal fistula: diagnosis and management. Indian J Surg 2014;76(2):131–6.
5. Capes T, Stanford EJ, Romanzi L, et al. Comparison of two classification systems for vesicovaginal fistula. Int Urogynecol J 2012;23(12):1679–85.
6. Beardmore-Gray A, Pakzad M, Hamid R, et al. Does the Goh classification predict the outcome of vesicovaginal fistula repair in the developed world? Int Urogynecol J 2017;28(6):937–40.
7. Goodwin WE, Scardino PT. Vesicovaginal and ureterovaginal fistulas: a summary of 25 years of experience. J Urol 1980;123(3):370–4.
8. Dwarkasing S, Hussain SM, Hop WC, et al. Anovaginal fistulas: evaluation with endoanal MR imaging. Radiology 2004;231:123–8.
9. Qureshi IA, Hidayaatullah AAH, Ashfag S, et al. Transvaginal versus transabdominal sonography in

the evaluation of pelvic pathology. J Coll Physicians Surg Pak 2004;14:390–3.
10. Kumar U, Albala DM. Fibrin glue applications in urology. Curr Urol Rep 2001;2(1):V79–82.
11. Muto G, D'Urso L, Castelli E, et al. Cyanoacrylic glue: a minimally invasive nonsurgical first line approach for the treatment of some urinary fistulas. J Urol 2005;174(6):2239–43.
12. Stovsky MD, Ignatoff JM, Blum MD, et al. Use of electrocoagulation in the treatment of vesicovaginal fistulas. J Urol 1994;152(5 Pt 1):1443–4.
13. Kursch ED, Stovsky M, Ignatoff JM, et al. Use of fulguration in the treatment of vesicovaginal fistula. J Urol 1993;149:292A.
14. McKay HA. Transurethral suture cystorrhaphy for repair of vesicovaginal fistulas: evolution of a technique. Int Urogynecol J Pelvic Floor Dysfunct 2001; 12(4):282–7.
15. Cruikshank SH. Early closure of post-hysterectomy vesicovaginal fistulas. South Med J 1988;81(12): 1525–8.
16. Raz S. Female urology. Philadelphia: WB Saunders; 1893. p. 373–7.
17. Lee D, Dillon BE, Lemack GE, et al. Long-term functional outcomes following nonradiated vesicovaginal repair. J Urol 2014;191(1):120–4.
18. Bodner-Adler B, Hanzal E, Pablik E, et al. Management of vesicovaginal fistulas (VVFs) in women following benign gynaecologic surgery: a systematic review and meta-analysis. PLoS One 2017; 12(2):e0171554.
19. Angioli R, Penalver M, Muzii L, et al. Guidelines of how to manage vesicovaginal fistula. Crit Rev Oncol Hematol 2003;48(3):295–304.
20. Enzelseberger H, Gitsch E. Surgical management of vesicovaginal fistulas according to Chassar Moir's method. Surg Gynecol Obstet 1991;173:183–6.
21. Carr LK, Webster GD. Abdominal repair of vesicovaginal fistula. Urol 1996;48(1):10–1.
22. Kapoor R, Ansari MS, Singh P, et al. Management of vesicovaginal fistula: an experience of 52 cases with a rationalized algorithm for choosing the transvaginal or transabdominal approach. Indian J Urol 2007;23(4):372–6.
23. Latzko W. Postoperative vesicovaginal fistulas: genesis and therapy. Am J Surg 1942;58:211.
24. Dorairajan LN, Khattar N, Kumar S, et al. Latzko repair for vesicovaginal fistula revisited in the era of minimal-access surgery. Int Urol Nephrol 2008; 40(2):317–20.
25. Ansquer Y, Mellier G, Santulli P, et al. Latzko operation for vault vesicovaginal fistula. Acta Obstet Gynecol Scand 2006;85(10):1248–51.
26. Martius H. Die operative Widerherstellung der vollkommen fehlenden Harnrohre und des Schliessmuskels derselben. Zentralbl Gynakol 1928;52:7.
27. Lee D, Dillon BE, Zimmern PE. Martius labial fat pad procedure: technique and long-term outcomes. Int Urogynecol J 2015;26(9):1395–6.
28. Raz S, Bregg KJ, Nitti VW, et al. Transvaginal repair of vesicovaginal fistula using a peritoneal flap. J Urol 1993;150(1):56–9.
29. Eilber KS, Kavaler E, Rodríguez LV, et al. Ten-year experience with transvaginal vesicovaginal fistula repair using tissue interposition. J Urol 2003; 169(3):1033–6.
30. Kochakarn W, Pummangura W. A new dimension in vesicovaginal fistula management: an 8-year experience at Ramathibodi hospital. Asian J Surg 2007; 30(4):267–71.
31. Hilton P. Urogenital fistula in the UK: a personal case series managed over 25 years. BJU Int 2012;110(1): 102–10.
32. Pshak T, Nikolavsky D, Terlecki R, et al. Is tissue interposition always necessary in transvaginal repair of benign, recurrent vesicovaginal fistulae? Urology 2013;82(3):707–12.
33. Gedik A, Deliktas H, Celik N, et al. Which surgical technique should be preferred to repair benign, primary vesicovaginal fistulas? Urol J 2015;12(6): 2422–7.
34. Malde S, Spilotros M, Wilson A, et al. The uses and outcomes of the Martius fat pad in female urology. World J Urol 2017;35(3):473–8.
35. Negro CL, De Stefanis P, Bosio A, et al. Transvaginal repair of neobladder vaginal fistula. Urologia 2010; 77(Suppl 16):11–5.
36. Rapp DE, O'connor RC, Katz EE, et al. Neobladder-vaginal fistula after cystectomy and orthotopic neobladder construction. BJU Int 2004;94(7): 1092–5.
37. Blander DS, Zimmern PE, Lemack GE, et al. Transvaginal repair of postcystectomy peritoneovaginal fistulae. Urology 2000;56(2):320–1.
38. Carmel ME, Goldman HB, Moore CK, et al. Transvaginal neobladder vaginal fistula repair after radical cystectomy with orthotopic urinary diversion in women. Neurourol Urodyn 2016;35(1):90–4.
39. O'CONOR VJ, SOKOL JK. Vesicovaginal fistula from the standpoint of the urologist. J Urol 1951;66(4): 579–85.
40. Miklos JR, Moore RD, Chinthakanan O. Laparoscopic and robotic-assisted vesicovaginal fistula repair: a systematic review of the literature. J Minim Invasive Gynecol 2015;22(5):727–36.

Abdominal Approach to Vesicovaginal Fistula

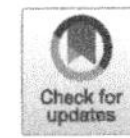

Elishia McKay, MD[a], Kara Watts, MD[b], Nitya Abraham, MD[b,*]

KEYWORDS

• Vesicovaginal fistula • Urinary bladder fistula • Vaginal fistula • Surgical procedures • Operative • Robotics • Laparoscopy

KEY POINTS

- Vesicovaginal fistula (VVF) is a devastating cause of morbidity and can be identified with physical examination and/or imaging.
- The abdominal approach to VVF repair includes a transvesical or extravesical technique.
- The same principles of VVF repair apply when using the robot-assisted laparoscopic approach.
- Shorter operative times, decreased blood loss, improved visibility, and similar cure rates with the minimally invasive approach have led to a rise in its popularity.

 **Video content accompanies this article at https://www.urologic.theclinics.com/.**

INTRODUCTION

Vesicovaginal fistula (VVF) is an abnormal communication between the bladder and the vagina resulting in continuous leakage of urine (**Fig. 1**). The term fistula was popularized in the sixteenth century. However, descriptions of these communicative tracts date back to 1550 BC and were first described in relation to obstetric injuries around 950 AD by physician and polymath Avicenna.[1] This article will briefly discuss fundamentals of VVF (etiology, presentation, evaluation, and diagnosis), followed by focus on abdominal approaches to VVF repair including open and minimally invasive techniques.

EPIDEMIOLOGY AND ETIOLOGY

Despite its long history of recognition, VVF remains a devastating cause of morbidity for women around the world. VVF incites inherent social stigma and emotional and psychological strain on its victims, as well as physical repercussions.[2] Causes include obstetric injury, postsurgical sequelae, radiation therapy, inflammation or infection, foreign body, and other trauma. Worldwide, these fistulas are most commonly related to obstetric complications, with prolonged labor being a predominant contributing factor. In countries with greater access to obstetric care, VVF is more commonly a complication of pelvic surgery or malignancy treatment, with the former most often preceded by inadvertent bladder injury or ureteral injury during abdominal hysterectomy. In the United States, the true incidence is not known but has previously been reported to be about 0.3% to 2%, with some studies reporting an overall incidence of 0.5% after simple hysterectomy and 10% after radical hysterectomy[3,4]

In general, fistulas occur when devascularized tissues become necrotic, leading to subsequent erosion through the urinary tract and the vaginal epithelium, thus allowing urine to escape through this channel. This avascularity can be caused by unrecognized intraoperative lacerations, crush injury of the bladder wall, suture impingement or

Disclosure Statement: None.

[a] Department of Obstetrics and Gynecology, Montefiore Medical Center, 1250 Waters Place, Tower 2, Suite 706, Bronx, NY 10461, USA; [b] Department of Urology, Montefiore Medical Center, 1250 Waters Place, Tower 2, Suite 706, Bronx, NY 10461, USA

* Corresponding author.

E-mail address: nabraham@montefiore.org

Urol Clin N Am 46 (2019) 135–146
https://doi.org/10.1016/j.ucl.2018.08.011
0094-0143/19/© 2018 Elsevier Inc. All rights reserved.

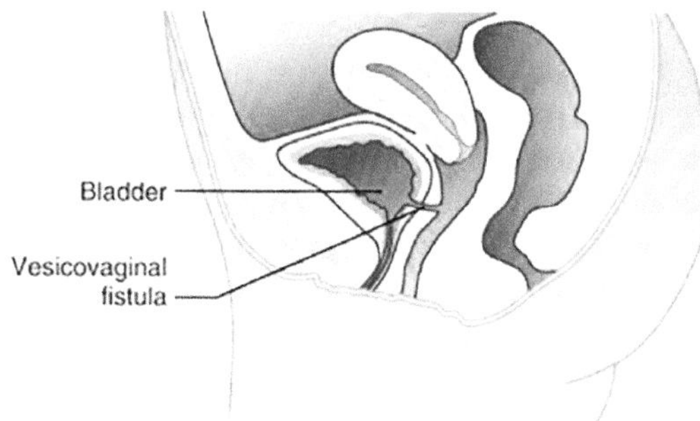

Fig. 1. Vesicovaginal fistula. (*From* Rosenman AE. Chapter 23: pelvic floor disorders: pelvic organ prolapse, urinary incontinence, and pelvic floor pain syndromes. In: Hacker & Moore's essentials of obstetrics and gynecology. 6th edition. Philadelphia: Elsevier; 2016. p. 291–303; with permission.)

kinking injury, electrocautery injury, or with dissection into an incorrect plane in the bladder.[5] Although it may take weeks for the tissues to break down completely and the fistulous tract to fully mature, symptoms are classically recognized 1 to 2 weeks after surgery (in the case of postsurgical etiology). Studies have demonstrated several intraoperative risk factors for subsequent VVF at the time of hysterectomy: surgery for benign disease, age less than 50 years old, uterus weight greater than 250 g, longer operative times (approximately 5 hours or more), and concurrent ureteral injury.[6]

DIAGNOSIS

A thorough history and physical examination are the first components of diagnosing a VVF. Women usually present with constant urinary leakage or may describe a thin vaginal discharge that began after their surgery. A high index of suspicion in this scenario may serve to decrease incorrect or delayed diagnosis.

Physical examination should commence with an external genital examination. A cough stress test should be done to rule out urinary incontinence from the urethral meatus, which can be a confounder.

Inspection should also include a speculum examination. Close evaluation of the vaginal wall tissue is imperative. A pinpoint opening on the anterior vaginal wall or vaginal cuff may be observed with obvious leakage. In presentations closer to the date of surgery, one may instead see a small area of erythema with granulation tissue, which is concerning for a newer fistula. In this case, a clear opening may not be visible.

If the previously described physical examination techniques are not diagnostic, a dye test can be performed. Retrograde filling of the bladder with indigo carmine or Methylene blue mixed with sterile water or saline will facilitate diagnosis of a urethrovaginal or VVF. After instillation of the mixture into the bladder via a Foley catheter, the examiner inspects the anterior vaginal wall for leakage while compressing the urethral opening to avoid incontinence. If no blue-tinged fluid is noted within the vagina, a tampon may be placed into the vagina and the patient asked to ambulate for a short time. The tampon can then be removed and examined for evidence of blue staining. Staining on the outlet of the tampon suggests urethral incontinence, whereas staining on the superior aspect of the tampon suggests a vesicovaginal or urethrovaginal communication. If no dye extravasates, or if clinical suspicion warrants, the presence of a ureterovaginal fistula can be tested by the addition of oral phenaozpyridine. The patient should take phenazopyridine about 30 minutes prior to the office visit. At the office, a tampon can be placed intravaginally, and the patient may ambulate. Orange staining of the tampon will capture ureterovaginal, vesicovaginal, or urethrovaginal fistulas.

Dye studies alone may not be sufficient to completely evaluate the number and location of urogenital fistulas. A computed tomography (CT) urogram and cystogram of the abdomen and pelvis or retrograde pyelogram and cystourethrogram can be used to evaluate for ureterovaginal and VVFs, respectively (**Fig. 2**). Recent evidence suggests

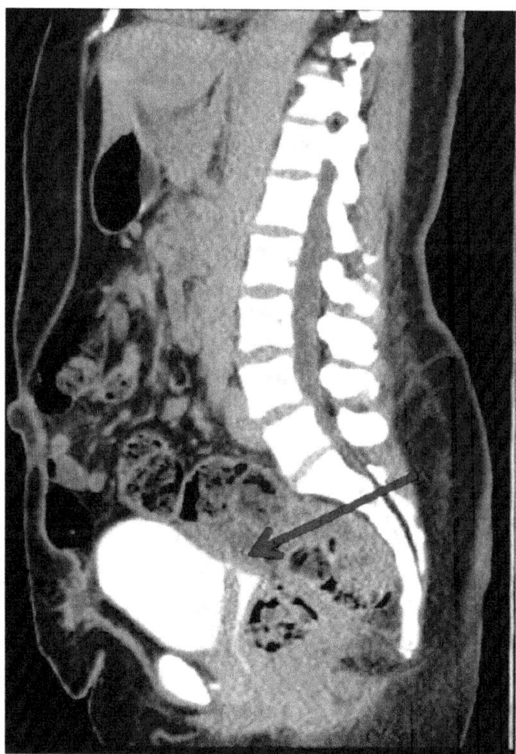

Fig. 2. CT cystogram demonstrating an apical VVF that could not be clearly visualized on pelvic examination.

that abdominopelvic MRI may also be of value and may have increased sensitivity compared with CT. MRI may better help to delineate borders of the bladder, urethra, and vagina, thereby helping with surgical planning.[7,8] Finally, cystoscopy should also be performed in order to identify potential involvement of the trigone and/or proximity to the ureters. Vaginoscopy can also be performed if speculum examination is inconclusive.

CLASSIFICATION OF FISTULAS

Fistulas can be further characterized into simple and complex based on size and tissue quality.

The term simple fistula is applied to a single fistula that is small (≤0.5 cm in diameter) and arising in nonradiated tissue. The term complex fistula denotes a fistula that has failed a prior repair attempt, is at least 2.5 cm in diameter, or which results from either chronic inflammatory disease or within radiated tissues.[3]

SURGICAL INTERVENTION

If a simple fistula is diagnosed shortly after surgery, conservative and expectant management is a reasonable initial therapeutic option. A Foley catheter should be placed into the bladder at time of diagnosis and left in place for 2 to 8 weeks with concurrent anticholinergic therapy. This has been shown to result in closure of the fistulous tract in approximately 10% of cases.[5,9]

If the patient is further out from surgery or if the defect failed to close with initial conservative management, then surgical intervention is recommended. The choice of surgical approach must take multiple factors into consideration, including the etiology of the fistula, desired timing of surgery, vaginal versus abdominal approach, concomitant procedures, excision of the fistulous tract, tissue interposition, sexual function, and adjuvant treatment.[4]

Surgical techniques to repair VVF have progressed over the years since Dr. James Marion Sims published the first report of a consistently successful method of repair in 1852.[1] Sims' emphasis on the critical importance of good exposure, continuous postoperative bladder drainage, and a tension-free closure remain fundamental to a successful repair. Surgeon skill and experience, as well as an accurate knowledge of the relevant surgical anatomy of the ureters and the anatomic relationships of the base of the bladder to the vascular pedicles of the uterus and vagina, are also integral.[8]

TIMING OF SURGICAL INTERVENTION

Timing of surgery is based upon the health of the surrounding tissue and optimizing chances of a successful closure. Traditionally, waiting 6 to 12 weeks was thought to allow granulation tissue to dissipate and thus increase success rates. Over the last several years however, earlier closures, within 1 to 2 weeks of injury, have been described with similar success rates.[10,11] Surgical intervention must be tailored to the individual circumstances of each case.

SURGICAL APPROACH

Vaginal Versus Abdominal Approach

In general, if either approach is acceptable, then the vaginal technique is preferred. Vaginal repair has demonstrated significantly shorter operative times, decreased blood loss, and shorter duration of hospitalization.[12] However, certain factors limit the feasibility of a vaginal approach in favor of an abdominal repair. Most notably, a small introitus, high or inaccessible fistulas, complex fistulas, a recurrent fistula after a failed prior repair attempt, fistulas with significant associated scarring, fistulas occurring in irradiated tissues, concomitant involvement of the uterus or bowel, or when the relative position of the ureters is seen as problematic or requires the need for ureteral reimplantation.[13]

The following section will focus on open and laparoscopic abdominal approaches to VVF repair looking at both transvesical and extravesical approaches. In all cases, early placement of a bladder catheter is recommended. Bilateral ureteral stents (if required) and a small gauge Foley or ureteral catheter for the fistulous tract can be placed cystoscopically or through the open bladder, if performing a transvesical approach.

OPEN ABDOMINAL APPROACH

Abdominal Incision

As in all open pelvic surgeries, one must first consider the risks and benefits of a lower vertical versus a transverse (Pfannensteil) abdominal incision. Benefits of a midline vertical infraumbilical incision include easier access to the upper abdomen, which facilitates later retrieval of the omentum for use as an interposition graft, and decreased blood loss. Risks include potentially worse postoperative pain and a less aesthetically appealing incision.

Alternatively, a low transverse incision limits access to higher abdominal structures but is often less painful and more easily concealed. If a transverse incision is deemed more appropriate, a muscle-splitting incision, such as a Cherney incision, will assist with increased access to upper abdominal structures (**Fig. 3**). Upon entry, exposure can be further facilitated with the use of

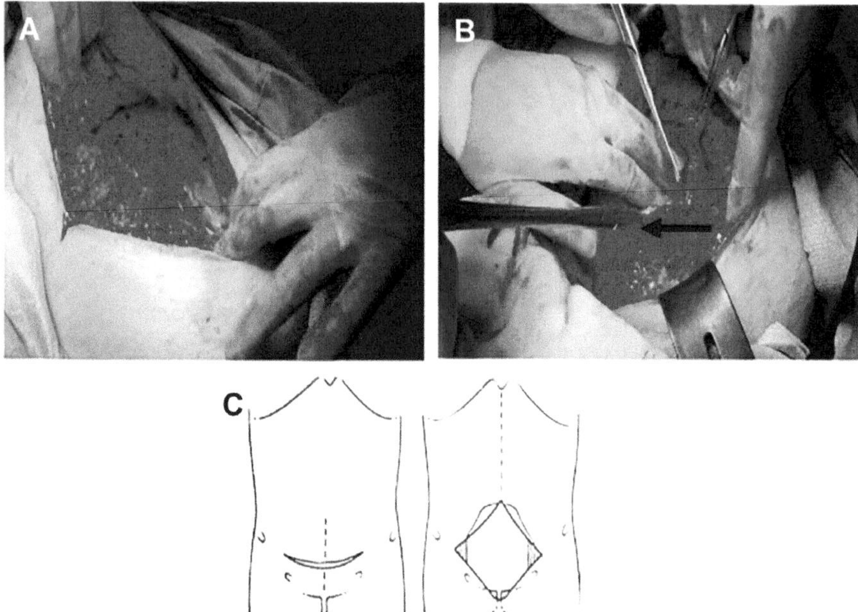

Fig. 3. Pfannestiel incision with vertical incision of rectus fascia. (*A*) Horizontal skin incision (*B*) Vertical incision of the rectus fascia (*C*) illustration of the desired view of the surgical field. (*From* Mangera A, Chapple C. Case discussion: vesicovaginal fistula following a total abdominal hysterectomy: the case for abdominal repair. Eur Urol Focus 2016;2(1):100; with permission.)

self-retaining retractors and packing the bowel up high, out of the pelvis.

Exposure of the Fistulous Tract

The fistulous tract can be visualized via a transvesical or extravesical technique.

Transvesical Approach

The transvesical approach is based on the technique described by O'Conor and Sokol as early as the 1950s, which remains a gold standard in the treatment of supratrigonal VVF.[14,15]

After excellent exposure of the pelvic structures is obtained, the bladder is mobilized.

An intentional, 4 to 5 cm high cystotomy is performed along the sagittal plane in the extraperitoneal portion of the bladder near the dome using either cautery or a scalpel[13] (**Fig. 4**).

The bladder incision is then extended down to the level of the fistulous tract. The cystotomy should be long enough to allow a thorough examination, with visualization of the fistulous tract and identification of both ureteral orifices. If excision of the tract is desired, a separate smaller-gauge Foley or vessel loop can be used to identify the tract course and ensure a full-thickness excision (**Fig. 5**).

Regardless of whether tract excision is desired, it is imperative to fully dissect and develop the vesicovaginal plane at least 1 to 2 cm beyond the fistulous tract. This will decrease tension on the repair and aid in layered closure for both the vaginal and bladder walls.[13]

Extravesical Approach

The extravesical approach, first described by Von Dittel in 1803,[16,17] focuses on targeted dissection, avoiding cystotomy, and preferentially dissecting to the fistulous tract via the vesicovaginal plane (**Fig. 6**). The superiority of either the transvesical or extravesical approach has not been established in the literature.[17] The authors recommend that the choice of surgical approach be determined by surgeon experience and individual fistula characteristics.

Excision of the Fistulous Tract

Classically, excision of the tract was described as an integral step for a good repair. However, this adage is now debatable.[18] Resection of tissue to provide healthy margins was thought to improve success rates.[19] However, excision with wide margins may result in a larger defect that ultimately can increase tension on the repair and risk of recurrence.[20] Presently, data suggest excision of the tract is comparable to no excision. Therefore, a decision should be made on a case-by-case basis.[21]

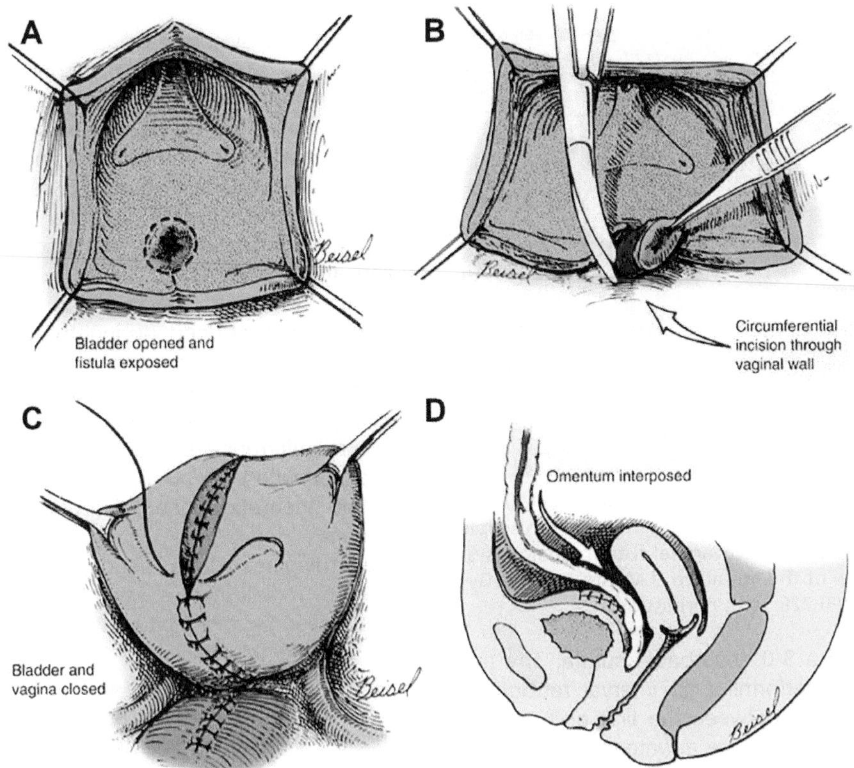

Fig. 4. Transvesical approach for VVF Repair (O'Conor technique). (*A*) Bladder opened and fistula exposed. (*B*) Circumferential incision through the vaginal wall. (*C*) Bladder closed in layers.Vagina closed. (*D*) Omentum interposed. (*From* Badlani GH, De Ridder D, et al. Chapter 89: urinary tract fistulae. In: Campbell-Walsh urology. 11th edition. Philadelphia: Elsevier; 2016. p. 2103–39.e9; with permission.)

To perform a fistulectomy, the surgeon should extend the cystototomy down to the threaded fistulous tract and circumferentially resect the tract. Care should be taken to ensure the margins are well vitalized.

Closure

A multilayered closure, with nonoverlapping suture lines, is generally preferred.[13,14,18,22,23]

Vaginal Closure

The vaginal defect can be closed in a single or double layer using interrupted or running 2-0 absorbable sutures.

Bladder Closure

The cystotomy should preferentially be repaired in 2 layers with either interrupted or continuous

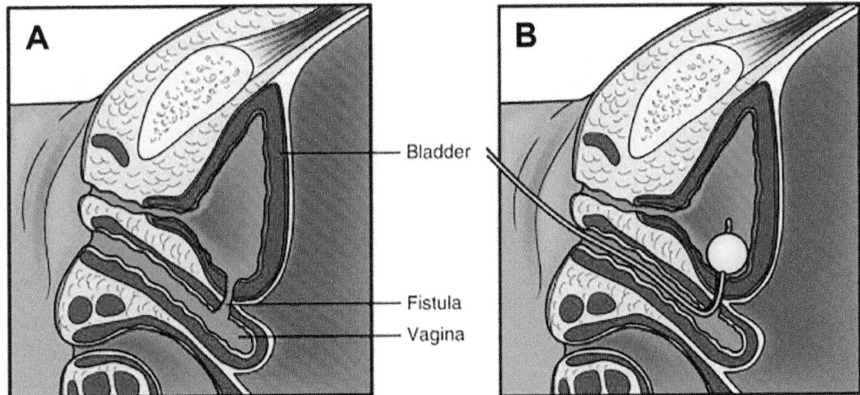

Fig. 5. Foley catheter in VVF to identify tract. (*A*) Fistulous tract between the bladder and vagina. (*B*) Foley catheter placed transvaginally into the bladder to visualize fistulous tract. (*From* Vasavada S. Chapter 65: transperitoneal vesicovaginal fistula repair. In: Smith JA, Howards SS, Preminger GM, et al, editors. Hinman's atlas of urologic surgery. 4th edition. Philadelphia: Elsevier; 2018. p. 484–7; with permission.)

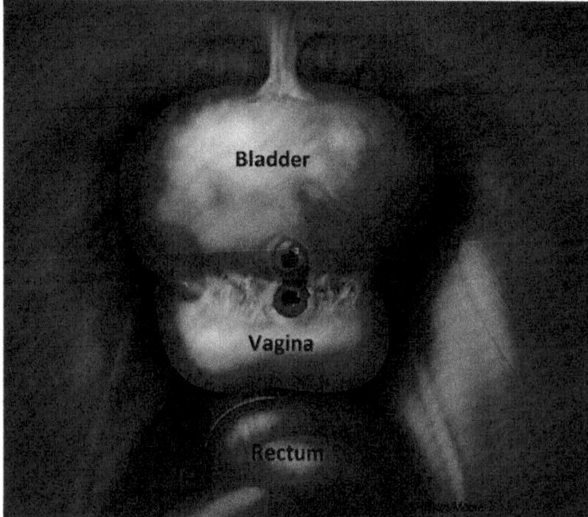

Fig. 6. Extravesical dissection to fistulous tract. (*From* Miklos JR, Moor RD, Chinthakanan O. Laparoscopic and robotic-assisted vesicovaginal fistula repair: a systematic review of the literature. J Minim Invasive Gynecol 2015;22(5):728; with permission.)

suturing using a 3-0 absorbable suture. The authors support performing an interval retrograde fill of the bladder between the first and second layer of closure to ensure a water-tight seal.[13,18] Some studies suggest ensuring the water-tight seal is more important to a successful repair than the number of layers employed.[17,18]

Tissue Interposition

Many surgeons performing repair of VVF support use of a tissue interposition graft. These grafts serve as barriers between the bladder and vaginal suture lines.

(**Fig. 7**) Use of omental flaps, epiploic appendices of the sigmoid colon, or peritoneal flaps has been reported. Tissue flaps are thought to provide another layer of well-vascularized tissue between the repair and surrounding tissue that could decrease failure rate. This technique has been described as early as 1937 and remains popular among surgeons. In addition to neovascularization of adjacent tissue, omental flaps are also thought to provide lymphatic drainage of exudates produced during the healing process, thus decreasing risk of infection and fluid collection.[15] However, Miklos and colleagues[17] demonstrated that omental interposition grafts made no difference in cure rates for VVF repairs compared with their no graft counterparts, making this theoretic benefit unproven in current literature.

Regarding technique, an omental flap is harvested by mobilizing a section of omentum, usually supplied by the right gastroepiploic vessels, and suturing this tissue to the anterior vaginal wall or the posterior bladder wall. Some surgeons argue that mobilization of the omentum increases operative time unnecessarily and prefer to use the often more proximate fatty sigmoid epiploica[24] (Video 1).

Nontissue grafts, such as fibrin glue, have also been used. However, available data are based on small sample sizes and, therefore, cannot be recommended.[25]

A Foley catheter should remain in place at the end of the case to keep the bladder decompressed and decrease tension on the repair site.

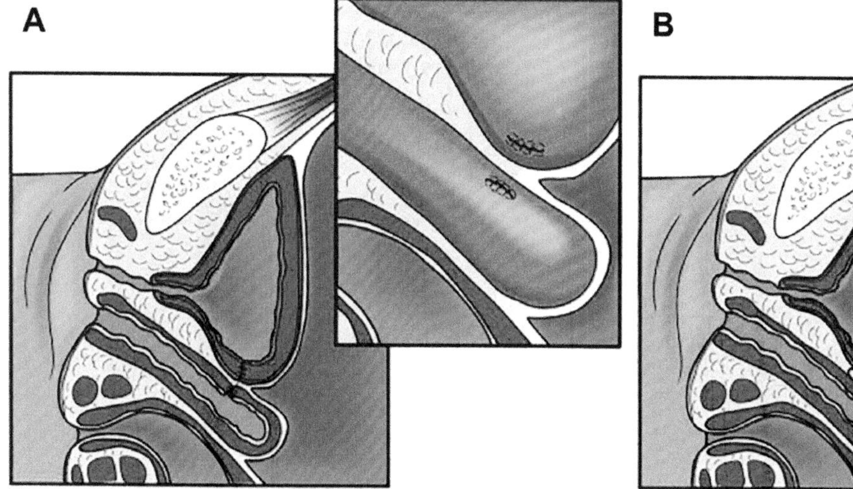

Fig. 7. Omental flap interposition. (*A*) Repaired vesicovaginal fistula. (*B*) tissue interposition. (*From* Vasavada S. Chapter 65: transperitoneal vesicovaginal fistula repair. In: Smith JA, Howards SS, Preminger GM, et al, editors. Hinman's atlas of urologic surgery. 4th edition. Philadelphia: Elsevier; 2018. p. 487; with permission.)

LAPAROSCOPIC AND ROBOT-ASSISTED LAPAROSCOPIC APPROACH TO VESICOVAGINAL FISTULA REPAIR

A laparoscopic approach to VVF repair was first described in the early 1990s. The first robot-assisted repair was reported in 2005.[24,25] These techniques employ similar steps to the previously described open abdominal practices. Comparable success rates have been demonstrated with minimally invasive approaches compared with the open approach but are associated with decreased blood loss and a shorter hospital stay by an average of 2 days.[17,24,26–28] Cure rates for the laparoscopic approach range from 75% to 98%, with most studies reporting success greater than 90% for primary repair. The failure rate for recurrent fistulas is about 10%.[29–31]

Application of robotic assistance to urogynecologic procedures is on the rise.[24] In regard to VVF, robotic surgery affords more facile lysis of adhesions, raising the question of superiority to either a laparoscopic or an open approach in this setting.[26,32] Compared with laparoscopic VVF repair, the addition of robotic assistance has demonstrated multiple benefits. The 3-dimensional view and magnification improve visibility of the fistula and surrounding structures. The ergonomic instruments allow for more accurate and precise movements, facilitating proper dissection and development of tissue planes, and aiding in knot tying and achievement of a tension-free closure.[26,27] The most commonly reported disadvantage of robotic surgery is the markedly increased cost compared with laparoscopy without robotic assistance.[17,26,27]

Notably, the fundamental steps of VVF repair are similar in regard to the laparoscopic and the robot-assisted techniques. Therefore the steps are discussed together with notation made for difference in approach.

TROCAR PLACEMENT

The patient should be placed in the dorsal lithotomy position. Early cystoscopy and placement of ureteral stents are recommended if the fistula is close to the ureteral orifices.[33] Most surgeons describe placing an open-ended ureteral catheter through the fistulous orifice cystoscopically for identification later (**Fig. 8**).

Standard laparoscopic trocar placement includes an infraumbilical port with 3 additional 5 mm accessory ports,[33] although there is no standard configuration. In general, trocars should be placed to allow optimal visualization and greatest range of motion for operating in the pelvis.

In robot-assisted repairs, multiple patterns of trocar placement have been described. Several articles describe using the same configuration typically used for robot-assisted prostatectomy.[25,34]

Melamud and colleagues[25] describe this method in detail. A 12 mm camera port is placed in the midline 20 cm from the pubis. The 8 mm robotic arm ports are placed 16 cm from the pubis lateral to the rectus muscles bilaterally and at least 10 cm from the midline camera port to avoid robotic arm collision outside the patient. A fourth 12 mm port is placed on the right side just above the anterior superior iliac crest. Finally, a 5 mm suction/assistance port is placed 7 cm cephalad and lateral to the midline camera port.

Gupta and colleagues report placing a 12 mm camera port in the midline at the level of the umbilicus, 2 lateral ports at either side of the pararectus location over the spinal umbilical line, and a 5 mm port on the right side 1 inch above and medial to the anterior superior iliac spine for assistance. Another 5 mm port is placed on the right side between the camera and the robotic port for suction.

An arch-type configuration and W configuration have also been reported (**Figs. 9** and **10**).

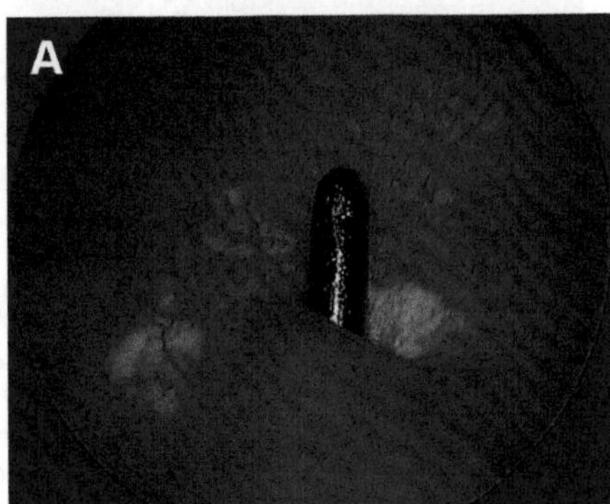

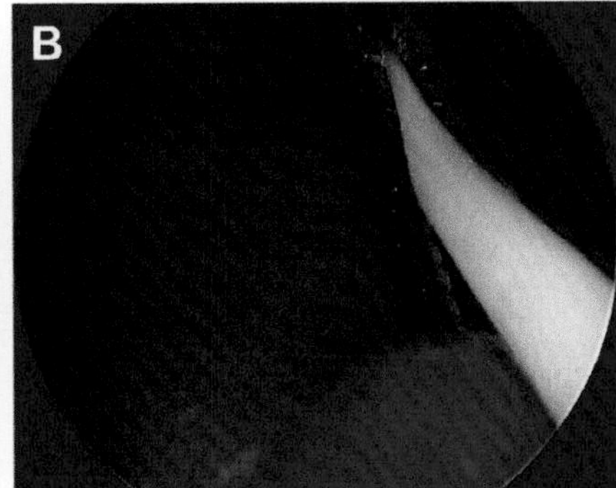

Fig. 8. (*A*) Supratrigonal fistula visualized cystoscopically. (*B*) Ureteral catheter placed through fistulous tract.

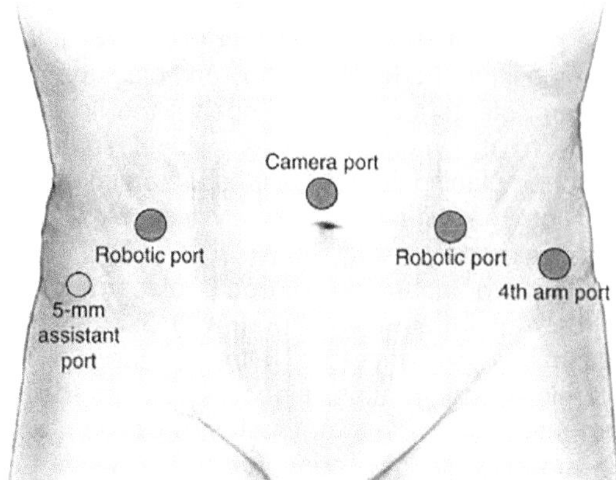

Fig. 9. Robotic port placement in an inverted U configuration. (*From* Badlani GH, De Ridder D, et al. Chapter 89: urinary tract fistulae. In: Campbell-Walsh urology. 11th edition. Philadelphia: Elsevier; 2016. p. 2103–39.e9; with permission.)

After trocar placement, the patient is placed in steep Trendelenburg position. The robot is then docked between the legs or side-docked depending on surgeon preference. The small bowel is tucked into the upper abdomen, allowing for adequate visualization of the pelvic anatomy.

A sponge stick or EEA sizer can be inserted vaginally for assistance with identification of the vaginal wall and dissection of the vesicovaginal plane. Additionally, retrograde filling of the bladder may aid in identifying the vesicovaginal reflection[17,29]

Next, a transvesical (**Fig. 11**) or extravesical (**Fig. 12**) approach to expose the fistula is performed in the same manner as previously mentioned. Notably, a literature review of 44 studies by Miklos and colleagues demonstrated success rates of transvesical and extravesical techniques as 80% to 100% and 97.67% to 100%, respectively (relative risk [RR], .98; 95% confidence interval [CI], .94-1.02). The previously placed fistula catheter will aid in identification of the VVF. The EEA sizer or sponge stick may be useful in providing a firm surface against which to dissect the retrovesical region. Upon identification of the fistula, resection of the tract may be performed but is not necessary.

Miklos and colleagues[29] demonstrated that success rates for single- and double-layer bladder closures range from 80% to 100% and 93.33% to 100%, respectively (RR, .98; 95% CI, .94–1.03). The first layer is closed with 3-0 absorbable suture in either an interrupted or continuous fashion (**Fig. 13**). Similar to the open abdominal technique, the bladder is retrograde filled to test for a water-tight seal. A second imbricating layer is then performed using either 2-0 or 3-0

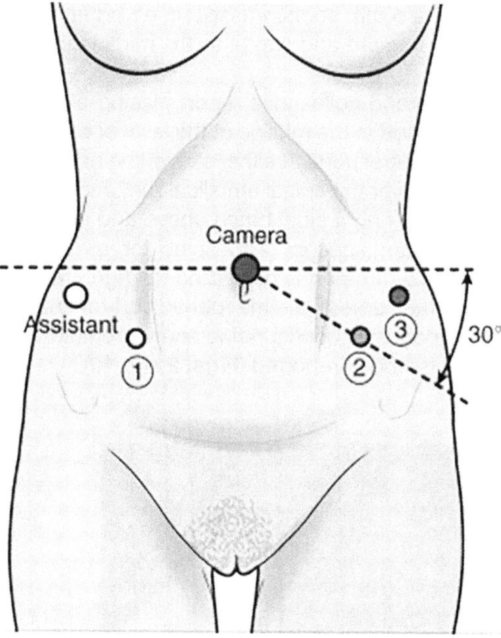

Fig. 10. Robotic port placement in a W configuration. (*From* Rosenblum N, Enemchukwu EA. Chapter 64: transvesical repair of vesicovaginal fistula. In: Smith JA, Howards SS, Preminger GM, et al, editors. Hinman's atlas of urologic surgery. 4th edition. Philadelphia: Elsevier; 2018. p. 482; with permission.)

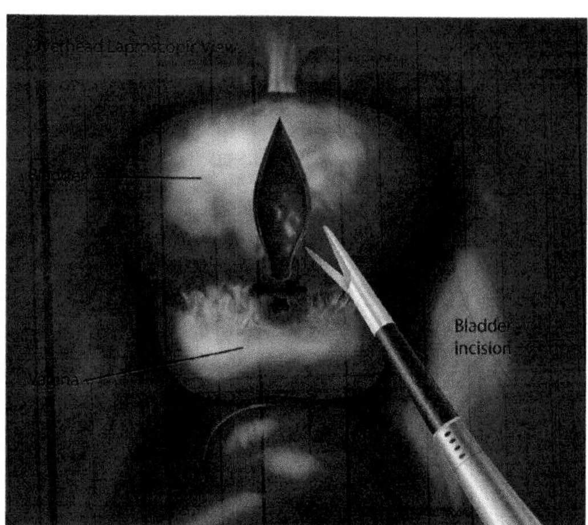

Fig. 11. Transvesical O'Conor technique used laparoscopically. (*From* Miklos JR, Moor RD, Chinthakanan O. Laparoscopic and robotic-assisted vesicovaginal fistula repair: a systematic review of the literature. J Minim Invasive Gynecol 2015;22(5):728; with permission.)

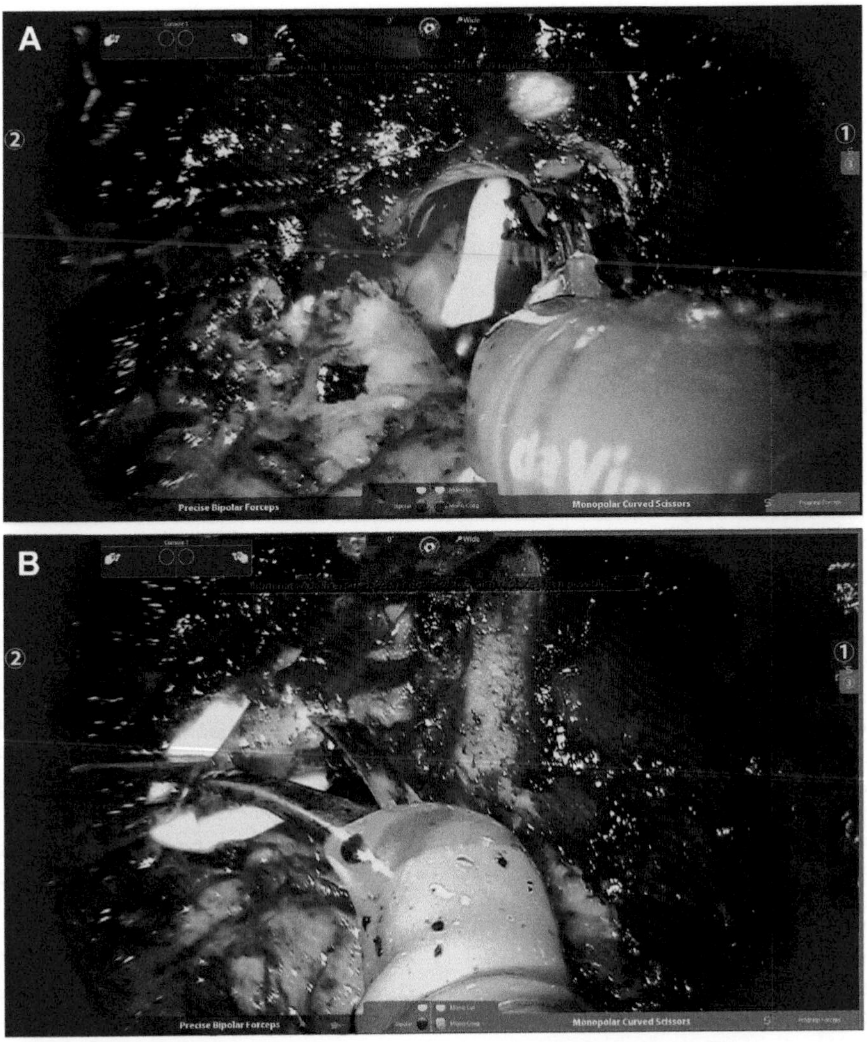

Fig. 12. (*A*) Extravesical dissection to fistulous tract. (*B*) Dissection of vesicovaginal space.

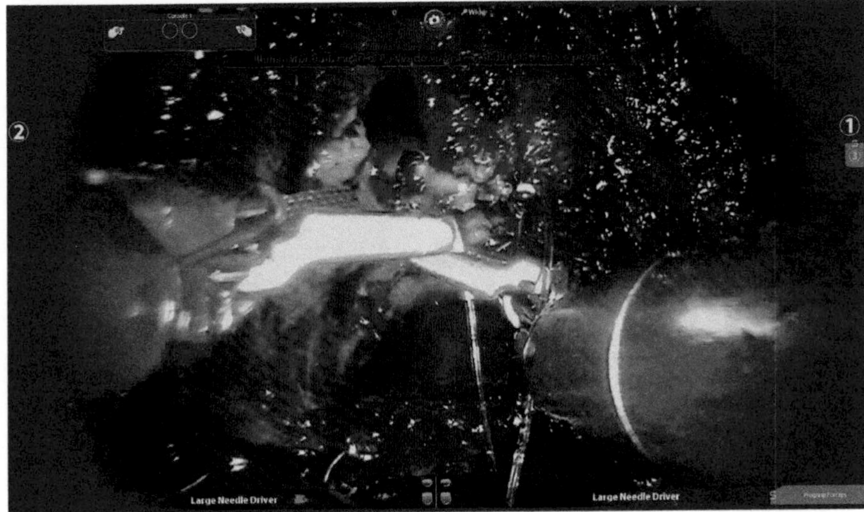

Fig. 13. Closure of bladder mucosa.

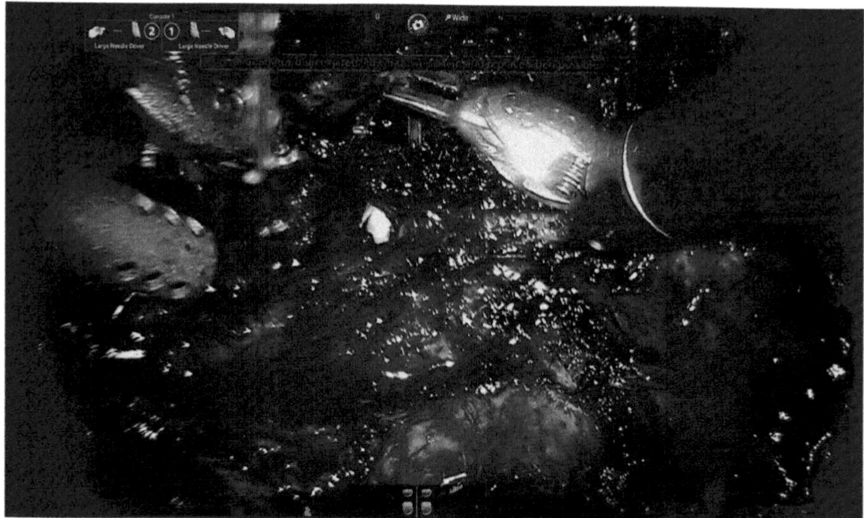

Fig. 14. Closure of vaginal opening.

absorbable sutures.[33] Stratafix is a barbed absorbable suture that can be used for bladder closure that offers the advantage of knotless suturing. The vaginal opening is closed using 2-0 Vicryl suture in a single layer (**Fig. 14**). V-lock is an absorbable barbed suture that can be used for vaginal closure.

Next, attention is turned to tissue interposition. The omentum can be harvested laparoscopically prior to starting the robotic portion of the case. If using the Da Vinci Xi platform, the omentum can be easily harvested robotically without redocking. The flap is sutured using interrupted stitches to the anterior vaginal wall (**Fig. 15**). Alternatively, sigmoid epiploica or peritoneal tissue may be used, as described previously.

After completion of the repair, a bladder catheter is placed to decrease tension on the closure. Foley duration varies by surgeon and ranges from 24 hours to 20 days, with an average of 7 to 14 days.[17,33,35]

A cystogram may be performed prior to catheter removal to confirm success of the repair.[12,35]

SUMMARY

Since O'Connor first described the open abdominal approach to VVF repair in the 1950s, surgical

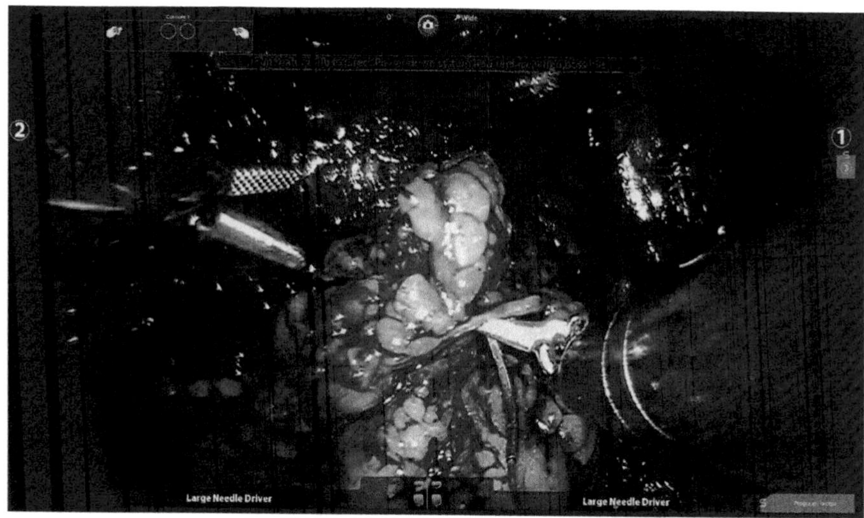

Fig. 15. Interposition of omental flap.

techniques have evolved. The principles of an effective repair include good exposure of the fistulous tract, double-layer bladder closure with intervening tissue, retrograde fill of the bladder to ensure a water-tight seal, and a tension-free closure with continuous postoperative bladder drainage. Minimally invasive approaches, particularly robot-assisted laparoscopy, have demonstrated shorter operative times, decreased blood loss, improved visibility, and similar cure rates without increased adverse events. These techniques are therefore rising in popularity among surgeons. Ultimately, surgical the approach to VVF repair depends upon the individual characteristics of the patient and fistula and the preference and experience of the surgeon.

ACKNOWLEDGMENTS

The authors would like to thank the many women who underwent various forms of this surgical repair without whom the safe and mostly efficacious methods in practice today would not be available.

SUPPLEMENTARY DATA

Supplementary data related to this article can be found online at https://doi.org/10.1016/j.ucl.2018.08.011.

REFERENCES

1. Zacharin RF. A history of obstetric vesicovaginal fistula. Aust N Z J Surg 2000;70(12):851–4.
2. Alio AP, Merrell L, Roxburgh K, et al. The psychosocial impact of vesico-vaginal fistula in Niger. Arch Gynecol Obstet 2011;284(2):371–8.
3. Angioli R, Penalver M, Muzii L, et al. Guidelines of how to manage vesicovaginal fistula. Crit Rev Oncol Hematol 2003;48(3):295–304.
4. Eilber KS, Kavaler E, Rodriguez LV, et al. Ten-year experience with transvaginal vesicovaginal fistula repair using tissue interposition. J Urol 2003; 169(3):1033–6.
5. Malik MA, Sohail M, Malik MT, et al. Changing trends in the etiology and management of vesicovaginal fistula. Int J Urol 2018;25(1):25–9.
6. Duong TH, Taylor DP, Meeks GR. A multicenter study of vesicovaginal fistula following incidental cystotomy during benign hysterectomies. Int Urogynecol J 2011;22(8):975–9.
7. Abou-El-Ghar ME, El-Assmy AM, Refaie HF, et al. Radiological diagnosis of vesicouterine fistula: role of magnetic resonance imaging. J Magn Reson Imaging 2012;36(2):438–42.
8. Chapple C, Turner-Warwick R. Vesico-vaginal fistula. BJU Int 2005;95(1):193–214.
9. Stamatakos M, Sargedi C, Stasinou T, et al. Vesicovaginal fistula: diagnosis and management. Indian J Surg 2014;76(2):131–6.
10. Hadley HR. Vesicovaginal fistula. Curr Urol Rep 2002;3(5):401–7.
11. Singh O, Gupta SS, Mathur RK. Urogenital fistulas in women: 5-year experience at a single center. Urol J 2010;7(1):35–9.
12. Alan D, Garely MJM Jr. Urogenital tract fistulas in women. 2018.
13. Michael S, Baggish MMMK. Atlas of pelvic anatomy and gynecologic surgery. Elsevier Saunders; 2006.
14. O'Conor VJ, Sokol JK. Vesicovaginal fistula from the standpoint of the urologist. J Urol 1951;66(4): 579–85.
15. Nesrallah LJ, Srougi M, Gittes RF. The O'Conor technique: the gold standard for supratrigonal vesicovaginal fistula repair. J Urol 1999;161(2):566–8.
16. Dittel LV. Abdominale Blasenscheidenfistel-operation. Wein Klin Wochenschr 1893;6.
17. Miklos JR, Moore RD, Chinthakanan O. Laparoscopic and robotic-assisted vesicovaginal fistula repair: a systematic review of the literature. J Minim Invasive Gynecol 2015;22(5):727–36.
18. Neeraj Kohli M, Miklos JR. Meeting the challenge of vesicovaginal fistula repair: Conservative and surgical measures. OBG Management 2003; 15(8):16–27.
19. McVary KT, MFF. Urinary fistulas. In: Gillenwater JY, Howards SS, Duckett JW, editors. Adult and pediatric urology. St Louis (MO): C. V. Mosby Co; 1996.
20. Tancer ML. Observations on prevention and management of vesicovaginal fistula after total hysterectomy. Surg Gynecol Obstet 1992;175(6):501–6.
21. Iselin CE, Aslan P, Webster GD. Transvaginal repair of vesicovaginal fistulas after hysterectomy by vaginal cuff excision. J Urol 1998;160(3 Pt 1): 728–30.
22. Phaneuf LE, Graves RC. Vesicovaginal fistula and its management; with a description of an intravesical operation for certain difficult cases. Surg Gynecol Obstet 1949;88(2):155–69.
23. Sokol AI, Paraiso MF, Cogan SL, et al. Prevention of vesicovaginal fistulas after laparoscopic hysterectomy with electrosurgical cystotomy in female mongrel dogs. Am J Obstet Gynecol 2004;190(3): 628–33.
24. Pietersma CS, Schreuder HW, Kooistra A, et al. Robotic-assisted laparoscopic repair of a vesicovaginal fistula: a time-consuming novelty or an effective tool? BMJ Case Rep 2014;2014.
25. Melamud O, Eichel L, Turbow B, et al. Laparoscopic vesicovaginal fistula repair with robotic reconstruction. Urology 2005;65(1):163–6.
26. Gupta NP, Mishra S, Hemal AK, et al. Comparative analysis of outcome between open and robotic

surgical repair of recurrent supra-trigonal vesicovaginal fistula. J Endourol 2010;24(11):1779–82.
27. Oehler MK. Robot-assisted surgery in gynaecology. Aust N Z J Obstet Gynaecol 2009;49(2):124–9.
28. Miklos JR, Moore RD. Vesicovaginal fistula failing multiple surgical attempts salvaged laparoscopically without an interposition omental flap. J Minim Invasive Gynecol 2012;19(6):794–7.
29. Miklos JR, Moore RD. Laparoscopic extravesical vesicovaginal fistula repair: our technique and 15-year experience. Int Urogynecol J 2015;26(3):441–6.
30. Kumar S, Kekre NS, Gopalakrishnan G. Vesicovaginal fistula: an update. Indian J Urol 2007;23(2):187–91.
31. Rovner ES. Urinary fistula. Veiscovaginal fistula. 2007.
32. Hemal AK, Kolla SB, Wadhwa P. Robotic reconstruction for recurrent supratrigonal vesicovaginal fistulas. J Urol 2008;180(3):981–5.
33. Ou CS, Huang UC, Tsuang M, et al. Laparoscopic repair of vesicovaginal fistula. J Laparoendosc Adv Surg Tech A 2004;14(1):17–21.
34. Pick DL, Lee DI, Skarecky DW, et al. Anatomic guide for port placement for daVinci robotic radical prostatectomy. J Endourol 2004;18(6):572–5.
35. Blaivas JG, Heritz DM, Romanzi LJ. Early versus late repair of vesicovaginal fistulas: vaginal and abdominal approaches. J Urol 1995;153(4):1110–2 [discussion: 1112–3].

Moving?

Make sure your subscription moves with you!

To notify us of your new address, find your **Clinics Account Number** (located on your mailing label above your name), and contact customer service at:

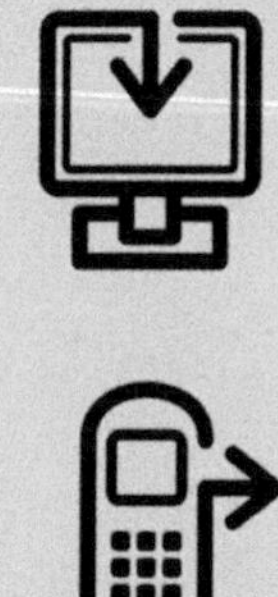

Email: journalscustomerservice-usa@elsevier.com

800-654-2452 **(subscribers in the U.S. & Canada)**
314-447-8871 **(subscribers outside of the U.S. & Canada)**

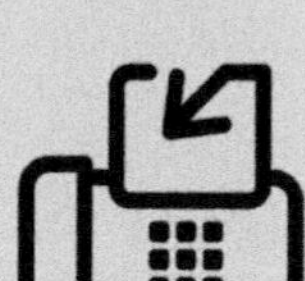

Fax number: 314-447-8029

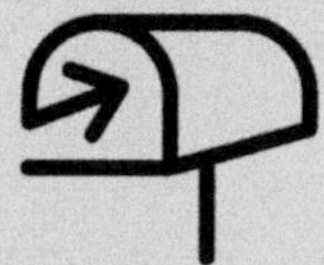

Elsevier Health Sciences Division
Subscription Customer Service
3251 Riverport Lane
Maryland Heights, MO 63043

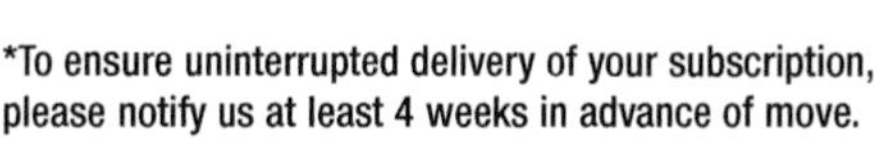

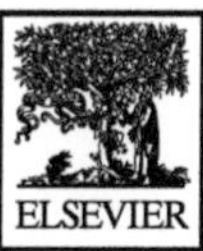

Printed and bound by CPI Group (UK) Ltd, Croydon, CR0 4YY
03/10/2024
01040372-0015